Unimagined Community

CALIFORNIA SERIES IN PUBLIC ANTHROPOLOGY

The California Series in Public Anthropology emphasizes the anthropologist's role as an engaged intellectual. It continues anthropology's commitment to being an ethnographic witness, to describing, in human terms, how life is lived beyond the borders of many readers' experiences. But it also adds a commitment, through ethnography, to reframing the terms of public debate—transforming received, accepted understandings of social issues with new insights, new framings.

Series Editor: Robert Borofsky (Hawaii Pacific University)

Contributing Editors: Philippe Bourgois (University of Pennsylvania), Paul Farmer (Partners in Health), Alex Hinton (Rutgers University), Carolyn Nordstrom (University of Notre Dame), and Nancy Scheper-Hughes (UC Berkeley)

University of California Press Editor: Naomi Schneider

1. *Twice Dead: Organ Transplants and the Reinvention of Death,*
   by Margaret Lock

2. *Birthing the Nation: Strategies of Palestinian Women in Israel,*
   by Rhoda Ann Kanaaneh (with a foreword by Hanan Ashrawi)

3. *Annihilating Difference: The Anthropology of Genocide,*
   edited by Alexander Laban Hinton (with a foreword by Kenneth Roth)

4. *Pathologies of Power: Health, Human Rights, and the New War on the Poor,*
   by Paul Farmer (with a foreword by Amartya Sen)

5. *Buddha Is Hiding: Refugees, Citizenship, the New America,*
   by Aihwa Ong

6. *Chechnya: Life in a War-Torn Society,*
   by Valery Tishkov (with a foreword by Mikhail S. Gorbachev)

7. *Total Confinement: Madness and Reason in the Maximum Security Prison,*
   by Lorna A. Rhodes

8. *Paradise in Ashes: A Guatemalan Journey of Courage, Terror, and Hope,*
   by Beatriz Manz (with a foreword by Aryeh Neier)

9. *Laughter Out of Place: Race, Class, Violence, and Sexuality in a Rio Shantytown,* by Donna M. Goldstein

10. *Shadows of War: Violence, Power, and International Profiteering in the Twenty-First Century,* by Carolyn Nordstrom

11. *Why Did They Kill? Cambodia in the Shadow of Genocide,*
    by Alexander Laban Hinton (with a foreword by Robert Jay Lifton)

12. *Yanomami: The Fierce Controversy and What We Can Learn from It,*
    by Robert Borofsky

13. *Why America's Top Pundits Are Wrong: Anthropologists Talk Back,* edited by Catherine Besteman and Hugh Gusterson

14. *Prisoners of Freedom: Human Rights and the African Poor,* by Harri Englund

15. *When Bodies Remember: Experiences and Politics of AIDS in South Africa,* by Didier Fassin

16. *Global Outlaws: Crime, Money, and Power in the Contemporary World,* by Carolyn Nordstrom

17. *Archaeology as Political Action,* by Randall H. McGuire

18. *Counting the Dead: The Culture and Politics of Human Rights Activism in Colombia,* by Winifred Tate

19. *Transforming Cape Town,* by Catherine Besteman

20. *Unimagined Community: Sex, Networks, and AIDS in Uganda and South Africa,* by Robert J. Thornton

Unimagined Community

*Sex, Networks, and AIDS
in Uganda and South Africa*

Robert J. Thornton

UNIVERSITY OF CALIFORNIA PRESS
Berkeley · Los Angeles · London

University of California Press, one of the most distinguished university presses in the United States, enriches lives around the world by advancing scholarship in the humanities, social sciences, and natural sciences. Its activities are supported by the UC Press Foundation and by philanthropic contributions from individuals and institutions. For more information, visit www.ucpress.edu.

University of California Press
Berkeley and Los Angeles, California

University of California Press, Ltd.
London, England

Library of Congress Cataloging-in-Publication Data

Thornton, Robert J.

Unimagined community : sex, networks, and AIDS in Uganda and South Africa / Robert J. Thornton.

p. ; cm. — (California series in public anthropology ; 20)

Includes bibliographical references and index.
ISBN 978-0-520-25552-4 (cloth : alk. paper)
ISBN 978-0-520-25553-1 (pbk. : alk. paper)
1. AIDS (Disease)—Uganda—Epidemiology. 2. AIDS (Disease)—South Africa—Epidemiology. 3. AIDS (Disease)—Social aspects—Uganda. 4. AIDS (Disease)—Social aspects—South Africa. I. Title. II. Series.
[DNLM: 1. Acquired Immunodeficiency Syndrome—epidemiology—South Africa. 2. Acquired Immunodeficiency Syndrome—epidemiology—Uganda. 3. Acquired Immunodeficiency Syndrome—prevention & control—South Africa. 4. Acquired Immunodeficiency Syndrome—prevention & control—Uganda. 5. Anthropology, Cultural—methods—South Africa. 6. Anthropology, Cultural—methods—Uganda. 7. Health Policy—South Africa. 8. Health Policy—Uganda. 9. Sexual Behavior—South Africa. 10. Sexual Behavior—Uganda. 11. Socioeconomic Factors—South Africa. 12. Socioeconomic Factors—Uganda. WC 503.4 HU4 T514u 2008]

RA643.86.U33T46 2008

614.5'993920096761 dc22   2007046954

Manufactured in the United States of America

15 14 13 12 11 10 09 08 07 06
10 9 8 7 6 5 4 3 2 1

This book is printed on Natures Book, which contains 50% post-consumer waste and meets the minimum requirements of ANSI/NISO Z39.48–1992 (R 1997) (*Permanence of Paper*).

To my father, Professor Givens Louis Thornton, with all my love. He took me to India and to Africa. He showed me how to see people and their ways with love and understanding. I miss him. He will be with me always.

Contents

List of Illustrations   xi

Acknowledgments   xiii

Note on Ethnic Names and Languages   xv

Preface   xvii

1. Introduction: Meaning and Structure in the Study of AIDS   1

2. Comparing Uganda and South Africa: Sexual Networks, Family Structure, and Property   33

3. The Social Determinants of Sexual Network Configuration   56

4. The Tightening Chain: Civil Society and Uganda's Response to HIV/AIDS   83

5. AIDS in Uganda: Years of Chaos and Recovery   100

6. *Siliimu* as Native Category: AIDS as Local Knowledge in Uganda   115

7. The Indigenization of AIDS: Governance and the Political Response in Uganda   130

8. South Africa's Struggle: The Omission and Commission of Truth about AIDS   149

9. Imagining AIDS: South Africa's Viral Politics   171

10. Flows of Sexual Substance: The Sexual Network
    in South Africa   195

11. Preventing AIDS: A New Paradigm for
    a New Strategy   220

   Notes   235

   References   257

   Index   275

Illustrations

1. Kamondo's family photo album, Mbarara, Uganda   20
2. The time of HIV/AIDS   26
3. Stoneburner and Low-Beer's epidemiological model of HIV prevalence change in Uganda   35
4. Comparison of HIV trends for Uganda and South Africa, 1985–2002   42
5. Comparison of HIV power-law trend lines in Uganda and South Africa, 1992–2002   43
6. Trend for changing HIV prevalence in Kampala, Uganda, 1985–2002   49
7. The earliest period of growing HIV prevalence in South Africa, 1982–1994   52
8. The bunga, or Buganda king's council building, in Mmengo, Uganda   67
9. The USAID pamphlet that popularized the ABC approach and gave oversimplified reasons for HIV prevalence decline in Uganda   88
10. Kamondo's grave in the family homestead   90
11. Median HIV prevalence among pregnant women in Uganda, 1986–2000   94
12. "Behave Responsibly to Avoid Getting AIDS" poster, circa 1989   128
13. *Theta News,* official newsletter of the Traditional and Modern Health Practitioners Together against AIDS and Other Diseases   141

14. Partial compilation of total condom imports and local
    distribution in Uganda, 1987–2003   144

15. Cumulative growth of Ugandan NGOs, CBOs, and FBOs
    dealing wholly or in part with HIV and AIDS   147

16. The minister of health, Manto Tshabalala-Msimang,
    defies court order requiring state provision of Nevirapine
    in cases of potential mother-to-child HIV transmission
    at birth   187

17. Exponential increase in number of South African NGOs
    and private organizations dealing with children and
    HIV/AIDS   189

18. Flows of sexual substance in social time and space   206

19. Sexuality as exchange of blood and gifts   209

20. The diviner's (*sangoma*'s) model of the body   213

Acknowledgments

My mother has been a constant source of inspiration as well as guidance. She read and edited the entire manuscript many times. In addition to providing me with material from her own reading, she helped me understand my project from the reader's perspective. Her help was immeasurable.

Pamela Nichols provided support and encouragement throughout the process of research and writing. By believing in my ideas, she pushed me through the difficult spots when I felt overwhelmed by the sheer mass of material on AIDS.

Of my anthropological colleagues, Keith Hart has been exceptionally encouraging and interested in my ideas and approaches. As always, I have benefited tremendously from his ideas and from the close reading that he gave the book in one of its earlier versions. I also thank Bettina Schmidt for her close reading and comments.

Fanie Enock Nkosi (known by his *sangoma*, or "healing name," Magodweni) of Umjindi, Mpumalanga, has given me deep insight into culture and healing in the South African lowveld. He aided my research in innumerable ways and contributed his knowledge and friendship without reserve. He died in January 2007 as I was finishing this manuscript, and I will miss him always. *Hamba kahle, buti wami.*

I also thank my research assistant, Zelda Gama, who has been with me throughout the research process in South Africa. Much of the research with traditional healers would not have been possible without her assistance in logistics, translation, and transcription of interview material. My former students Shado Dludlu, Kereng Kgotleng, Josephine Malala, Joseph Nkuna, Zodwa Radebe, Gloria Rafobane, and Nokuthula Skhosana also participated in aspects of this research. I have benefited from our discussions of ideas over the years. The help, understanding, and friendship I have received from many traditional healers during my research into AIDS, sex and sexuality, healing and concepts of health, disease and the body have been invaluable.

I am grateful to Elisabeth Hsu of the Institute for Social and Cultural Anthropology, Oxford, for providing me with an opportunity to spend a couple of months in Oxford in order to complete the book. I thank Green-Templeton College, Oxford, for providing me with a space to work that allowed the sort of concentration and focus that finishing a book requires.

Thanks to "Zapiro" (Jonathan Shapiro) for his cartoon (figure 16), which is at once trenchant and sympathetic.

Research work for this book was conducted from early 2002 to mid-2006. Funding and support came from a number of sources. Primary funding was provided by the South African National Research Foundation, under grant no. 2054123. Research in Uganda during 2003 was made possible through a research contract from AIDSMark/USAID as part of the ABC Study directed by Douglas Kirby, ETR Associations, Scotts Valley, California. According to terms of the USAID contract, the statutory notice of acknowledgment follows:

> This publication was [partly] made possible through support provided
> by the AIDSMark project sponsored by the U.S. Agency for International
> Development, under the terms of Award No. HRN-A-00-97-00021-00.
> The opinions expressed herein are those of the author(s) and do not necessarily reflect the views of the U.S. Agency for International Development.

Finally, the opinions expressed in this work are entirely my own and do not necessarily reflect the views of any of the funders or my collaborators.

Note on Ethnic Names and Languages

With minor exceptions, Ugandan and South African languages belong to two broad families: the Bantu family and the northwestern branch of the Indo-European family of languages. Thus, all of the languages within these families have basic grammar in common.

Southern Uganda represents the northernmost reach of the Bantu languages, while South Africa represents their southernmost reach. Bantu languages use prefixes to designate specific meanings for general, or root, terms. Thus *Ganda* is the root name of the largest ethnic group and kingdom in southern Uganda, and prefixes denote its various aspects. For example, *Luganda* is the Ganda language, *Buganda* is the Ganda kingdom or territory, and *Baganda* is the plural for Ganda people, or the Ganda nation or tribe.

Similarly, in South Africa, *Zulu* is a root name from which other terms are derived. For example, *IsiZulu* is the Zulu language, and *AmaZulu* is the Zulu people or nation (especially the followers of the Zulu king, particularly those living in the northern part of the province of KwaZulu-Natal). These prefixes vary somewhat from language to language. Thus, *SeSotho* is the name of the Sotho language, where the *se-* prefix is cognate to the *isi-* prefix in *IsiZulu*.

Besides Luganda, English is the other dominant language in Uganda. In both South Africa and Uganda, English is the primary language of education, especially at the secondary school and university levels, and the primary language of commerce. In everyday practice, however,

South African language use involves considerable mixing of at least four languages: IsiZulu, English, Afrikaans, and SeSotho. Although there are officially eleven languages in South Africa, all others are either closely related to these four or are mutually intelligible. Most South Africans and Ugandans use multiple languages in daily life.

Preface

I did not want to study AIDS, but as an anthropologist in Africa, I could not avoid it. Anthropology has been called the study of mankind in context. HIV/AIDS is now part of that context, especially in sub-Saharan Africa. It touches on the deepest of human concerns: sex, health, death, kinship, family, language, and culture. Because these are also the core areas of anthropology, my concern with HIV and AIDS is thus an anthropological concern. This anthropological approach departs significantly from standard epidemiological, public health, medical, and sociological perspectives and methods.

Anthropology is holistic, integrative, and, where appropriate, comparative. I offer here a holistic comparison of Uganda and South Africa—two countries with radically different trends in HIV prevalence—using methodological tools that integrate mathematics, sociology, demography, epidemiology, and traditional anthropological approaches and techniques. Uganda and South Africa are part of a broadly similar cultural area—Bantu-speaking sub-Saharan Africa—and thus suitable for comparison. I compare them across a broad range of cultural and social features in order to explain the differences in the epidemiology of AIDS in a way that is not reduced to the biology of a single body (or cell) or to the psychology of the individual who "behaves" sexually, or encounters "risk." In other words, my approach links the world of individual meanings, motives, and understandings to increasingly large scales of organization in a way that is neither individualistic nor sociological but genuinely anthropological. My emphasis is on process, structure, and linkage across differing scales of action and experience and on interaction between domains of meaning, whether we understand these as cultures, discourses, or worldviews. The social fabrics that transmit HIV have for the most part escaped the grid of sociological theory until now.

I focus on the concept of the sexual network. By their nature, sexual networks cannot be *seen* either by those who participate in them or, usually, by the social sciences. People involved in sexual networks—that is, those who are sexually active—do not represent the extent, size, pattern, or even existence of these networks either to themselves or to social scientists. Thus, unlike the explicit networks of friendship or kinship, the sexual network is an invisible community; it is *unimagined*.

Although sexual networks are necessarily subsets of friendship networks and supersets of kinship networks, they are rarely traced as a genealogy is or as one might construct a guest list for a wedding. They do not constitute social categories. The social sciences have little grasp of sexual networks because they are not institutions or social structures in the normal sense. While we have elaborate theories about social institutions, we have only the most limited understanding of social networks, especially sexual networks. They remain essentially untheorized and largely undescribed.

AIDS is not only a professional but also a personal concern for me. I have lived in both Uganda and South Africa for long periods and throughout most of my adult life. My personal and family history is bound up with their national histories. I was a young man in Uganda, and I raised a family in South Africa. My perspective on AIDS is based in part on my own experience and the sense that I have made of it. Not everyone will agree with this perspective. For instance, in this book I present South Africa as a radically egalitarian society compared to Uganda. Given South Africa's history of apartheid, some will find this ironic or even plain wrong. I also largely ignore race. It appears to me that with respect to sex and choice of sexual partners, race does not predict or determine significant social differences. The success of apartheid, in fact, was to convince South Africans that they were more different from one another than they in fact are. Its failure sprang from the fact that this belief was empirically, not just morally, wrong. I treat South Africa as an African country and do not distinguish South Africans by race.

Anthropologists are less concerned with what people do as instances of generalized categories—class, race, ethnicity, nationality—or as manifestations of supposed universal psychological or neurological processes than they are with real people doing real things in concrete contexts. They attempt to understand the meanings people give to their own actions—what motivates them—and to the actions of others. This involves a kind of philosophy, but it is "philosophy with the people left in."[1]

The channels through which HIV travels in the human population are, as I see it, social structures of a special sort, the sexual network. Infection by HIV occurs during moments of the most profound meaning, moments of sexual intimacy. Without understanding sex as a relation, we cannot grasp this elementary fact. And without seeking to understand the social and cultural values attributed to sex itself, we fail to understand the basic motives that drive the epidemic at the human level. For this reason, as an anthropologist I have not been able to avoid the study of AIDS.

AIDS can, of course, be ignored or denied. We have seen this in the responses of members of the South African government and of churches and other moral and political leaders. Malaria, tuberculosis, and violence, some point out, kill more people across all of Africa than AIDS does. Also, talk about AIDS requires talk about sex, and this presents insurmountable moral barriers to many people. Yet even the denial of AIDS is an acknowledgment of its fierce presence. Denial rises from powerful anxieties about sex, death, and the knowledge that HIV infection occurs at the moment of sexual intimacy. To know about AIDS is to possess an almost unbearable knowledge.

The impact of AIDS is much deeper than that of other diseases or even of violence: these merely kill. Although violence and other diseases cause suffering, they do not challenge fundamental values of the self, society, and culture. These causes of death have been around long enough that their economic, cultural, and social effects are well known. They are fully comprehended by indigenous medical systems and well understood by biomedicine. Violent deaths are also comprehensible in terms of local knowledge and traditions of violence, through the moral knowledge of religion and humanism, and by politicians and social scientists who study violence. Violent causes of death can be cured or stopped, albeit with great difficulty; AIDS cannot. For those who suffer from AIDS and die, and for their families, friends, colleagues, and communities, the disease is tinged with a kind of moral mystery. Especially in eastern, central, and southern Africa, AIDS is now a part of everyone's life and loves. More people are infected with HIV here than anywhere else in the world. The epidemic in this part of the continent is characterized as mature, heterosexual, and pervasive, which means that no one is immune from infection or at least from its effects. Although there are marked regional differences, HIV exists in virtually every corner of the southern continent, in all communities and in all age groups. It weighs on the consciousness and conscience of every endeavor and penetrates all aspects of life.

AIDS presents challenges to the constitution of community and to the very grounds of knowledge in a way that no other disease or epidemic has ever done. In particular, it challenges people's ability to imagine the set of relationships that transmit HIV and that are the only means for halting its spread. The community of AIDS is almost unimaginable. Because of the nature of its transmission, because of the long delay between infection and its manifestation, and because there is no cure after a quarter century of effort to find one, our knowledge of AIDS creates immeasurable anxiety.

The moral dimensions of AIDS—summed up in the somewhat awkward words *stigma* and *denial*—have often made it difficult to acknowledge or to create either a moral or a political community with and for those who are HIV-positive. The knowledge that a sister, a lover, a parent, a friend, a coworker, or even an enemy is HIV-positive creates anxieties and uncertainties with which many struggle to cope. It is not possible for any single lover, anyone who has been involved sexually with another, to imagine the vast sexual networks in which they are unknowing participants. This unknowing is as fundamental to the nature of sex as are its pleasures and intimate knowledge of another. Although HIV is transmitted through sexual networks—more or less efficiently depending on their configuration, timing, and extent—it is a purely occult community, one we can never see or imagine.

The title of this book, *Unimagined Community*, points to these facts while gesturing to the political community of the nation, which, according to Benedict Anderson, is necessarily an *imagined community*, owing its existence to national languages fostered by print capitalism; its members can never participate in it directly.[2] By contrast, the community of the sexual network is never imagined and never represented by those who do in fact participate in it. The *un*imagined community of those who carry the virus, who suffer with AIDS, or who have lost their parents, children, and loved ones to it bears a deeply problematic relation to the imagined community of the nation.

The latter part of this book deals with the uneasy relationship between the community of AIDS and the HIV-positive and the political community of the nation. Though vexed, this relationship determines the course of both AIDS and the nation because effective action against HIV infection must be collective and communal. It can take place only within a community of values and with a spirit that *values* communities. Trust, mutual knowledge, connection, commerce, and communion—the very values on which the sense of community rests—are undermined by the presence of HIV within it.

This study plunges into a deep anthropology of AIDS, sex, and sexual networks. I hope that it will provide new understandings on which to base better preventive measures. The anthropological inquiry presented here explores the basis of the anxiety surrounding our knowledge about AIDS and attempts to create an image of the communities that we have so far failed to imagine or to which we have often failed, morally, intellectually, and politically, to make a commitment.

CHAPTER I

Introduction

Meaning and Structure in the Study of AIDS

AN ANTHROPOLOGICAL APPROACH TO AIDS

This book offers an anthropological, or "ecological," approach to the study of acquired immunodeficiency syndrome (AIDS). It departs from epidemiological and demographic approaches expressed in statistical measures and from the behavioral approaches expressed in tables of behavior change. I examine the dimensions and processes of everyday life in order to understand how sexual networks that transmit the human immunodeficiency virus (HIV) are formed and work. My principle finding is that change in HIV prevalence is primarily determined by the differences in the configuration of large-scale sexual networks rather than by the cumulative effects of behavior change, a necessary but not sufficient condition.

This is also a comparative study, focusing on two African countries, Uganda and South Africa, that appear to be diametrically opposed in the way AIDS has progressed and in their respective social, cultural, and political responses to AIDS. Comparisons between South Africa and other countries in Africa are rare largely because South Africa is taken to be an exception. Here, I treat South Africa as an African country among other African countries. In an effort to explore and explain the differences between South Africa and Uganda, I compare the structure of sexual networks and the factors that shape these networks, thus promoting or inhibiting the transmission of HIV. In doing this, I assume that South Africa is indeed part of Africa and generally comparable in other respects to Uganda. As a long-term resident of both countries, I believe that this is the case.[1]

Although this is not a policy study, it presents a way of understanding AIDS in its specifically African context that may help us shape effective policy in the future. I sketch some new directions for policy in chapter 11.

In southern Africa today, it has become a truism that even if one is not *infected* by HIV, one is certainly *affected* by it. In South Africa alone, well over two million people, most of them in the prime of their lives, had died as a result of HIV infection by mid-2007.[2] Some died slowly after painful illnesses that left them wasted and too ill to speak. Others died quickly from coinfections such as diarrheal diseases, tuberculosis, or malaria. All have left a gap in the lives of their families and in their communities. In South Africa, AIDS currently accounts for almost 50 percent of all deaths.[3] In 2006, nearly one thousand people died each day of AIDS,[4] and these numbers continue to increase.

In South Africa, which has the best health and economic infrastructure on the African continent, life expectancy will drop to fifty years of age by 2010.[5] Child and maternal mortality rates are rising, largely because of AIDS, with most of the increase since 1970 occurring from 2000 on.[6] On weekends in South Africa, the cemeteries are the busiest places in town. The dead already fill to capacity twenty-seven of Johannesburg's thirty-three cemeteries, and city managers worry about where future dead will be buried.[7] In Uganda, by comparison, death rates fell in the early 1990s, around the time HIV prevalence started to fall, and have remained stable,[8] although by 2007 there were indications that HIV prevalence was beginning to rise again.[9]

Yet South Africans continue to deny the impact of AIDS on the country. The president, Thabo Mbeki, formerly claimed that HIV did not cause AIDS or death and thought that it was a plot by major international drug companies to poison his people with dangerous medications. Now he mostly remains silent about the threat of HIV. The minister of health, Manto Tshabalala-Msimang, steadfastly advocates vitamins and a healthy diet as a cure for AIDS while overseeing the slowest and most bureaucratically encumbered medical response to AIDS in southern Africa. President Mbeki's silence on HIV and AIDS in the past several years makes it difficult to determine whether the president is following the will of the people or they are following his lead. By consensus across the country, few will speak about AIDS. When people die from what must certainly be AIDS, the survivors say, "We don't know why he/she died." This denial does not necessarily mean that they suspect witchcraft or even malicious harm caused by those who are jealous. Many are also fully aware that the cause of death is AIDS, and the very *act of denial* is itself taken to be an acknowledgment that the death was caused by AIDS. But few say this directly. South African denialism is not merely a refusal to acknowledge reality. By not speaking about AIDS, South Africans airbrush it out of the picture. But their silence is a statement that points to another cultural reality. This alternative reality, this silence, is one of the issues this book explores.

The shadow of AIDS, the great unmentionable, creeps quietly across the face of the country. And yet there is scarcely a person in the country who does not actually know what is going on. The devastation is obvious, but only a few HIV activists choose to make it an issue. They bring lawsuits against the government's Department of Health and win their cases, but little changes in the administration. Some provincial and municipal administrations go ahead, regardless of government policy, in seeking to provide antiretroviral medications for those who are already infected. Most prevention campaigns have been glitzy, costly failures, if judged in terms of prevalence rates. The most notable, LoveLife, with the support of the South African government, has sponsored huge billboards and other costly advertising campaigns with little evidence of success. Such campaigns have been a great boon to advertising companies, now partly owned by the rising black business elites, but the prevalence of HIV has continued to increase. Countless nongovernmental organizations and church and educational organizations have also rallied to care for those who are afflicted and to deliver prevention messages to those who are not, but their efforts are uncoordinated and often at cross-purposes.

As if to highlight matters, the former deputy president, Jacob Zuma, awaiting trial on charges of corruption, was alleged to have raped an HIV-positive AIDS activist and family friend in Durban, on or about 4 November 2005.[10] He was tried and eventually found not guilty. Although it is difficult to avoid seeing this incident as symbolic of the conflict between the government and people of South Africa today, in fact, it seems to have been much more banal than that. Zuma testified in court that he knew his victim was HIV-positive. But, he declared, since HIV was more likely to be passed from male to female, and since he was HIV-negative, he did not think the risk was great enough to deny himself the pleasure. The problem was not lack of knowledge:

indeed, as the chair of the government's AIDS program and the leader of a "moral regeneration" drive, he used his superior knowledge of the statistical probabilities to excuse the alleged rape and justify his decision to have unprotected sex with the victim. Moreover, he told the court, he took a shower after raping the woman because he believed this would protect him against HIV. All of this, he testified, was a consequence of his deep commitment to Zulu traditional culture, which required that men and women satisfy their sexual desires whenever they became apparent. The case reflected the complex interplay of sex, money, violence, and politics . . . but also of love, trust, joy, and relationship-building that characterizes contemporary South Africa.

There is nothing simple about this case. The problem of AIDS and the spread of HIV throughout southern Africa involve every aspect of life, love, and the pursuit of happiness. No single approach is capable of comprehending it all because of its human complexity. A comprehensive summary of most of the research on AIDS in Uganda noted in July 2006 that the reasons for the decline in HIV prevalence in Uganda are still "complex and not yet completely understood."[11] An anthropological approach is likely at least to shed the most light on the problem. Effective response is another matter. That depends on how the problem is represented in popular culture and in political discourse, on whether there exists a political will to make the necessary changes, and on how the myriad institutions and social networks are able to respond. To understand these processes, to know AIDS, is a complex task indeed.

KNOWING AIDS

I was twenty years old when I first arrived in Uganda, in 1969. The country seemed a miracle of beauty and calm. The population then numbered less than ten million but has nearly trebled since. I lived with my parents, brother, and sister in an airy white house with dark parquet floors and lush gardens all around. From the deep red soil of the small vegetable patch planted by my mother and tended by James Atieno, our feckless gardener, we had a constant supply of fresh lettuce, tomatoes, peppers, and eggplants. The nearby markets supplied a cornucopia of sweet fruit and other vegetables. The staple food, *matooke*—a starchy green banana that was steamed and mashed—literally grew on trees. Eaten with a handful of beans or a bit of chicken, *matooke* made a nutritious and filling meal. Both beans and chickens seemed to grow naturally in every banana grove. In the rainy season, rains seemed to arrive just as one sat down to lunch and were generally over by the time the meal was finished, leaving the air fresh and clean. The altitude was high enough for the air always to be fresh and never too hot or dry. It was perfect.

I taught science and geography at a Catholic girls high school in Kampala and attended Makerere University. My father was deputy director of the U.S. Peace Corps and my mother taught at the teacher training colleges. My brother and sister attended high school. In the evenings, I went to the many nightclubs that featured Congolese jazz, or to one of the downtown hotels, and danced and drank Bell beers until late. During the holidays I traveled to all corners of the country, sleeping wherever I could, often in small country *hoteli* that were really just bars with a few rooms with beds in back. Roads were mostly dirt, with one paved highway from the Kenyan border to Kampala and on to the western border through Mbarara to Kigezi, and to the mining town of Fort Portal on the Congo border. The only other main road made a loop to the north through Mbale on the slopes of Mount Elgon along the Kenyan border, then across the lower part of the northern districts, and back again to Kampala from Gulu.

Uganda is deeply divided by strong ethnic differences. The southern half is inhabited by people speaking languages of the Bantu family. Politically, they were well organized into several ancient kingdoms with royal lines and histories stretching back five centuries or so. Buganda was the central kingdom, which had eventually conquered and dominated most of the rest of the southern part of the country by the time Europeans arrived in the late nineteenth century. With the help of Europeans, the kingdom of Buganda brought the northern part of the country under its control, and eventually the whole country became a protectorate of the British Crown. The northern half of the country, however, was inhabited primarily by loosely organized tribes of warrior-pastoralists and small agriculturalists without large-scale political organizations like those in the kingdoms of the south. Uganda, fashioned from these varied kingdoms, chiefdoms, and territories, became independent in 1962.

The 1960s were the glory days of Uganda's short history as an independent country. Everything appeared poised to move from good to better. In some respects, things seemed as if they could scarcely be better. Ugandans themselves were apparently happy and content. They partied and danced freely. University students and people in the villages were openly sexual and seductive. For most, the land provided a good living. Communities were often self-contained economic entities with limited need for commodities from outside. The few things that were purchased—cloth, salt, cooking oil, lanterns, candles, and paraffin—were always locally available from trading shops run almost exclusively by Indian traders. Villages were wholesome places with little apparent hunger—except perhaps in the far north near the Sudanese border and in the dry regions of northeastern Uganda. With long spears and shields, the Karimojong and Jie herdsmen continued their age-old fight over cattle when they were not grazing their large herds. Although they were the poorest of Uganda's people, from the several months I spent in their large wood-fenced homesteads, or *manyattas,* I could see that they also were fully self-sufficient, proud, and happy with their lot. For the vast majority of Ugandans, money was scarce, but food, most of it home grown, was not. People stayed close to their lands and villages as a result.

All of that changed in 1971 when Idi Amin Dada, then commander of the armed forces, staged a coup that overthrew President Milton Obote. Shooting started early on the morning of the coup, just before elections were to be held. By first light, it was clear that the rosy future that had once seemed certain would not dawn. Radio Uganda played the same British military marches all day, and the BBC repeated the line, "Heavy fighting in and around Kampala; it is not known if the European population is safe." We did not know either. Later that day, I ventured from the Makerere University campus into Wandegeya market with a Sudanese friend of mine to see if we could find out what was happening. Large-caliber machine gun fire soon drove us back. I wanted to run, but at the urging of my friend, already used to battle in his native Sudan, I stood quietly behind a bush until the shooting stopped and we were able to retreat without raising suspicion from the undisciplined troops. Cordite smoke and fog already filled the valleys of the many hills on which Kampala is built. We later found out that Idi Amin had routed the forces of the president.

A few years earlier, Obote and Amin together had attacked the palace of the king of Buganda, Edward Muteesa, ending the kingship, which had endured for five centuries on the shores of Lake Victoria. Muteesa had fled to England, where he died of alcoholism a few years later. Now it was Obote's turn to flee the country. He took shelter in neighboring Tanzania under the protection of the Tanzanian president, Julius Nyerere. Most of the small population of people of Indian and European origin were driven out of the country, and for the next fifteen years all areas of Uganda plunged deeper and deeper into the chaos of warfare, coups, economic collapse, and the decay of infrastructure, farms, industry, and governance. Ugandans moved from their villages in desperation, and soldiers freely roamed the country. The soldiers raped women where and when they pleased and pillaged the country. Ostensibly to alleviate the ravages of the Amin regime, Nyerere's Tanzania attacked Uganda in order to restore Obote. Obote returned in 1980 and set up a new government in Uganda. He turned out to be even more ruthless and despotic than Amin, and the country continued its decline into complete social collapse and barbarism.

Most Ugandans blamed the arrival of AIDS in the country on the violence and social dislocations of this era. A new disease, or an older disease that the locals called by a new name, "slim" or *siliimu* (in Luganda and other Bantu-family languages in southern Uganda), was gradually taking hold in southwestern Uganda. It was first perceived in the area where Tanzanian troops first crossed into Uganda, and it continued to spread along the shores of Lake Victoria as smugglers in boats carried goods across the Uganda/Tanzanian border in the army's wake. A large trade in contraband goods developed along the border in the extreme northwest corner of Tanzania and the southwest corner of Uganda in the Rakai District. Smuggling, trade, and raids took place especially across Lake Victoria, involving the previously isolated fishing communities on its shores and on the islands. Even today, the Rakai District, neighboring Masaka, and the communities along the lake shore and on the islands have the highest HIV prevalence in Uganda. This may not be due entirely to the violent conflict, unrestricted smuggling and raiding, and outright warfare that gripped this area for nearly a decade, but this set of conditions is likely to be at least an important factor in the rise of HIV infection in this area. By the end of the 1970s, AIDS was already noticeable in this corner of Uganda.

Exactly fifteen years after Idi Amin overthrew the first Milton Obote regime, the National Resistance Army (NRA) led by Yoweri Kaguta Museveni marched into Kampala. As the final battles ended, Museveni was sworn in as president on 27 January 1986 in the Lubiri, the old palace of the former king of Buganda. The place was as significant as the event since it signaled the return of respect for the old kingships of the southern part of the country, and the end of fifteen years of chaotic and brutal rule. Although Obote had been duly elected after the 1980 elections returned his party, the Ugandan People's Congress (UPC), to power, his efforts to defeat Museveni's NRA were brutal. He was

removed again in mid-1985 by the military, and briefly replaced by
Tito Okello as president months before the NRA's successful attack on
Kampala.

Museveni was born sometime during 1944 in Ankole District of—in
his words—the "Bahima nomads of southwestern Uganda." His illiter-
ate parents remembered only the approximate time of his birth since it
occurred about the time that Kahaya II, the Ankole king or *omugabe*,
died.[12] Museveni was named after the Seventh Battalion (*Abaseveni*,
"the sevens") of the King's African Rifles, the colonial African army to
which Idi Amin had belonged. Museveni's family was aristocratic and
belonged to the cattle-keeping Hima tribe, a Ugandan ethnic group
that shared a historical genealogy with the more widely known Tutsi of
neighboring Rwanda and Congo, and who are known for their unique
breed of gentle, long-horned red cattle. His parents had converted to
Christianity during the first years of his life. His mother became a
born-again evangelical Anglican, while his father remained more traditional in his outlook but was an enlightened modernizer. Museveni
himself believed that "it was good to have this dichotomous religious
existence."[13] He emphasized these points in his autobiography, *Sowing
the Mustard Seed,* whose title was drawn from the Bible story in
Matthew 13:31–32. The mixture of Ugandan tradition and evangelical
Christianity was later to direct his approach to HIV.

By his own description, Museveni had a long history of advocacy
for social and cultural change, first in his attempts to modernize cattle
keeping and health practices in his own Hima tribe in his early teens,
and later in various political action groups in high school and at university in Dar es Salaam. He came to power ready to tackle a complex
social problem such as HIV/AIDS with firm grounding in Ugandan
tradition and Christianity, and with a strong background in activities
directed toward social and cultural change.

After leaving Uganda in 1972, I completed a PhD in anthropology at
the University of Chicago, spending two years in a village in central
Tanzania to do my doctoral research. In 1979, I became a lecturer in
anthropology at the University of Cape Town in South Africa. South
Africa was very different from Uganda. The land was drier, the people
better dressed and more businesslike, the lifestyle urban and often
more European than African. During the years that I had lived and
worked in East Africa, South Africa had never seemed to me to be part
of Africa. We could buy the South African *Drum Magazine* in Uganda

and Kenya, and this showed an Africa that seemed modernized in ways East Africans could only dream of. Photos of black South African models decorated the walls and cupboards of many young Ugandans in those days. South Africa seemed like a place I would one day like to visit, and I finally had my chance: a three-year teaching contract that would acquaint me with a part of Africa that none of my teachers at Makerere, Stanford, or Chicago had deigned to mention in my many African studies and anthropology courses. Several of my Makerere lecturers were refugees from South Africa, but they did not talk about it to their students. It was also off the map of Africa according to African studies in the United States.

South Africa in 1979 was still in the grip of apartheid, but after thirty years of National Party rule that grip was clearly failing. The population, at twenty-five million, was little more than half what it is today (forty-eight million), and similar to Uganda's current population of twenty-eight million. In Cape Town, racial segregation had never been as rigid as in the rest of the country because the large "colored" population formed a sort of racial middle ground. I bought a house in an area that had never been fully segregated, and my family became integrated into the South African lifestyle.

South Africa was not what I had expected as an anthropologist. During my years in Chicago, racial segregation was virtually absolute, though informal and illegal. Certain streets marked racial dividing lines that few dared to cross. Black and white people did not, in the main, work together or visit one another's houses. Although they spoke the same language, there was very little communication, and that little was often tinged with fear and misunderstanding.

In South Africa, although racial segregation was formal and legally sanctioned, black and white people were in constant daily contact. Many white people had black servants living in their houses, with whom they interacted at close quarters in the daily domestic routine. The great majority of nonwhite people worked in white-owned businesses or in government, or had other sorts of daily contact with people of other races. Unlike in Chicago, where a white person might rarely meet a black person who lived nearby and spoke the same language, daily social interaction in South Africa was ordinary, uncomplicated, cordial, and routine despite linguistic differences. In contrast, political and economic inequalities between what were then called "races" or "population groups" in South Africa were apparently absolute. Despite the daily social reality, perceived transgression of legal separation could result in long imprisonment or even death. These contrasting and unjustified realities made South Africa a "very strange society," as Alan Paton remarked in *Cry the Beloved Country*.

It was clear by the beginning of the 1980s that these social arrangements could not endure. The apartheid state began desperate efforts to save itself, efforts that gradually segued into endgame politics. Two new "separate but equal" parliaments were set up, one for "colored people," and one for Indians. Colored and Indian politicians emerged who were willing to play the game, and some people voted for them. Although illegitimate except in terms of the local legal game, these events brought increasing numbers into a normalized political process. In one of the more grotesque political burlesques of those days, the South African state granted independence to the separate homelands of Transkei (homeland of the Xhosa people), Ciskei (also Xhosa), Venda (Venda), and Bophutatswana (Tswana). This had the overall effect of highlighting the absurdity of the system, and it was an absurdity that no one could miss.

By 1985, however, internal resistance groups became bolder and violence began to increase. When I was a lecturer at the University of Cape Town, it became routine to administer examinations in Pollsmoor Prison for those students who had recently been arrested for protest action. Police attacks and tear gas on campus were regular occurrences. Ironically, the overall effect was to cause widespread interaction across most political and social barriers and to convince most South Africans that change was inevitable. In the late 1980s, South Africa looked as though it, too, would descend into political chaos and violence as the apartheid government struggled to remain in power and as several democratic resistance movements sensed that apartheid's denouement was approaching. A few years later, in 1990, Nelson Mandela was released from prison and, contrary to most people's expectation, South Africa began a rapid transformation to political freedom, universal voter franchise, democracy, and the peaceful integration of all aspects of government and civil society. By the time the new African National Congress – dominated government formed in 1994, apartheid was already long over in the minds of the vast majority of South Africans.

At the beginning of the 1990s, HIV infection in South Africa was still barely noticeable. But by 1994, when the African National Congress (ANC) took power under the new constitution and after the first fully democratic elections in South African history, the HIV prevalence rate was already at 7.6 percent among women attending prenatal clinics. There were large differences in HIV prevalence between South African subregions. KwaZulu-Natal Province, predominately Zulu-speaking and home to Durban, South Africa's third largest city, had a prevalence rate of 14.4 percent. The Western Cape Province, predominately Afrikaans- and English-speaking and home to Cape Town, the second largest city, had a reported prevalence rate of only 1.2 percent.[14] Shortly after the new government was sworn in, it drew up a comprehensive national health plan in collaboration with the World Health Organization and the United Nations Children's Fund (UNICEF).[15] The plan was never effectively implemented.[16] With all of the political and other work that had to be done to ensure that the transition to democracy and an open society remained peaceful, Nelson Mandela, the first president of the New South Africa (as it was called), effectively ignored the hidden AIDS crisis. He did not speak openly about AIDS until more than a decade later, following the death from the disease of his own son by his first marriage.

By then, President Mbeki's beliefs about AIDS meant that there would be no leadership from government on this issue. Mbeki stated his reasons in an infamous monograph awkwardly titled "Castro Hlongwane, caravans, cats, geese, foot & mouth and statistics, HIV/AIDS and the struggle for the humanization of the African."[17] Primarily circulated within the ANC at first, the document was not signed but was widely attributed to President Mbeki and several of his close associates. It begins with an epigram from John Le Carré's novel *The Constant Gardener,* and expresses concern that

> there are many people and institutions across the world that have a vested interest in the propagation of the HIV/AIDS thesis, because they have too much to lose if any important element of this thesis is proved to be false. . . . [T]hese include the pharmaceutical companies, which are marketing anti-retroviral drugs that can only be sold, and therefore generate profits, on the basis of the universal acceptance of the assertion that "HIV causes AIDS."[18]

Above all, the document accuses those who "accept the assertion that HIV causes AIDS" of holding a position that "is also informed by deeply entrenched and centuries-old white racist beliefs and concepts about Africans and black people." Suspicions of racism and drug profiteering apparently drove the ANC government's rejection of what it called "normal science." Again, the South African denialism did not come from any lack of knowledge about AIDS; quite the opposite.

Thus, twenty years after President Yoweri Museveni had come to power in Uganda with the attack on AIDS at the top of his nation-building agenda, the new South African government continued, as much as possible, to avoid the issue. Unlike Uganda, where the struggle against AIDS could be integrated into a program of political development, the South African leadership apparently feared that open talk about AIDS and sexuality would be divisive. President Thabo Mbeki, in particular, expressed the view that discussion of AIDS implied that black people were sexually promiscuous and "uncivilized." For these and other reasons, he failed to lead a struggle against the progress of HIV infection in the population. By 2007, HIV prevalence was pushing toward 50 percent among young women in some parts of the country, and continued to rise in most other segments of the population.

Unlike in most of the rest of Africa, specific ethnic or other group identities of any kind are no more than two centuries old in South Africa. The Afrikaners and the Zulu kingdom, perhaps the best known of South Africa's ethnic communities, came into being only in the 1820s and 1830s; before then they did not exist as self-conscious political entities. At about the same time, many white English-speaking and other Europeans began to settle there in larger numbers. Other African identities and political communities—Tswana, Sotho, Swazi, Xhosa, Venda, and others—began to emerge only around the time that Tswana, Sotho, and Swazi states were carved off in the late nineteenth century. Bechuanaland (which later became Botswana at independence in 1966) and the kingdoms of Swaziland and Lesotho, however, were not formally constituted until the early twentieth century, after the Anglo-Boer War. Widespread warfare and pervasive migration of virtually all of the population in the 1830s and 1840s, the rise of gold and diamond mines and labor migration in the 1860s to 1880s, and the Anglo-Boer war from 1898 until 1910 served both to mix the population and to formalize ethnic, linguistic, and political boundaries.

The country of South Africa finally emerged as a single entity in 1910. The struggle against apartheid had much the same effect as the wars of the nineteenth and early twentieth centuries. By the end of the twentieth century, South Africans continued to live and work together in a single nation and a single national economy in which everyone was dependent on one another in a highly complex, modern, globalized capitalist economy. The inescapable irony of South African life is that the same processes that led to racism, ethnic divisions, and apartheid also created an ethos of equality, an unremarked daily routine of integration, and a tightly knit single national economy and society.

Unlike in Uganda, in South Africa very few people lived directly from the land (that is, by subsistence agriculture or even small-scale farming). Legally, most of the land was owned by a small class of white male farmers, who were effectively local chiefs in charge of large tracts of deeded land. Farm owners of other races (today, approximately 16 percent of owners) managed their farms in the same way as local chiefs. In 2005, 82 million of South Africa's total 122 million hectares were classified as commercial farmland and owned by only forty-five thousand people, most of whom were white. Approximately one million hectares of this land have been restored to nonwhite (mostly black African) claimants under the Restitution of Land Rights Act of 1994. Although this includes some urban land, usually in residential plots, most of it is rural farmland. The bulk of this has been restored to claimant communities under the terms of communal property associations that do not permit private ownership. Much of the rest of South Africa is too arid or mountainous for any form of agriculture. The remaining portion is urban land or roadways and transportation facilities, state- and company-owned forests or game reserves, protected watersheds or parks, mining reserves, and government land. Although the privately owned tracts are called farms in South Africa, they bear little resemblance to farms in Europe, the United Kingdom, or the United States. Most of the land of these farms is simply bush or pasture, with active intensive farming restricted to small parts of their holdings.[19] Large populations of Africans live on most of these farms, some as labor, some as tenants with small fields of their own, some as labor managers or tradesmen, and others just as residents. Households of other family members, helpers, and employees of all races often live on these lands as well. But "farming" is almost exclusively commercial and in 2005 it contributed no more than 3.4 percent to gross domestic product (GDP). Throughout the twentieth century, farming was capital intensive, often depending on large "loans" from government that were frequently written off in order to keep the farms successful and under white ownership. Food was either purchased or—on the farms—doled out sparingly as wages-in-kind.

Another large portion of the country was communal tribal trust land in the so-called homelands. These were run by chiefs similarly to how owners ran private farms, but the chiefs in these cases were called traditional authorities and had a sort of loose legitimacy rooted in the precolonial political order. The chiefs, like the farmers, had been recruited by the apartheid regime to regulate movement of people around South Africa. Indeed, the movement of people was perhaps the most urgent concern of the entire apartheid state apparatus, with most legislation directed to its control.

Also unlike in Uganda, few people in South Africa owned land. The pervasive and constant movement of people across the face of the land was both motivated and constrained by the peculiar political and economic geography. Work opportunities existed primarily in the areas owned by mines, the state, and farms, and in urban areas, whereas most people still lived in the communal homeland areas and specially designated periurban areas called "townships" or "locations" to distinguish them from "towns" and "cities," where, officially, only white, Indian, and colored people could live in separate segregated suburbs. In fact, however, almost as many black people lived in these areas, working as domestic helpers, laborers, and other sorts of assistants. During most of the twentieth century—not just under the apartheid regime of the National Party, which held sway for forty-four years from 1948 to 1992—huge efforts were devoted to concentrating most of the white, Indian, and colored population in the so-called urban areas and most of the black population in townships and rural native reserves or, later, homelands.

State policy aimed to encourage the development of local and ethnic differences, while social, political, and economic forces drove the people of the country toward social integration and the breakdown of ethnic barriers. All South Africans participated in the same national economy as consumers, purchasing food and necessities for cash rather than producing it themselves. Production was the preserve of large commercial farms and industry (some of it state-owned), while transportation, roads, and utility services (water, electricity, sanitation) were exclusively the domain of the state. A highly efficient paved system of roads linked all but the most remote parts of the country in a common network for those with access to cars and trucks, and extensive rail and bus links serviced the rest. It was possible to travel anywhere in South Africa in little more than a day or two, and people traveled extensively. The number of bus tickets to and from Transkei (one of the homelands) sold in Cape Town in one year in the 1980s was equivalent to the city's entire population.

In the end—the end of the twentieth century and the end of apartheid—the unintended consequences of government policy won out over its explicit intentions. South Africa entered the time of AIDS as a highly mobile, largely urbanized population with few significant ethnic, regional, or linguistic barriers to social interaction. One of the most enduring legacies of apartheid, and perhaps its greatest success during its existence, was to convince South Africans, and much of the rest of the world, that South Africans were divided far more than they actually were, by race, language, ethnicity, and class. This was possible partly because virtually no South Africans had experienced life in the rest of Africa, and for those who aided or participated in the struggle against apartheid, explicit comparison between South Africa and the rest of Africa was effectively forbidden for complex political reasons. There is, consequently, almost no explicit comparison between South African society and the rest of Africa even today. This still hampers our understanding of the radically different regional HIV epidemics in the continent.

Well into the first decade of the twenty-first century, South Africa has the most vibrant economy in sub-Saharan Africa. It is the power-house of the southern half of the continent. A great deal of the trade and almost all of the financial business from central and eastern Africa comes through South Africa. The South African economy is begin-ning to dominate those of countries as far north as Uganda. Where once Ugandans were puzzled by depictions in *Drum Magazine* of the strange land to the south, today South African retail, transportation, banking, and tourism businesses have begun to take hold, especially in Uganda and Tanzania. The characteristic branding of South African mega-retailers such as Pick 'n Pay, Shoprite, and Protea Hotels is highly visible in East African capitals.

Formal unemployment remains high in South Africa, but it has become clear in my ethnographic work in South Africa's small towns and villages that there is a huge underground or informal economy involv-ing most of the "unemployed" in enterprises that produce a reasonable living for most people. For instance, the South African government has built 1.7 million housing units for the poor and homeless throughout the country.[20] This has created a huge underground (illegal) economy in rentals, price speculation, bribery, services (renovation, expansions, decorating, furniture, repairs), and other activities that seem to absorb much of the time of the unemployed. Thus, while formal statistics show South Africa far ahead of other African countries in terms of its GDP, its real wealth is even greater.

This does not mean that South Africa has become a fully integrated classless society; far from it. As in the rest of the world, the rich got richer and the poor got poorer, but the racial mix of rich and poor has changed rapidly from the 1990s on. By 2005, there were significant numbers of exceptionally wealthy black business people and professionals and an increasing number of poor and indigent whites. Colored and Indian populations, for the most part, held their own somewhere in the middle-income levels, with growth of Indian incomes and wealth increasing much more rapidly than those of all other ethnic groups.

But even when I arrived in South Africa in 1979, I found that South Africans of all colors and social positions were relatively wealthy compared with Ugandans or Tanzanians. Even the urban poor in South Africa lived more comfortably than most of the Ugandans or Tanzanians I had known. Above all, South Africans interacted intensively across most social categories in one way or another. Although South Africans were divided in many ways, informal networks based in common language (mainly Zulu, English, Afrikaans, and Sotho), religion (Christian, Muslim, Jewish, and Hindu), place of employment, sports team support and participation, and other activities and shared interests brought South Africans of all categories into daily contact. The informal economy, especially during sanction busting under apartheid, created further networks of exchange that crossed most boundaries, national, racial, or other. Where ethnic or tribal differences were strong and unambiguous in Uganda or Tanzania, in South Africa these identities were most often shifting, negotiable, and varying, depending on context.

AIDS was just beginning to be noticed in southwestern Uganda by the time I arrived in South Africa. The causal agent, HIV, had not yet been identified by science. In my new home, however, there was no awareness of the disease that would kill two million people in the next twenty-five years, and infect five million or more out of a population that was estimated at about forty-six million in 2005. Its impact was first noticed on the West Coast of the United States, and then, as doctors noticed similarities in symptoms between gay men in California and patients in Uganda, it became apparent that HIV was becoming "the ultimate global disease."[21] No one then knew how bad it might be. In South Africa no one was even thinking about it yet.

My first contact with AIDS came in the mid-1980s. A colleague at the University of Cape Town was invited by his cousin to scout the possibility of making a film about the anthropologist and primatologist Diane Fossey, whose pioneering work on the mountain gorillas of Rwanda had brought them to the world's attention. She had died, or been murdered, under mysterious circumstances in her house in the Parc des Volcans in Rwanda. Her earlier swashbuckling style and unorthodox methods had brought her personal notoriety. Some five years earlier, my brother had been shocked to meet her deep in the Kigezi forest in Uganda with two pearl-handled revolvers strapped to her hips. Now she was dead, and my colleague, Andy Sillen, and I were engaged to investigate the circumstances of her death in case the story proved filmworthy.

I met Andy in Kigali, the capital of Rwanda, and we began to travel around the country making inquiries. After a couple of weeks, Andy developed a mysterious illness that did not seem life-threatening but became increasingly debilitating. We returned to Kigali and eventually found a Belgian doctor who told us that Andy had contracted trypano-somiasis (sleeping sickness) from the bite of a tsetse fly. Worse, he was about to go into a coma from which it was unlikely he would recover. The doctor refused to treat him in Kigali, saying that the treatment she had available would in all likelihood kill him, and if it did not, in the course of treatment he would almost certainly contract a new disease that was only then becoming known: AIDS. She advised us to get back to South Africa as quickly as we could, adding that, even so, his chances of survival were not good. We barely made it to Nairobi, where he was successfully treated. There we saw a picture of the Kigali Hospital in *Time* magazine. The caption read: "Rwanda's 'AIDS Central,' the Kigali Hospital."

At home in South Africa, there was still no indication that HIV would travel that far south. By the end of the 1980s, however, some notice was taken. At the time, AIDS was still thought of in South Africa as a disease of homosexual men. One of the vilest of the South African government-aligned news reporters, Cliff Saunders, traveled to Uganda to ask questions about the epidemic. His report, broadcast on the television evening news, showed him asking a Ugandan man if he had had sex with other men. "Eh?" the Ugandan responded incredulously as the microphone was thrust in his face. "But there are so many women!" Cliff Saunders smiled and shook his head in comical resignation. At that time, the government-controlled South African Broadcasting Corporation was presenting AIDS as a joke.

The HIV epidemic began to take off in South Africa around 1990. Paradoxically, in that same year, HIV prevalence began to fall dramatically in Uganda. Once it was clear that the epidemic was headed in radically different directions in the two countries, a few people began to ask why. But not in South Africa. There were too many other issues at stake and problems to solve. Mandela's initial failure to deal with the epidemic segued into Mbeki's staunch denial of its impact. Remarkably, it was not until the beginning of the new millennium that AIDS began to focus the minds of the country's leaders. By then, it was no longer possible to halt the epidemic in its early stages.

In my own research in the small towns and rural areas of South Africa during that time it had become apparent that carrying on as usual was impossible. AIDS was everywhere; all aspects of society and culture were beginning to be affected, and my attention as an ethnographer turned, perforce, to AIDS, sex, and sexual behavior. My study of traditional healers in the South African lowveld (formerly known as the eastern Transvaal) provided access to traditional and popular ideas about HIV and its associated syndromic diseases and symptoms. It also gave me a different point of access to attitudes about sex and its practice in the small towns and rural areas.

In 2003, I had the opportunity to return to Uganda for the first time in thirty years. I was invited to be a member of a team that would study the reasons for the decline in HIV prevalence in Uganda while it continued to increase in the rest of the world. Funded by the U.S. Agency for International Development (USAID), the project as originally conceived would examine three countries selected from those where HIV prevalence had fallen (Uganda, Thailand) or where there was some evidence of local declines in prevalence (Lusaka, Zambia). These would be compared with three countries in which prevalence was still rising (Zimbabwe, Cameroon, and Kenya).

Arriving in Kampala in July, I felt as if I had come home again. I was able to find many of my old familiar places despite the vast changes that had taken place over thirty years. I was able to make my way back to our old house on Mbuya Hill. It was still as lovely as I remembered it, even though goats were now stabled in my old bedroom. The science laboratory that I had set up at Rubaga Girls High School during my first adventure in education was still almost as I had left it, despite the growth of the school and vast changes everywhere else. Notably, the many nightclubs and bars where I had once hung out, and where sex had always been available for the price of a beer, were gone. In their place were huge evangelical and Pentecostal churches in tents and buildings. The music one heard in the street was no longer Congolese jazz, but born-again Christian pop music. Much of this activity, it turned out, was funded by wealthy American Christian missions.

Our research began, and we soon found that Ugandans everywhere were overwhelmingly aware of AIDS and that huge changes had happened in many aspects of their lives as a result. USAID's hidden agenda gradually became apparent, however. President George W. Bush and his administration had been convinced by some researchers that sexual abstinence and churches had played the major role in reversing the AIDS trend in Uganda. Our project was meant to prove conclusively that this was the case. As our interviews, focus groups, and textual research progressed, however, it became clear that this was not the case; at best, it was only part of a very complex story. It appeared that USAID believed that the Ugandan president, Yoweri Museveni, had insisted on abstinence, especially in the military, which he commanded when he came to power in January 1986. We were therefore surprised when a colonel in the medical corps told us, "Thank God, Museveni never told us not to have sex! He would have been laughed out of the country!"

Instead, Museveni had promoted what he called "zero grazing." Based on the colloquialisms and metaphors of Museveni's own pastoral tribe, the Hima, this phrase meant, in practice, "carry on having sex, but keep it local and close to home." The slogan referred to the practice of tethering a cow to a peg in the middle of a patch of good grazing. As the animal ate the grass that its tether permitted it to reach, it would clear a circular area around the peg. This was the zero of "zero grazing." It did not mean abstinence—zero sex—as some earlier researchers, and President Bush's advisors, seemed to think. It simply meant, "Eat (have sex) as much as you like, but don't roam too widely." As it turned out, this simple rule may have turned the tide in Uganda because it altered the configuration of the sexual networks on which the spread of HIV depends, *not* because it increased sexual abstinence. But the misunderstanding in Washington eventually killed the research. Alarmed by the fact that our research was not producing the desired results, a USAID manager came to Kampala from Washington. He sent the research collaborators away and prematurely ended the research. Appeals resulted in our being allowed to finish a curtailed project in Uganda, but the overall project involving other countries was canceled. Another dimension of the politics of AIDS was brought forcibly to my attention.

After thirty years of devastation by warfare and AIDS in Uganda, I did not expect to find many old friends from the late 1970s alive. Apart from Makerere student colleagues who had left the country, I had lost touch with everyone from those times. My mother had not. She

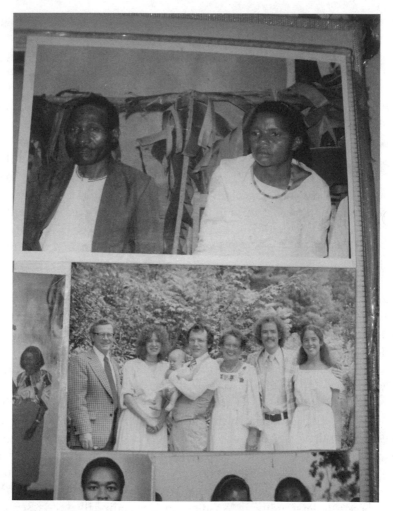

FIGURE 1. Kamondo's family photo album, Mbarara, Uganda, shows the Thornton family's picture from 1978 (below) and Kamondo with his wife (above). The author is in the middle with his newborn son. (Photograph by R. Thornton)

emailed me to try to find the family of Kamondo, one of her favorite students from Ggaba Teacher Training College. He had become the headmaster of a school in Mbarara and had stayed in touch with my parents, who now lived in the United States. For thirty years, my father had kept beside his bed a spear that Kamondo had given them. Other friends had explained to me that in western Uganda, a husband would jam his spear across the doorframe while he was having sex with his wife so that no one would interrupt them. But, by the same token, if he came home and found someone else's spear across the door to his wife's quarters, he must be polite and leave quietly. The gift of the spear had been a joke, meant to indicate how fond Kamondo had been of my mother. My father had taken it in good humor. But, perhaps because of these same western Ugandan customs, Kamondo had died of AIDS many years before my arrival. I managed to track down his wife, now the headmistress of the school where Kamondo had taught. We walked past his grave as we entered the house, where family members still felt the loss of Kamondo and his brothers, who lay buried in the courtyard of the family compound. All may have died of AIDS.

Inside the house, we talked of old times and paged through the family's photo album. On one page I found my own picture. In it, I am standing with my first-born son in my arms with my parents, siblings, and wife. The picture was taken in 1979, the year we moved to South Africa. My mother had sent it to Kamondo's family sometime after that. Above the picture was a much more recent picture of Kamondo with his wife. Kamondo is dressed in the traditional Ganda formal attire of a *kanzu*, a white floor-length gown that had originally been introduced by the Arabs in the nineteenth century, and a gray suit jacket, introduced by the English at about the same time. Behind them is a traditional banana leaf screen. In the picture, Kamondo already looks ill (see figure 1).

Back home in South Africa, colleagues, friends, and friends of friends were also beginning to be infected by HIV in larger numbers. Some were dying; others managed to obtain antiretrovirals and were having varied degrees of success in beating back the infection. As in Uganda in the early 1990s, a decade later in South Africa it was not possible to ignore the impact of AIDS on friends, colleagues, and family. Still, the president and other members of the South African government continued to downplay the issue or ignore it altogether. And things began to go wrong again in Uganda. President Bush had managed to recruit Ugandan president Museveni into his "coalition of the willing" in the prelude to the American attack on Iraq. Museveni was heavily dependent on American funding for AIDS programs and for his own efforts to stay in power beyond his constitutional term limit. To protect that funding, he needed to follow Bush's line on AIDS, sex, and the war on terrorism. Museveni's wife was a born-again Christian in sympathy with the Bush administration and its policies that promoted abstinence even in the face of overwhelming evidence that it did not work, and deemphasized condoms despite all the evidence of their effectiveness. As a consequence, Ugandan HIV prevalence is creeping up again.

My long and intimate acquaintance—indeed, affection—for these two countries, Uganda and South Africa, gives me a special perspective as well as a personal motive to understand the progress of this epidemic. It has convinced me that AIDS must be seen in the broadest possible cultural and social perspective, over time, and across space.

TEMPORAL AND SPATIAL ASPECTS OF THE HIV EPIDEMIC

The HIV/AIDS epidemic is, of course, a medical fact. The temporal and spatial aspects of this pandemic, however, are largely social and cultural. The growth of the epidemic, the processes by which it is transmitted from one person to another, the huge regional and local differences in prevalence and in the types of the virus that are responsible, are, for the most part, the consequence of social and cultural factors.

In the first place, there are actually multiple epidemics. Each country and each region of each country manifests different characteristics that either predispose it to rapid spread of the infection or tend to retard the spread. Transportation networks and travel among regions link different regions in different ways. Moreover, economic differentials among regions and countries tend either to encourage or to discourage travel and other contacts among them, thus leading to different rates of transmission in different regions and countries. Sexual practices, numbers of sexual partners, rates of prostitution, and other practices also differ spatially and create different spatial distributions of HIV. Above all, however, the specific configuration of sexual networks determines much of the landscape of HIV transmission and AIDS morbidity.

This, in itself, is not enlightening. All pathogens are transmitted from one person to another (or, rarely, from some nonhuman source to a human), and if we could draw a graph or diagram of who infected whom for any pathogen, it would look like a network. This would be true for any pathogen that is transmitted directly from person to person, such as the pathogens responsible for leprosy, tuberculosis, warts, or mononucleosis. Pathogens that cause diseases like cholera and flu, by contrast, are transmitted through the common medium of air or water, and thus use channels that can affect anyone who breathes or drinks these common resources.

Effective public health regimens can offer protection from both kinds of pathogens. So can wealth, because it permits a degree of filtering of the common resources (air, water, food) and limits the networks of contact with others through customs and behaviors associated with what may be called "class" or other social differentials. In principle, the pattern of infection could be represented as a network if we were able to trace who, when, and what in all cases. Of course, we cannot do this because most of these pathogens are invisible. Instead, we resort to statistical methods that assume a more or less equal chance of infection for all members of a vulnerable population—that is, a population of people who are susceptible to the disease and who have not (yet) built up immunity. In the case of HIV, this gives us a measure of prevalence, or the proportion of the population that is infected. It tells us virtually nothing about how HIV is transmitted.

This is because, unlike other epidemics, HIV is not transmitted randomly but rather primarily through sexual networks. Sexual networks are a specific kind of social structure. Sex has a value, and this value is what is "transacted," exchanged, revalued, and "consumed" through the interactions that constitute the sexual network. Moreover, sex, for the most part, takes place only under highly constrained and structured social conditions—especially in the context of what we call intimacy or privacy. It is a social act unlike any other, despite its everydayness and normality. It is, in fact, a kind of foundational social relation on which many other social relations are built.

These facts make HIV infection and its consequence, AIDS, different from any other disease, and, at the population level, different from any other epidemic. This difference is wholly apart from the fact that HIV infections cannot, so far, be cured or prevented through natural or induced immunity (vaccination). It also is a social disease like no other because it moves through and by means of social structures and because only social and cultural measures can (so far) prevent it or slow its progress.

Thus, the sexual network, although largely invisible, is unlike the invisible networks that link people in other epidemics. The networks through which the virus flows are not easily disrupted by public health initiatives, and wealth alone has no impact on its spread. Only humans are potential threats to others, and only, for the most part, when engaging in what is among the most fundamental and valuable of human pursuits. The process of transmission of HIV is therefore imbued with deep meanings, fundamental values, and all the complexity of society as a whole.

HIV/AIDS is an infection of society, of social structures, and of culture itself, as much as of an individual. It is not enough to treat it merely as a medical condition, as an epidemic, or as "behavior." In this book, I try to find ways to view AIDS as a characteristic or emergent property of the social domain—especially with respect to sexual networks as a type of social structure—and to understand its cultural and social-structural dimensions. This involves the examination of AIDS in relation to all of civil society and the state. The way in which people absorb the knowledge of AIDS into their cultural repertoires also determines the kind and quality of their response to it. This approach requires a reexamination of the meaning and value of sex itself. It amounts to a broader ecology of AIDS in which the large-scale systematic and environmental aspects are taken into account.

TIME AND AIDS

As we seek to develop responses to AIDS, we make the social and cultural context of the epidemic ever more complex. Medical and social interventions have different effects on different regions, and differ from individual to individual. Prevention and treatment methods evolve over time, and their efficacy and possibilities for implementation depend on the degree of development of delivery infrastructures, receptivity of the population, educational and media interventions, cultural responses, and social structures. The high cost of treatment means that there is a strongly marked differential in the ability of regions, countries, or continents to afford treatment. The nature and severity of stigma associated with the infection and its manifestation as AIDS, and the ability of the society to respond effectively and creatively to death and dying, are also factors that distinguish different responses in spatial terms. After the death of parents, siblings, and other household members and of members of the various productive units of society (such as farms, industry, transportation firms, and so on), it is clear that different regions are affected in different ways.

These factors are related in complex temporal ways as well. The epidemic has changed its spatial distribution over time as sexual networks link up or break over time. It is most likely that HIV has been endemic in human populations since the 1940s or 1950s,[22] and perhaps for generations.[23] For many years, it remained unnoticed, accounting for a few deaths in western and central Africa. It was an endemic infection that seems to have remained under some sort of control or limit. Today, it is probably impossible to say precisely where or how it began, or how it was previously contained in small isolated populations. It did not become an epidemic until it was already global.[24] Thus, an epidemic that seems to have begun in rural western or central Africa eventually appeared no later than 1979 in the United States, where it was first recognized as a distinct disease or syndrome in the early 1980s.[25] At first, it appeared only among small populations of homosexual men.[26] But it soon began to appear elsewhere and in other populations. It spread to the Caribbean[27] and began to be recognized across Europe. By July 1982, 452 AIDS cases had been reported to the Centers for Disease Control (CDC) in Atlanta, and in August the syndrome acquired its name.[28] Eighteen months later, the number of cases known to the CDC had increased by a factor of seventeen. By late 1984, the CDC had recorded 7,699 cases in the United States alone, and 3,665 deaths.[29] A group of doctors and researchers first noted instances in Uganda at this time and soon took the lead in the Ugandan response to the crisis.[30]

From the early 1980s, then, HIV spread rapidly but differentially to other parts of the world. As it spread, apparently the types of sexual and other activities that were most likely to spread the infection also shifted from early concentration in homosexuality and intravenous drug use to heterosexuality. By the beginning of the twenty-first century, heterosexuals were responsible for the bulk of transmissions.[31] Clearly, different social and sexual practices in different areas led to greater or lesser degrees of vulnerability and thus to different rates of transmission in different regions. The geographies of other epidemics and endemic infections such as tuberculosis, malaria, pneumonia, and other coinfections influenced the rate of transmission within and between regions and greatly affected the speed with which the viral infection gave rise to AIDS.

Thus, we need to understand the AIDS epidemic in both spatial and temporal terms and in the context of complex cultural and social structures. We can divide the temporal progression into three broad periods:

- The time before AIDS (which remains indefinite, but roughly before 1979),
- The time of AIDS, and
- The time after AIDS, a time that may never come.

We are now in the second of these periods. The third period is notional—we might say cultural—because it does not yet exist, and as

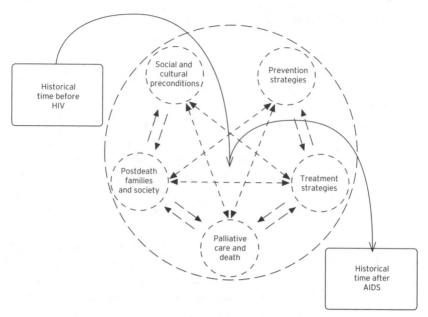

FIGURE 2. The time of HIV/AIDS: Subprocesses are linked in complex feedback and feed-through loops, although situated in historical time.

far as we know it may never exist. It is nonetheless an essential part of the temporal process, because this is what must motivate social action in response to AIDS. It fulfills the function of the Second Coming, the dream of salvation, the notion of the final stage of capitalism, the pure market, or the once-promised coming of the pure communist paradise. It may never happen—indeed, many may declare it an impossible dream—but it is still essential to our well-being and to the social imaginary.

The first period is real but merely antecedent. In the period before AIDS, societies already had developed and entrenched multiple factors—ideas and ideologies, values and practices, social forms and cultural norms, demographic densities and distributions—that influence the vulnerability of the society to HIV infection. This influences, in turn, the rate of transmission as well as the rate of progression from HIV infection to full-blown AIDS and death. These are the social preconditions for the epidemic. Once the virus has become fully endemic to a population in the second period, each group responds differently and meets the crisis of disease and death in different ways. The ability to acknowledge the severity and to deal with it either effectively or dysfunctionally differs dramatically. The second period is the current empirical reality and context of this book.

Within the second period, there are an additional five or so phases in a cycle (see figure 2). In the first phase, the virus begins to take hold of the sexual network that supports and transmits it. The preexisting cultural and social features of the demographic landscape that it will inhabit determine how and to what degree it takes hold. In the second phase, there is a response. An effort must be made to cope with the infection and its consequences. Here, the political and social structure of a community, society, or country must begin to change in order for its sexual networks to change. It must seek to cope with fear, stigma, and public health crises of many sorts. In some cases, there are political demands for effective action. In the third phase, several different types of treatment strategies must be formulated. It has become clear that single or isolated responses, no matter how effective each might be in isolation, do not work. The Ugandan multisectoral approach demonstrates the effectiveness of the integrated approach, and the fragmentation and conflict that have characterized the South African response are reflected in its ineffectiveness. Treatment strategies include medical interventions such as antiretroviral therapy, but in addition ways to change sexual behavior and sexual networks must be found and implemented. In the fourth phase, as people begin to sicken and die, there must be responses that aim to ameliorate suffering, to ease the passing of those who will not survive, and to arrange for death itself. This must include dealing with orphans, the consequence of broken and damaged webs of kinship and support, and, in some cases, changes in the way we deal with death. Finally, in the fifth phase there is the emergence of a social framework in which AIDS exists as a more or less permanent unpleasant fact. In other words, as AIDS becomes endemic, and not merely epidemic, its consequences become part of the cultural and social landscape. As new frameworks of belief, knowledge, and action emerge, people must come to terms with living in a different way.

In a mature AIDS epidemic, these temporal periods and phases eventually exist together. Although we can think of the social and cultural preconditions as existing before the epidemic—as they certainly did—they continue to exist, both for the individual and for the larger communities and society, as other stages develop. Each set of conditions, strategies, and outcomes develops at its own speed but also in response to the other processes.

Each also manifests different temporal scales. The preconditions—the entrenched traditions and social forms—change very slowly,
if at all. Meanwhile, the disease is transmitted and progresses at a much
greater rate than social institutions and cultural responses can change
to meet the challenge. Both prevention and treatment issues evolve at
different rates relative to one another, and with respect to the overall historical process of the epidemic. Responses to death and dying,
like the social preconditions for infections and transmission, are also
likely to change slowly, but since they must meet the absolute volume of
increasing mortality with limited resources, increasing mortality must
force a change. Overall, however, there is also a broad historical trend
in which the epidemic has developed from nothing to its current stage
at which it constitutes a significant threat to the health, well-being, and
lives of large numbers of people. Eventually—we must assume—HIV,
too, shall pass. This must occur in the scale of historical time that
subsumes the temporal scales on which each subprocess takes place
and can be measured. The key to this lies in understanding, first of all,
the unique properties of sexual networks that are responsible for HIV's
spread.

TOWARD A THEORY OF SEX AND NETWORKS

In order to develop an anthropological approach to AIDS—a holistic
or ecological approach that integrates understanding of the person with
the full social context and system—the problem of AIDS must be conceptualized as a problem of understanding historical process and social
process in cultural terms. This is a kind of historical anthropology.[32]

The problem of HIV/AIDS involves change in cultural meanings,
norms, and social action. It is clearly not enough to see it merely as
a problem of knowledge and/or behavior without seeing, as well, the
broader context. Decreasing prevalence—or, for that matter, a plateau
or stasis of the epidemic—is as much a *problem* in these terms as is
increasing prevalence. From a public health perspective, a fall in prevalence—such as occurred in Uganda—is a success and therefore *not* a
problem. Seen in the perspective of sexual networks and the kinds of
unique social structures they entail, however, a decline in prevalence is
equally problematic. The question that is raised has to do with a logic
of social structure and its role in shaping the history (or process) of the
epidemic. Since HIV is transmitted in the context of deep, explicit, and
intimate meanings, this approach entails grappling with the problem

of meaning in the *process* of transmission that leads to new infections (incidence). Although AIDS has generally been understood as a biological phenomenon, or as one that will cede eventually to a practical reason, the structure of the epidemic has to do primarily with meaning and culture. While many have addressed the question of meaning, this has been in the context of *response* to HIV—stigma, denial, representations in popular culture and in public discourse, declaration of one's "status," knowledge, attitudes—rather than an exploration of the meaning of sex and the values and motives that are deployed in the social organization of the sexual network. This problem is one of the primary concerns of this book.

But there is a fundamental theoretical difficulty with this approach, one that no amount of empirical knowledge or ethnography can amend. This difficulty has to do with the way we conceptualize sex itself, and with how we might understand the special types of networks that are built through sexual relations. This difficulty arises especially from the difficulty in trying to understand sex as social action and sexual networks as social institutions. In terms of the canonical theory of social action, we must seek to interpret what people do (action) in terms of the *social* meanings that motivate it. Social meanings are, however, public, shared, negotiated with other members of society—the social groupings to which we belong as humans—and therefore properties of culture and/or society that exist at a scale larger than the individual. This theoretical perspective presents problems when we seek to understand sex because it is private, specifically not public or shared by groups, and apparently motivated by biology (the drive to procreate), desire, pleasure. These motives are apparently psychological or are properties of the person. Similarly, sexual networks are invisible to social theory, as they usually are to their participants. They are what I call *unimagined communities*.

These problems must be taken seriously since they seem to lie at the root of the failure of a great deal of effort to change sexual behavior by means of methods that are apparently very effective in changing other kinds of social behavior. Advertising, political rhetoric, and public discourse of all kinds are evidently highly effective in changing consumption patterns in modern consumer societies, as the vast wealth of the major corporations that use them shows. Coke is preferred worldwide, despite the evidence of blind taste tests that show that people actually prefer the taste of other drinks such as Pepsi. Nike shoes offer no measurable physical advantage apart from status display. Apple computers are clearly better products, but personal computers that run Microsoft operating systems sell in far greater numbers. Political parties that are obviously corrupt and offer few, if any, services or advantages to the people who elect them maintain power through rhetoric against all odds. Despite the success of political rhetoric and advertising in these other contexts, however, it seems that they do not work in changing *sexual* "consumption" behaviors.

Sexual action, as opposed to social action, has a number of special qualities that make it resistant to public discourse, rhetoric, advertising, and other means of public persuasion. Sex has some of the qualities of ritual or of ritual process,[33] that is, it is enacted within the context of intimacy—what I call the space of the dual. This unique space of the sexual couple/coupling lies between the psychological space of the person and the social space of the many. Like the healing rituals that Victor Turner studied among the Ndembu people of what is now northwestern Zambia, sex is not public, proceeds in stages, distinguishes the experienced from the virgins (uninitiated), and entails status and conflict. The values of sex extend well beyond the values of desire, its fulfillment in pleasure, and procreation. Indeed, entry into sexual activity is a life crisis handled in many different ways by different cultures and different ages. These features have scarcely been theorized in cultural terms, primarily because the field has been monopolized by psychological, medical, and biological understandings of sex. In order to intervene effectively and where necessary, we must first understand the cultural value of sex. What we seek in the case of AIDS is an understanding of how the meaningful act of sex—quintessentially private, personal, intimate, local, and familial—is magnified by the presence of a new lethal virus to worldwide historical proportions. In other words, we seek to account for the fact that intimate acts of sex, under certain conditions, have historical and structural effects that are public, political, global, and demographic in their scope.

Viewed as social action, sex has properties of motive, intention, unintended consequences, and "working misunderstandings,"[34] but unlike theory of social action,[35] it is not public. In the public domain of HIV/AIDS, discussion of sex and sexuality and rhetorics of intervention constitute a kind of *theater of sexuality and AIDS*. Uganda has made this literal by developing a huge cultural industry around "AIDS theater" in churches, schools, government departments, workplaces, and villages (see chapters 6 and 7). The theater of sexuality and AIDS in South Africa has been of a much different sort, played out in courtrooms, on the street in demonstrations, and in the press. While in Uganda theater has been collaborative and part of the entire nation-building project after the installation of the new government under Museveni—and after the fifteen years of postcolonial collapse from 1971 to 1986—the South African theater has been oppositional, combative, and often secretive. In this sense, the Ugandan approach seems to reflect and demand a social integrationist or even functionalist approach, while South Africa demands an approach that understands conflict as a fundamental part of the "normal" social process, as integral to social integration, and as "peace in the feud."[36] Indeed, as I have argued elsewhere,[37] the anthropologist Max Gluckman's theoretical perspective—which emphasized the political process and conflict—is essentially a South African perspective. Max Gluckman's influence on anthropology, especially political anthropology that examines process and conflict at the local level, has been profound, but he was a South African and brought a South African perspective to anthropology. It reflects the way things work in South Africa, even in the time of AIDS. Other approaches are more appropriate elsewhere, for instance in Uganda, where the contemporary political order forbids political parties altogether.

African "local knowledge"[38] is explored here in some depth because this knowledge gives us access to the structures of knowledge. For instance, the early development of an indigenous cultural category for AIDS in Uganda, slim or *siliimu,* went a long way toward making it possible for Uganda to develop an early indigenous response. In South Africa, deep cultural values of what I call flows of sexual substance provide an alternative way of seeing HIV in the body for traditionalists in South Africa (especially traditional healers, *sangoma*s, and their clients).

The central problem of this book, then, concerns the structure of the social and cultural context of HIV transmission. I attempt to go beyond the issues that the sociologists of AIDS have addressed, that is, to show how it related to the macrocategories of wealth/poverty,[39] gender,[40] region,[41] age, race—and even economy[42] and politics[43]—in order to look instead at the social structure of HIV/AIDS transmission and sexual networks in particular.

The first step involves acknowledging that sex is a social relation, not (simply) a behavior. This is deceptively simple and seems obvious once stated, but for the most part sex acts have been understood as acts of individuals that take place in the context of other kinds of social relations characterized as economic, sociological, political, or ethnic/ racial. But to take sex as a social relation entails seeing sex as autonomously creative of other social relations and cultural categories. The sexual relation is not merely *influenced* by culture,[44] or *constrained* by political-economic factors, but is itself a fundamental building block of society as a whole and is a social relation sui generis. This theoretical step amounts to revaluing the sexual act for the sociological enterprise. The empirical problem lies in trying to understand how some sexual networks are pervasive and extensive (as in South Africa), while in other areas and countries they are more fragmented, fragile, and susceptible to interruption (as in Uganda). Clearly, HIV transmission is much more efficient in a maximal, cross-linked, pervasive, and extensive network than in a fragmented, limited set of smaller networks or clusters. Nevertheless, the sociological causes and coordinates of differing configurations of sexual networks have so far eluded researchers. This book offers some answers to the questions of how and why the specific configuration of sexual networks differs and, in particular, why there is such a vast difference between South Africa and Uganda in patterns of HIV prevalence.

CHAPTER 2

Comparing Uganda and South Africa

Sexual Networks, Family Structure, and Property

South Africa and Uganda have been at the center of attention in the HIV/AIDS pandemic.[1] The first evidence of the HIV epidemic in Africa emerged in Uganda in the early 1980s.[2] It is the only African country that has shown an overall and sustained decrease in prevalence (until recently, when prevalence has apparently begun to rise).[3] By contrast, South Africa was not forced to deal with the epidemic until the 1990s, and today has an HIV prevalence that is among the highest in the world. Since 1992, HIV trends in the two countries have moved strongly and consistently in opposite directions. This cannot be due simply to levels of sexual activity, since Uganda had a total fertility rate (TFR) of 6.9 in 2001[4] and 7.1 in 2005,[5] the highest in eastern and southern Africa. Uganda's TFR has remained roughly stable at least since 1955. South Africa's fertility, in contrast, has been relatively low and is declining,[6] with a TFR of 2.7 in 2005,[7] the lowest in Africa.

The explanation for the difference in the prevalence trends lies in differing *configurations of sexual networks* in the two countries. To demonstrate this, this chapter develops a mathematical model of prevalence trends and shows how this allows us to see differences in the topology of sexual networks. (A certain amount of mathematics is required here, but this is separated from the rest of the text and a reader who is not interested in the mathematics can skip over these sections.) Chapter 3 shows how sexual networks are embedded in and shaped by differing social contexts, especially with respect to marriage, reproduction, the development of households, and the transfer of wealth and property. Together, these approaches help to explain the radical differences between HIV prevalence trends in Uganda and South Africa.

It is clear that in Africa, sexual networks are responsible for transmitting the virus in almost all adult cases of HIV infection. It is also increasingly clear that the configuration and dynamics of sexual networks—such as their periodicity or timing, their density, and their randomness or clustering—are as important as individual sexual behavior in understanding the dynamics of HIV transmission, incidence, and prevalence.[8] For instance, it has been estimated that newly infected people with high levels of HIV in their blood are up to ten times more likely to infect others than are people with older infections.[9] This estimate is based on research by Maria Wawer and her team on a sample of ten thousand people ages 15 to 49 living in forty-four villages near Uganda's border with Tanzania. If newly infected people with high levels of HIV in their blood have sexual contact with multiple partners during this time, they become extremely efficient transmitters of HIV in the overall sexual network.[10] The efficiency with which HIV is transmitted in sexual networks is highly sensitive to its periodicity and to the number of links (sexual contacts) between participants.

The concept of *sexual networks,* as it is developed here, introduces a social dimension into research that has, for the most part, focused previously on the individual (knowledge and attitudes) and on behavior and practices. This involves a change in the scale of analysis: large-scale social formations as compared to small-scale individual behavior. It also involves a conceptual shift toward a social-epidemiological model that is able to accommodate society-level structures rather than simply statistical aggregates of individual behavior in so-called populations. If we take sexual relations to be *social relations* (not just behavior), and sexual networks to be types of *social structures,* we can see that HIV is transmitted at the population or national level by specific types of large-scale social structures, that is, sexual networks.

This approach constitutes a significant methodological departure from the standard statistical medical-epidemiological approach, and from those social-scientific approaches to HIV/AIDS that focus on the individual.[11] This can be seen by comparing the standard epidemiological model (shown in figure 3), produced by Rand Stoneburner and Daniel Low-Beer[12] with the model based on power-law curves shown in figure 5 (to which we turn later in this chapter). Stoneburner and Low-Beer use a Gaussian model (called a bell curve because of its shape) to

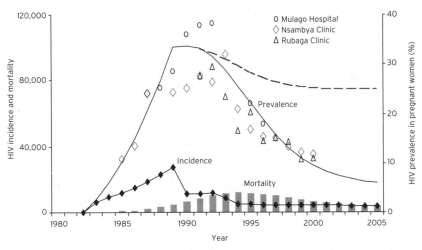

FIGURE 3. Stoneburner and Low-Beer's epidemiological model of HIV prevalence change in Uganda. (Based on Stoneburner and Low-Beer 2004: 717, fig. 3A)

approximate the empirical data. This model probably represents the best fit between the observed data (all from Kampala, drawn from the principal antenatal sentinel surveillance sites at Rubaga, Nsambya, and Mulago hospitals) and the standard epidemiological model.

Stoneburner and Low-Beer explain their model as follows:

> Simulations of HIV incidence and prevalence in pregnant women, and mortality in the population aged 15 to 59 of Kampala, Uganda, from 1981 to 2005, showing simulated HIV prevalence under HIV incidence "intervention" (solid line) and "baseline" (broken line) scenarios compared with empirical HIV data from antenatal clinic sentinel surveillance sites in Nsambya (diamond shapes), Mulago (circles) and Rubaga (triangles). The intervention scenario, in which incidence rates are reduced by 80% over a 2-year period among 15- to 24-year-olds beginning in 1992–1993, produces declines in HIV prevalence consistent with empirical data. In the baseline scenario, incidence rates remained unchanged after 1990 and prevalence remains stable.[13]

Several problems are immediately apparent. In order to make the standard epidemiological model approximate a fit to the empirical data, the authors have had to assume that incidence (new infections) declined suddenly by 80 percent between 1989 and 1990.[14] This is extremely unlikely and does not correspond to any of the recollections and stories about this period that Ugandans told us during research conducted in 2003. The reduction in incidence shown in this model is only hypothetical, introduced in order to make the standard epidemiological model achieve a closer fit to the data. In fact, the decline in prevalence is such that even if incidence had been zero—extremely improbable—it still would not account for the data.[15] Some researchers, however, have taken the hypothetical decline in incidence to be real. For instance, the authors of the influential 2002 U.S. Agency for International Development document *What happened in Uganda?* do this (repeating it again in 2006) when they argue that "it is most probable that HIV incidence in Uganda peaked sometime during the late 1980s."[16] In other words, to make the data (observed HIV prevalence) fit the model (a standard epidemiological curve) we have to assume that four out of five of all sexually active people suddenly stopped having unprotected sex for a couple of years.[17] Without this sudden, dramatic, and improbable collapse in incidence, for which no confirming data exist, the dashed line wildly overestimates the actual HIV prevalence.

Indeed, *incidence actually increased annually* from 0.9 percent 1993 to 2.3 percent in 2003, even as prevalence was falling for those who tested at voluntary counseling and testing centers.[18] The rise in incidence is consistent with a falling HIV prevalence only if incidence is rising in relatively small, isolated networks. If incidence were in fact rising across a randomly selected population that is widely linked in a common sexual network—as the standard epidemiological model assumes—then prevalence would also necessarily rise. This is not the case in Uganda. Instead, incidence is stable or rising in relatively isolated subnetworks (lately, especially among women and middle-aged people) within which HIV prevalence may rise quite rapidly, but outside of which prevalence may remain stable or fall. This is also consistent with the fact that Uganda has a very high TFR.

Indeed, since there are no population-based estimates of HIV in Uganda or hard evidence of behavior change before 1989, all must be conjectural.[19] Even so, at the end of the Stoneburner and Low-Beer curve, the calculated hypothetical trend line (solid line) considerably *underestimates* HIV prevalence, which in reality levels off at a higher level than the standard epidemiological model would suggest. Furthermore, the curvature of the estimated (or fitted) curves tends in the opposite direction to the easily observable curvature of the actual data. The estimated curve in the period 1982–1992 is concave, or negative, but the actual data appear to trend in a convex way. In the period 1992–2002 the estimated curve shows a typical down-sloping logistic or sigmoid form tending toward zero, whereas the actual data suggest a concave downward trend that levels off well above zero. It appears that the epidemiology model is simply of the wrong form (cf. figure 4 later in this chapter).

In Uganda, HIV remains endemic at higher prevalence levels than other virus infections even following the collapse in prevalence after the peak of an epidemic. This is because HIV does not confer immunity to infection on survivors (because there are none) as recovery from other viral infections does, and because the period of active viral infection (viremia) is much longer in the case of HIV (and generally bimodal or multimodal, rising at the beginning of infection and at the end). More important, however, the standard epidemiological model is based on the "normal" (Gaussian) probability curve,[20] which assumes that infection is randomly distributed in the population. Although this is roughly true for most infectious agents that are dispersed by water, air, and food supplies, it is not true of sexually transmitted pathogens, which rely on "wet" person-to-person genital contact. In other words, HIV is transmitted primarily through a social network of a special kind, the sexual network. This error has had much greater consequences, however, than the difficulty it presents to those who seek to develop mathematical models of the epidemic.

This problem in modeling HIV prevalence was noted in the early 1990s by two molecular biologists at the University of California, Berkeley.[21] Peter Duesberg and David Rasnick argued that because HIV epidemiology did not fit the normal epidemiological patterns characteristic of almost all other viral and bacterial epidemics, it must not, therefore, be a viral epidemic at all. Basing their argument at first on data from the United States and Europe, they pointed out that "AIDS is highly non-random with regard to sex (86% male); sexual persuasion (over 60% homosexual); and age (85% are 25–49 years old). . . . From its beginning in 1980, the AIDS epidemic progressed non-exponentially, just like lifestyle diseases."[22]

They also pointed out that AIDS has no single defining disease[23] but is a syndrome, like obesity or illnesses caused by smoking, and that the vast majority of people who died of AIDS had a history of recreational drug use, or had taken antiretroviral (ARV) drugs. Since HIV infection in the population they had studied was also nonrandom, they concluded that HIV does not cause AIDS but was a product of toxicity arising from recreational drug use, lifestyle choices (especially ones that often accompanied the gay lifestyle in the United States and Europe in the 1980s), and the drugs that were then used to treat HIV, especially AZT. If HIV were an infectious virus, they reasoned, it should infect people more or less randomly (that is, there would be a Gaussian distribution of infections), and should grow exponentially at first. HIV infections did not do this. In a 1996 publication, Duesberg and Ellison claimed—correctly at the time for U.S. data, but ignoring African data entirely—that HIV was still not heterosexually transmitted "outside of drug addicts" and that "by any measure, the war on AIDS has been a colossal failure."[24]

The core of Duesberg and Rasnick's argument was the fact that the observed HIV trends in the data they examined did not conform to expected epidemiological patterns for viral pathogens such as flu virus or poliomyelitis.[25] Instead, it looked much more like the linear progression of illnesses caused by environmental factors such as pollution, illnesses caused by toxins, or lifestyle diseases.[26] Based on these and the other differences they observed, their conclusion that HIV was not a cause of AIDS seemed reasonable. Their conclusions were eventually shown to be wrong, but their critical observation about the shape of HIV prevalence trends was accurate.

Unfortunately, their findings reached the attention of the president of South Africa, Thabo Mbeki, a year or so later.[27] This was to have tragic consequences. Their logic convinced President Mbeki. In October 1999 he told the National Council of Provinces that AZT was poisonous,[28] and in early 2000 he set up the Presidential International Panel of Scientists on HIV/AIDS in Africa, which included Duesberg and Rasnick (see chapter 9). Then, in April 2000, in a strongly worded and very personal letter to United Nations secretary general Kofi Anan, U.S. president Bill Clinton, and British prime minister Tony Blair, Mbeki came close to saying that HIV did not cause AIDS, and urged world leaders to pay particular attention to the differences in the African HIV epidemic.[29] Mbeki's position was drawn fully and directly from Duesberg's work, although this was not directly acknowledged by the South African president. In a briefing paper for Mbeki that must have been received immediately before Mbeki penned his letter to world leaders, Duesberg stated the kernel of his argument that HIV does not cause AIDS, drawing on earlier work with Rasnick and Ellison. Duesberg wrote, "the African AIDS epidemic is not following the bell-shaped curve of an exponential rise and subsequent sharp drop with immunity, that are typical of infectious epidemics. Instead it drags on like a nutritionally or environmentally caused disease."[30] Duesberg also specifically warned Mbeki in his briefing document about those who opposed his views. Citing Mbeki's own letter to world leaders, which had been published by the *Washington Post* on 19 April, Duesberg wrote,

> President Mbeki must also be warned about Dr. Joe Sonnabend's answer to the president's question about the epidemiological discrepancy between the "heterosexual" AIDS epidemic in Africa and the non-random, 85%-male epidemic in the U.S. (Mbeki's letter to U.S. President Clinton, *Washington Post*, April 19, 2000). According to Sonnabend's hypothesis, Africans acquire HIV heterosexually, because they simultaneously suffer from a long list of diseases, including "tuberculosis, malaria, other protozoan infections, bacterial diarrhoeal infections, pneumonia, plasmodium, Leishmania" etc. However, the very low AIDS risk of an African HIV-positive, compared to an American, calls this hypothesis into question. If the Sonnabend-hypothesis were correct, African HIV-positives should develop AIDS much more readily than their American counterparts. But the opposite is true. In fact according to Sonnabend most Africans should already have AIDS by the time they pick up HIV "heterosexually."[31]

This is remarkable logic by any measure, and wholly tendentious. But, by this time, Mbeki was fully and personally committed to what came to be called the dissident position. Duesberg and Rasnick had convinced him through their topsy-turvy logic (a) that the drugs used to treat AIDS were in fact the cause of it,[32] and (b) that because of parasites, other bacterial and viral infections, and a generally higher disease load that Africans carried as a result of poverty, they probably already had AIDS by the time they contracted HIV!

Accordingly, in his address to the World AIDS Conference in Durban in April 2000, Mbeki declared that poverty was the real cause of AIDS. Predictably, this unleashed a storm of protest and dismay, but up to the time of this writing (early 2008) Mbeki has yet to renounce any of these beliefs. All of the dissident documents and his own dissident writings are still available on the Internet,[33] some of them through official African National Congress Web sites. The controversy, however, has succeeded in stopping him from expressing his views publicly. It has not prevented a rearguard action from the President's Office and the Department of Health aimed at delaying provision of ARV therapy and mother-to-child transmission protection.

The root of this tragedy lies originally in Duesberg and Rasnick's perfectly valid observation that the HIV prevalence curves are not typical of epidemics caused by other pathogens. They cited one example of an attempt to predict HIV prevalence that appeared in the *Journal*

of the American Medical Association in 1990.[34] This lack of fit to
the "normal" curve is due to the fact that HIV is transmitted through
sexual networks and is not randomly distributed. As we shall see, there
are good reasons for this divergence from normal epidemic processes,
reasons that do not mean that HIV does *not* cause AIDS, or that it is a
disease of poverty or lifestyle.[35] It simply shows that, like environmental toxins and lifestyle diseases, HIV is spread through social structures
(sexual networks) and is shaped by them.

Previous social research on HIV/AIDS has concentrated on the
behavioral responses of individuals, especially their knowledge, attitudes, beliefs, and practices (KABP) with respect to sex and reproductive health. Work on sexual networks has previously focused on iden-
tifying risk factors and tracing contacts, and, in any case, is virtually
absent in Africa. By contrast, the approach taken here directs focus
away from individual behavior and risk in order to focus on the sexual
network as a form of social structure, not simply contacts occurring as
the result of behavior.

Unfortunately, while we have some data on sexual behavior in Africa,
we mostly lack specific data on the details of sexual networks.[36] As
early as 1992, Caldwell, Caldwell, and Orubuloye noted, "The AIDS
epidemic in sub-Saharan Africa has revealed the inadequacy of our
knowledge of the extent of sexual networking in the region."[37] This
was still true in 2006: empirical data on sexual networks in Africa,
with a few exceptions,[38] do not exist. There are, however, ways to study
the structure of networks indirectly in other ways.

A NEW APPROACH TO NETWORKS

Recent discoveries—many of them since the late 1990s—in computer
science and mathematics about the behavior of networks provide new
conceptual tools that can help us to illuminate the hidden processes
in sexual networks.[39] Researchers have examined large-scale complex
networks of many kinds, including the Internet (the physical infrastructure), the World Wide Web (the hyperlinks that make the Internet
work), networks of neurons, food webs in small ecosystems, secret communication networks among terrorists, and citation networks among
physicists. They have found that there are a number of invariant rules
that govern how networks are configured and, more important, how
they change and evolve. For instance, research has shown that these
and other networks, irrespective of their size, have a "small world"

configuration in which all members of the network are linked with, on average, as few as two or three links between any two nodes in the network, and at most six links—known as "six degrees of separation" in social networks.[40]

These findings can be usefully applied to the study of sexual networks. Analysis of how HIV prevalence changes over time—the trend—can provide information about the gross structure of sexual networks for which we lack detailed empirical data. This chapter uses these new models to examine the shapes of the trend lines based on least-square approximations to a power-law model of changing HIV prevalence in order to show that the shape of these trends suggests differences in the structure of sexual networks in Uganda and South Africa. Findings from trend-line analysis are supported by analysis of differences in social structure that seem most likely to have an impact on the configuration of sexual networks, including patterns of kinship, marriage, household structure, inheritance, and wealth.

COMPARING HIV TRENDS IN UGANDA AND SOUTH AFRICA

HIV prevalence in Uganda rose very rapidly in the 1980s and early 1990s until 1992, when it began to decline very rapidly.[41] When it first began to be measured in 1985, it was already above 10 percent at antenatal clinics. It is likely that HIV had been endemic at a low level in Uganda for at least a decade, and possibly for generations, before it was first tentatively measured in 1982.[42] By 2002, the decline in HIV prevalence had stabilized at around 7 percent, fell slightly, and then possibly crept up again by 2007.[43] The direction of the trend after 2002 is still not clear.[44] On the other hand, South Africa has seen a steady rise in the prevalence from the beginning of the 1980s until the present, with as yet little evidence of a leveling off.[45] In 1992, the overall prevalence in Uganda was around 24 percent, with rates as high as 29 percent in Kampala and averaging 20 percent in the four other major towns in Uganda.[46] In 2005, the overall prevalence in South Africa nationally was similar to that in Kampala, Uganda, thirteen years earlier. Prevalence in some age and sex groups and in some regions in southern Africa now exceeds 30 percent, a level never reached in Uganda.

The vast difference between the two countries is illustrated most starkly in figure 4. This simply shows the temporal relationship of changing trends in the two countries. The data on which these trends are based are, of course, much messier. There is also a large margin of error associ-

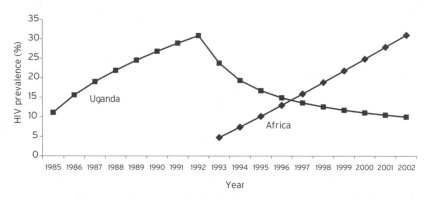

FIGURE 4. Comparison of HIV trends for Uganda and South Africa, 1985–
2002. Prevalence trends in Uganda and South Africa are starkly different.

ated with each data point. Since we are concerned only with longer-term
trends, however, the margin of error associated with each point can be
eliminated as a concern.[47] The fact that these trends are highly consistent
with each other for different data sets within each country also increases
the reliability of these findings. Since we are trying, first of all, to compare two countries in the broadest possible strokes, however, elimination
of the noise in the data allows us to see the overall relationships in time
and in the shape of these trends. In the following analysis, it is necessary
to separate out different periods for close analysis.

We first compare these trends for the eleven-year period (1992–2002
inclusive) when South African and Ugandan trends were moving in
opposite directions. When we plot these two different national trends
against each other, several significant patterns emerge during that
decade.[48] Figure 5 shows the trend for South Africa as a whole against
two sets of data for Uganda.[49] The triangles represent aggregated data
for Kampala (drawn from the same antenatal HIV surveillance sites
used in Stoneburner and Low-Beer's model, shown earlier in figure
3). In this plot, median values for these three sites have been used,
because each set of data alone shows a broadly similar trend. Squares
represent the data from Uganda's four largest cities with antenatal
clinic sentinel sites: Mbarara in the southwest, Jinja in the south central area, and Tororo and Mbale in the east. Diamond-shaped mark-
ers represent data points for antenatal clinic sentinel sites in South
Africa.

For each set of data, a power, or power-law, trend line is calculated
and plotted (see explanation boxes). Curves of this sort are associ-

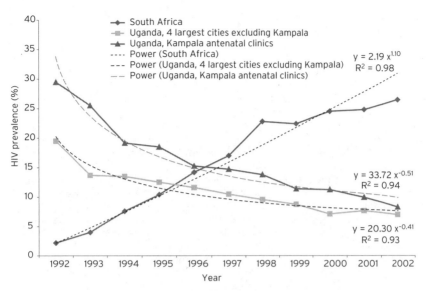

FIGURE 5. Comparison of HIV falling and rising power-law trend lines in Uganda and South Africa, 1992–2002.

ated with complex network systems.[50] The remarkable fact that the Ugandan data follow a power-law trend much more closely than it does the standard epidemiological model, shown in figure 3, suggests that efforts to understand the HIV epidemic in the same terms we use to model and visualize other epidemics is likely to fail. Something else is at work here. Since power-law trends are closely associated with networks of all kinds, it suggests that we might gain insight by examining the social networks that transmit HIV. Power-law trends are also associated with the sudden changes in chemical and physical systems called phase changes, such as when water (a liquid) suddenly turns to steam (a gas) at the boiling point, or when it turns to ice (a solid) at the freezing point. It turns out that phase changes are analogous to the changes in HIV prevalence in Uganda.

Where sexual networks are infected with HIV, the prevalence of infection will be a function of the number of sexual contacts (links) between people (network nodes) in a network of a specific configuration, and, over time, may behave in different ways depending on how the network is structured. For Uganda, it changes in a nonlinear way that is characteristic of highly structured complex networks with hubs and/or clusters and of networks that exhibit fractal structures. This is distinctly different from a linear growth that would be seen in simple

THE MATHEMATICS OF THE TREND LINE

The trend line (heavy dark line imposed over the data points) shows the closest fit of the data to a curve described by a power-law equation of the form $y = ct^a$. Here y is *HIV prevalence* expressed as percentage. The t is *time* in years, for this is how the available data are given to us. The symbol c is a proportionality constant that simply adjusts the scale of the graph, and a is the calculated exponent that allows the trend to fit the data.

The R^2 value estimates the closeness of fit, with values approximating 1 indicating a close fit. Here, the trend lines fit the data very closely, with values approximating 1.

When $a = 0$, the curve is simply a horizontal line in which $y = c$, a constant value. When $a = 1$, we have a simple linear relation, that is, a straight line. The South African data show an exponent close to 1, in which $y = ct$.

Fractional exponents where the absolute value of a lies between zero and one, $0 < |a| < 1$, however, yield curves like those seen in the Uganda case. If the exponent is negative, the curve has a concave shape with what is called a fat tail: the prevalence, y, declines rapidly at first and then tails off very slowly without reaching zero, as in figure 5. Positive values of the exponent yield the inverse "growth" pattern, shown by the trend line from 1985 to 1992 in figure 6.

This plot uses Microsoft Excel's built-in least-squares fit to the power-law model.

diffusion models of transmission, or exponential growth of unbounded biological systems, or the sigmoid curves of growing populations ultimately constrained by the carrying capacity or saturation of their environments. Specifically, the Ugandan curves lie halfway between stability ($a = 0$) and linear growth ($a > 1$) that would be characteristic of simple diffusion. This behavior is the signature of complex network organization that is fractal, or similar at different scales.[51]

The two trends for Uganda—one for Kampala, the capital of Uganda (comprising median values for antenatal clinics at Rubaga, Nsambya, and Mulago hospitals), and one for the other four major cities for which we have good data—both show approximately equal declines during this period.[52] Both curves conform closely to each other, with the curve for Kampala reflecting higher HIV prevalence in the city than in the smaller regional cities. Trend curves for rural data and smaller towns (Moyo, Mutolere, Masindi, Hoima, Kilembe, Pallisa, Aber, Lwala, Soroti, Matany, Kagadi, Arua, Lacor, and Nebbi) are similar in shape, but lower in magnitude. Data for these sites are incomplete and therefore not presented here. The trends drop steeply for the first several years from 1992 to 1995, and then begin to level out toward an overall prevalence of around 6–7 percent. This is confirmed by the preliminary results of a national survey of HIV prevalence in Uganda based on voluntary blood tests conducted on a representative statistical sample for the entire population that also shows an overall prevalence of about 7 percent.[53] Equally significant is the fact that HIV levels stabilize but do not tend toward zero as ordinary viral epidemics would. This fact is accurately modeled by the power law, but not by the "normal" (Gaussian) distribution curve.

The decline follows a period from the early 1980s to 1992 in which HIV prevalence rose rapidly in Uganda toward a peak in 1992. The transition from rapid escalation of HIV rates in Uganda from the early 1980s up to 1992 was as remarkable as their decline. The period of increasing prevalence is also closely modeled by a power law. The transition between increasing HIV prevalence and decrease is very rapid (see figure 6 later in this chapter).

By separating the period of increasing prevalence (1985–1992) from the period of decreasing prevalence (1992–2002), we can calculate two discontinuous trend lines that show similar but inverted patterns.

The fact that these two trends were inverses of each other, with closely similar absolute values of the power-law exponent, suggests that whatever was happening in the overall sexual network to cause an increase in HIV was also happening during the period of decreasing HIV prevalence, but in a way that was somehow inverted. Moreover, this trend-line analysis suggests that the changes in HIV prevalence were functions of the configuration of the overall sexual network, rather than simply statistical changes in human sexual behavior. In other words, we do not have to assume that 80 percent of the sexually active population stopped having sex between 1991 and 1992, as Stoneburner and Low-Beer are driven to assume, given the nature of their model. As we shall see, it is very likely that what was happening during the period of increasing HIV prevalence in Uganda was an increase in the number of links (sexual contacts) between persons or groups of people (such as within villages, around nightclubs or bars, or at funerals or other ritual events), and especially an increase in the links between highly infected persons or clusters that were highly linked to other persons or clusters, such as soldiers, transportation workers, "sugar daddies/mamas," and others. During the period of decreasing prevalence, overall connectivity decreased, but especially the links between highly infected persons or groups in the network and the general population decreased. This would explain the power-law shape of the trends since these are the signature of networks connected in this way.

POWER LAW:
THE MATHEMATICAL DETAILS

Unlike an *exponential* prevalence curve, the *power-law* curve is simply a function of time, *t*, raised to a constant power. The exponent is a real number; that is, it may be a positive or negative whole number or fractional number. By contrast, the exponential curve expresses a situation in which the prevalence is a function of itself: that is, the higher the prevalence, the faster the rate of increase, or the lower the prevalence, the lower the rate of increase, usually (in real-life systems) up to some limit imposed by the availability of resources.

The trend of the decline in Uganda conforms to a power-law decay from the peak reached in 1992. The decline in HIV prevalence (P_{HIV}) as a function of time (*t*, in years, in accordance with the data sets) is estimated by the expression

$$P_{HIV} = 0.3372t^{-0.5087}$$

for Kampala antenatal center test sites, and by

$$P_{HIV} = 0.203t^{-0.4129}$$

for the four other large cities (where *t* is time in years, in accordance with the data). The two trends are very similar, and both have a negative noninteger exponent *a*, $0 < |a| < 1$. The trend for the period of *increasing* HIV prevalence, 1985–1992, for Kampala (figure 6) is estimated by

$$P_{HIV} = 11.09t^{0.4912}.$$

All power-law exponents (−0.5087, and −0.4129 for the period of decreasing HIV prevalence, and 0.4912 for the period of increasing prevalence) are approximately of the same magnitude, $|a| \approx 0.5$. The similarity in these values suggests that we are dealing with the same form of network. In the first period (1985–1992), links were rapidly forming, making the sexual network an increasingly *efficient* transmitter of HIV. In the second period, links were rapidly breaking, resulting in a *decreasing efficiency* of HIV transmission in the sexual network.

Previous work on networks has assumed that they are static and can be represented adequately by graphs (drawings) that represent the links between nodes at some arbitrary time or over some arbitrary period of time.[54] This is not adequate for our purposes, however. Sexual networks are dynamic, not static: over time, they grow or shrink, their configuration may change, and the number of links in them may increase or decrease. We need a model of networks that takes this into account.

Fortunately, the power law describes just such changes in a network. Research on the evolution of the hard-wired Internet and software-based World Wide Web (WWW) has shown that "the networks are becoming *denser* over time, with the average degree [the average number of links] increasing (and hence with the number of [links] growing super-linearly in the number of nodes). Moreover, the densifi-

THE NETWORK POWER LAW

Leskovec, Kleinberg, and Faloutsos (2005) have found that "as the graphs [of networks such as the Internet and World Wide Web] evolve over time, they follow a version of the relation":

$$l(t) \approx n(t)^a$$

where $l(t)$ and $n(t)$ represent the number of links (l) and the number of nodes (n) at some time t, and a is the power-law exponent. The expression $l(t)$ simply states that the number of links is a function of time. This is a power-law relation that means that the number of links in these networks increases in proportion to the number of nodes raised to some power represented by the exponent a. This expression describes the growth of a network. Leskovec, Kleinberg, and Faloutsos (2005) call it the "densification power law" or the "growth power law." Since their research concerns the Internet (the physical electronic infrastructure that connects computers) and the World Wide Web (the software links connecting users that are followed by browsers such as Netscape, Firefox, and Internet Explorer), both of which are growing rapidly, they do not consider the case in which networks shrink by losing links. This is what happens when HIV prevalence declines. In this case, the inverse of the "growth power law"—in other words, a "decay power law"—exists when the exponent is negative, as follows:

$$l(t) \approx n(t)^{-a}$$

This relation says that the number of links between nodes decreases more rapidly (sublinearly) than the number of nodes (persons). This relation closely models the period of decreasing prevalence in Uganda.

HIV prevalence in the population, then, will be proportional to the number of links (sexual contacts) that connect the nodes (persons) in the sexual network as a whole, itself a subset of the entire population. Thus, HIV prevalence will vary according to the number of links, which, in turn, is proportional to the number of nodes raised to the power a, the "densification exponent" that is characteristic of all such complex preferential attachment networks. Accordingly, a power law that describes HIV prevalence trends emerges:

$$P_{HIV} \approx l(t) \approx n(t)^a$$

cation follows a power-law pattern."[55] What this means is that empirical observation of very large networks such as the Internet and WWW shows that the number of links between nodes increases more rapidly (superlinearly) than the number of nodes. This is caused by what has been called preferential attachment, or a "rich get richer" phenomenon.[56] According to this, the establishment of links to new nodes tends to favor those that are already highly linked. Nodes that are already popular, such as Yahoo.com or AOL.com, attract more links than other Web sites do. This is also true of neurons in simple organisms, networks of Hollywood actors, or famous scholars whose works are most often cited. According to Barabási, these patterns, "potentially present in most networks, could explain the power laws we spotted on the Web and in Hollywood," among many others.[57] In the case of sexual networks that transmit HIV, clusters of intensive sexual contact produce higher likelihoods of HIV transmission. In other words, with respect to HIV, the "rich" (highly infected clusters) get "richer" (that is, prevalence increases more rapidly than it does in sexually less well-connected clusters or categories of people).

THE POWER-LAW MODEL AND HIV TRENDS

It is intuitively obvious that HIV spreads through links in the sexual network. Thus, nearly all seropositive people will be members of the sexual network, in which some people overall, and *all* seropositive people, necessarily have direct or indirect sexual contact with more than one other person. In fact, the set of HIV seropositive people is a subset of the network of all sexually active people in the larger population. Infected individuals constitute a sample or subset of the set of all members of the sexual network that has been "selected" by HIV infection. Within the network, all HIV-positive people are necessarily linked by some set of links to all other HIV-positive people, and to some HIV-negative people. Some members of the set of HIV-positive people are likely to have many sexual contacts with others, especially during periods in which HIV prevalence is increasing. They may constitute hubs in the network, and are efficient transmitters of HIV. In fact, there may be clusters of HIV-positive people whose links with one another and with some HIV-negative people are quite dense. These persons or clusters can act as transmission centers or hubs. Sexual networks, however, usually have long filaments of contacts with cross-links to other filaments and to hubs. These filaments can act as transmission lines in the way electrical power lines do. The efficiency with which HIV is transmitted overall, then, will depend on the specific configuration of the network. This is what we find in the data for Uganda. The overall picture of increasing *and* decreasing HIV prevalence for Kampala data is shown in figure 6.

It is important to note that the pattern observed here does not look like the patterns seen in other types of epidemics caused by "normal" bacteria or viruses. The composite curve in figure 6, which fits the data quite closely, shows a remarkable and sudden reversal. Such trends suggest that the dynamics of the system are unstable, and that something

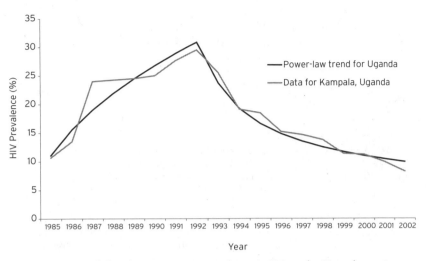

FIGURE 6. Trend for changing HIV prevalence in Kampala, Uganda, 1985–2002.

like a phase transition or catastrophe event occurred in 1992. A sudden shift of this sort—a tipping point[58]—is most likely to be caused by a rapid reorganization of the overall structure of the sexual network that transmits HIV rather than by incremental and local changes in HIV incidence caused by behavioral change, morbidity, or death alone. Much recent work in the mathematical analysis of networks shows that nonrandom networks (such as the Internet, but also social networks, scholarly citations, networks of neurons, and food chains in ecological systems) all show power-law patterns. Steven Strogatz, one of the leading innovators in this field, remarks, "Power laws hint that a system may be organizing itself. They arise at phase transitions, when a system is poised at the brink, teetering between order and chaos. They arise in fractals, when an arbitrarily small piece of a complex shape is a microcosm of the whole."[59]

This analysis of the Ugandan HIV data strongly suggests that just such a phase transition occurred. It also suggests that the structure of the network is fractal, that is, it exhibits a similar structure at different scales of analysis. This would be consistent with a highly clustered network in which different clusters of sexually active and therefore interlinked individuals are further grouped into larger clusters, and so on. In such a network, each cluster has fewer links to other clusters, both within the same order of magnitude (sections of a village) and at higher orders of magnitude (regions, language groups, age groups)

WHY A POWER LAW LOOKS LIKE
A STRAIGHT LINE IN THE CASE
OF SOUTH AFRICA

The trend line equation for the South African data is approximated by the power-law equation

$$P_{HIV} = 0.0219t^{1.1048}$$

where the exponent is close to 1.

As we have seen, where the exponent in the power law is 1 or close to 1, the graph of the equation approximates a straight line because any value raised to the power of 1 is simply that value:

$$f(t) = t^1 = t.$$

In the South African case, this corresponds to a more or less straight line sloping upward over time, meaning that the increase in prevalence is simply directly proportional to time, with a small multiplication factor of 0.0219 that increases the slope ever so slightly upward.

than it does within itself. This structure permits what amounts to the phase transition that we see in figure 6, in which the network suddenly became much more resistant to transmission of HIV virus around 1992. *This would be consistent with a model in which a highly clustered network with limited links between clusters suddenly lost those interlinking long-distance connections, resulting in a phase transition of the network.* Through a process similar to water freezing and suddenly becoming "lumpy" with ice crystals, and then becoming hard as it freezes to a solid, it seems that beginning about 1992 the Ugandan sexual network returned to a lumpy, clustered state. In other words, while people continued to have sex, possibly with multiple partners, persons or clusters that acted as hubs in the network largely disappeared. This is consistent with the data on changes in sexual behavior in Uganda.

By contrast, the trend for South Africa (figure 5) is approximated by a straight line. This would not immediately suggest that networks were involved, except for the fact that we know they are. What it does suggest is that the South African sexual network permits a more or less unimpeded flow of HIV through it, roughly like liquid paraffin diffusing through a wick in a lamp, or a strong smell diffusing through a room from its source. It takes a bit of time, but it moves at a constant rate. It would seem that something like this was happening in the South African sexual network.

NORMAL EXPONENTIAL GROWTH
OF EPIDEMICS

In their early stages, epidemics normally grow exponentially, that is, the rate of change in prevalence of some infectious agent (for example, a flu virus) in the population is at first proportional to the number of persons infected: the greater the number of people already infected, the greater the rate at which more people will become infected. This relation can be expressed mathematically by the ordinary differential equation

$$\frac{dy}{dt} \approx y$$

meaning that the change in y with respect to time, t, is proportional to y. This has as its solution in y the simple exponential growth equation,

$$y = ce^{kt},$$

where c is the initial value (in this case 1), k is the proportionality constant, and t is time represented on the x-axis. The e, a constant value, is a special type of number, called a transcendental number, like π; $e = 2.7183\ldots$. It can be thought of as the limit on the returns from compounding interest (versus simple interest) as the number of periods of compounding interest are increased. It is thus a natural value for the base of the exponential function.

The South African data show an approximately linear progression during the period 1992–2002. A linear progression would mean, in this case, that HIV prevalence (the y-axis) is simply a function of time (the x-axis), or, in other words, that prevalence is growing steadily with time and that the *rate* of change was not itself changing. We must keep in mind that the data do not preserve spatial characteristics, so what they show is a gradual trend toward saturation of the *entire sexual network* with HIV infection. This in turn suggests that the sexual network is relatively homogeneous and randomized, that is, that all members are likely to have contact with people both close and far away, or within some category (linguistic, cultural, age) as well as with others outside this category. It has been shown that people in multilingual communities in Uganda are far more likely to have extramarital sexual contact than those within monolingual communities.[60] Since virtually all South Africans live in multilingual communities and almost all speak several South African languages, this may predispose them toward greater sexual contact across the network. It also suggests that most sexually active people have multiple partners, and that most have more or less the same number of

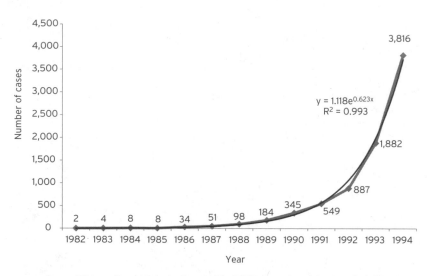

FIGURE 7. The earliest period of growing HIV prevalence in South Africa, 1982–1994. (Data source: United Nations Programme on HIV/AIDS 2002)

partners (links) in the sexual network. The behavior of the trend during this period suggests a nearly free diffusion of HIV through the population, as if the growth of the epidemic is a function of time alone, rather than—what is usually the case in epidemics—prevalence over time being a function of the number of infected people already in the population. Furthermore, it suggests that the system (all sexually active people linked in the HIV transmission network) is not yet close to saturation or phase transition.

But the growth of HIV prevalence in South Africa did not suddenly begin as a linear increase. In its earliest stages, it grew exponentially, as it did in the earliest periods of infection in the United States and other places for which we have relatively complete data. (We do not know what happened in Uganda at first, because HIV and AIDS were unknown and not tracked before HIV had already infected up to 10 percent of the population in certain parts of the country.)

Further analysis of South African data shows that the earliest period of the HIV epidemic is most accurately described as *exponential*. In its earliest stages, HIV prevalence increased freely, as if it encountered no barriers, that is, as if it were like a virus that could be spread by and infect anyone. This could be true only if the sexual networks in which it was propagated were multiply and randomly connected. Viruses and bacteria that are free to move easily, and where there is no previous immunity, grow exponentially in a population before they either evoke immunity in previously infected people, or die off as their hosts succumb to lethal pathogens (in which case, they decline exponentially to zero or near-zero levels).

Exponential curves generally emerge in natural systems where growth is unrestricted, such as the growth of any population (dividing cells or free growth of viruses, bacteria, or other organisms) that is not limited by resources (food, light, or space). Such trends occur where the rate at which prevalence changes is a function of prevalence itself, that is, the more infections that already exist, the greater will be the increase, up to some limit such as death, recovery from infection, or lack of vulnerable individuals. The earliest South African data show precisely such a trend (the R^2 value of 0.9935 is a virtually perfect fit to the exponential trend line), as illustrated in figure 7. This trend, taken together with the later data, describes an almost perfect growth curve in which limits to growth have not been reached. It also strongly suggests that HIV transmission in South Africa occurs in a fully connected and randomized network without internal structural limits such as clustering or formation of core groups of endemic but limited infection.

(Re)Organization of Sexual Networks and Prevalence Change

The patterns we see in prevalence trends strongly suggest that sexual networks in Uganda are highly clustered or lumpy, with many locally dense subnetworks that have fewer connections between them. In South Africa, networks appear to be randomized and highly interlinked. The catastrophe event or phase transition in the Uganda prevalence trend resulted from a fairly sudden reorganization of the sexual network, during which the density of links between local high-prevalence, high-density networks—clusters or lumps in the network—and the rest of the population were suddenly reduced. In South Africa, this has not happened because the network is much more uniform, with large numbers of people multiply connected to one another.

In Uganda, the centers of infection were either clusters of highly interlinked and infected persons around a bar or night club, for instance, or else highly sexually active persons such as soldiers or truck drivers. People involved in culturally sanctioned networks of sexual exchange (e.g., wife-sharing, or sexual cleansing after the death of a spouse) are also likely hubs. In terms of this model, it does not matter whether these links were severed by behavior change (using a condom or reducing the number and/or frequency of sexual contacts) or by death or other factors. The result was the same: fewer links between highly infected hubs, clusters or filaments and the rest of the population. Since infected and highly sexually active hubs (whether individuals or groups/clusters) are highly efficient in spreading HIV, reducing links from these hubs creates a nonlinear decline in the transmission of HIV. If some percentage reduction in sexual links occurs (say, r percent), then this will have little effect within densely connected subnetworks, but it will have a significant effect on linkage between clusters. In fact, r percent reduction of cross-cluster links will effectively isolate some parts of the population from infection. The effect overall will be a reorganization of the total sexual network in which prevalence will be nonlinearly related to r. This can be described as a phase transition. In other words, the rate of change in HIV prevalence was not directly proportional (linear) to the sum of changes in individual sexual behavior or death but was instead a function of the change in the organization of the overall network, which had the effect of accelerating the decline in HIV prevalence.

The structure of the South African sexual network appears, from this analysis, to be quite different. In particular, it seems that the sexual network spans the nation (and probably also much of the southern African region, including, at least, Botswana, Lesotho, and Swaziland, which share languages, culture, and population freely with South Africa). There appear to be few clusters or hubs in a relatively homogeneous network of sexual relations that ultimately incorporates most sexually active people (and certainly all those with more than one partner). In such a network, HIV spreads according to normal growth curves (logistic or exponential) and has so far not reached a natural limit. In fact, we cannot, as yet, say what that natural limit might be.

Given the lack of actual empirical data on sexual networks, then, it appears that analysis of trends may serve as a proxy measure for the structure of sexual networks. Since we know that the configuration of sexual networks is critical to the transmission of sexually transmitted infections, it follows that such knowledge can be crucial in understanding the progress of the epidemic. This, in turn, can help us to create and implement interventions that might be more effective than what we have seen so far in Africa.

Perhaps the most important lesson that we may derive from this new understanding of networks and HIV transmission is that significant change in HIV prevalence is a property of the social network rather than of individual behavior. We must redirect our attention, then, from the scale of the individual—behavior, psychology, risk assessment, and so on—to the scale of the social. This represents a radical shift in perspective.

CHAPTER 3

The Social Determinants of Sexual Network Configuration

EXPLAINING THE DIFFERENCES

We have seen that the different configurations of large-scale sexual networks—in particular, their self-organizing behavior due to structural characteristics—is the primary factor in the radical differences between HIV prevalence trends in Uganda and South Africa. I turn now to consider the social-structural causes for these differences in the configuration of the sexual networks. Rather than seeking explanation at the level of individual choice and behavior—what is usual in epidemiological studies—we look for explanation at the social level. Indeed, differences between the two countries in statistical aggregates based on surveys of individual sexual behavior—that is, the so-called ABC factors (abstinence, being faithful, using condoms)—are much smaller than the empirical differences in HIV prevalence. Differences between Ugandan and South African political and social structures are, however, quite large.

Comparisons that neglect the larger differences in social structure in favor of the small differences in sexual behavior appear confounded. For example, one group of leading researchers working in Uganda noted in 2006 that "although HIV prevalence declined in 1990s, we cannot disaggregate the contributions of specific behavioral change (abstinence, monogamy, condom use), postwar social stabilization, the direct effects of government prevention programs, and the natural evolution of the epidemic (i.e., declines in prevalence due to mortality exceeding incidence, and declines in transmission as fewer people were in the early, highly infectious, stages of disease)."[1] The problem here is that although all of these factors certainly contributed to the decline, the statistical methods that have been used do not allow them to be disaggregated.[2] Statistical methods do show, however, that none of them, either singly or together, can fully account for the rapidity of the decline. By taking a larger "ecological" or systemic view, we can see that this remarkable fact was a property of the entire sexual network, itself part of (or a sample of) the entire social network. This allows us to examine the social-structural features of Ugandan and South African societies in order to show how other social factors shaped the sexual network and, in the case of Uganda, caused its collapse.

In fact, differences in knowledge about HIV, education campaigns, and aggregate statistics of sexual behavior and behavior change are not as helpful as we might expect in explaining the differences. Both countries have implemented extremely extensive educational campaigns, with more than 90 percent of their populations being aware of AIDS and how to prevent it.[3] Both have provided condoms free of charge or cheaply to large numbers of people[4] and have intervened in numerous other ways, with significant involvement of all aspects and levels of government and civil society (with the exception of the president and the minister of health in South Africa). Surveys show, too, that sexual behavior has changed by similar amounts in both countries.[5] Moreover, statistical aggregates of sexual behavior data show that Uganda and South Africa are not abnormal compared with countries in the rest of the world.[6] It has proved extremely difficult to evaluate the effect that knowledge, sexual attitudes, and beliefs have on sexual behavior, and the effectiveness of condoms has also been difficult to assess. The report of a large and comprehensive metastudy of global trends in sexual behavior remarked that "the apparent absence of an association between regional variations in sexual behavior and in sexual-health status [prevalence of HIV and other sexually transmitted infections] might also be counterintuitive. In particular, the comparatively high prevalence of multiple partnerships in developed countries, compared with parts of the world with far higher rates of sexually transmitted infections and HIV, such as African countries, might hold some surprises."[7] Thus, it appears unlikely that much of the difference in the shape and direction of HIV trends between the two countries can be successfully attributed to this set of factors. The differences remain puzzling even after years of research and analysis.

As we saw in chapter 2, prevalence trends, especially in Uganda, do not conform to expected, standard demographic growth or logistic curves, or to standard epidemiological models based on these. In their attempt to fit an epidemiological model to the data, Stoneburner and Low-Beer had to assume an extremely rapid—and unrealistic—drop in incidence between 1989 and 1994.[8] More problematic is the fact that the simulation predicts further rapid falls in prevalence after 2000. This would conform to normal viral epidemics in which the viral infection eventually falls to near zero as patient recovery, increasing population-level immunity, and possibly death raise the epidemiological threshold to a point at which the virus can no longer propagate. This evidently does not happen in HIV epidemics. Instead, judging from current evidence, HIV prevalence may stabilize, and may continue to decrease but does not trend toward zero. This is consistent with a power-law model but not with standard epidemiological curves that are based on Gaussian bell-curve or exponential models.

Thus, the behavior of the curves depicting increases and decreases of HIV at the population level suggests that the configuration of the sexual network is a causal element in prevalence trends over time. This is because HIV transmission is not randomized as aerosol transmission of flu or cold viruses generally are. It is therefore difficult to explain these differences on the basis of statistically randomized survey data on sexual behavior and behavior change, or by using ordinary epidemiological methods alone.

In mature, generalized, heterosexual HIV epidemics such as these, many factors affect choice of sexual partners and the frequency and periodicity of sexual contact. Accordingly, sexual networks that transmit HIV infection can take on different configurations. These configurations have different properties with respect to the efficiency of transmission of the virus and their vulnerability to interruption or breakage.[9] Where networks break, through any form of limitation or cessation of sexual activity or use of a barrier (condom), HIV transmission is interrupted, and therefore further incidence of HIV infection is hindered. The overall effect that different degrees of such interruption will have on the efficiency of transmission in the overall network, however, is a property of the configuration of the entire network, not simply of the statistical frequency of interruptions (that is, the overall sum of numbers of broken links, or nontransmitting nodes). In other words, the magnitude of behavior change—use of condoms and changes in number of partners and frequency of sexual contact—affects HIV prevalence differently depending on the specific architecture of the sexual network.

This observation shifts attention away from personal sexual *behavior* to the level of the *social*—specifically, to social and sexual networks. It forces a shift in the scale of observation and suggests that interventions that fail to take into account the configuration of the overall sexual network are likely to have limited or unpredictable effects, or no effect at all. Since the only measures we have for describing and predicting the development and future trajectory of the epidemic are behavioral, it is not surprising that we are still searching for answers after more than twenty years.

SEXUAL NETWORKS, FAMILY STRUCTURE, AND PROPERTY

Notable efforts have been made to develop historical, cultural, political, and sociological explanations for the characteristics and magnitude of the HIV/AIDS epidemic in Africa.[10] It is clear, first of all, that there have been significant differences in the way the state has responded, and in the type and level of civil society involvement.

Uganda had exemplary leadership from President Yoweri Museveni and from his government, in general, in the fight against AIDS, whereas South Africa has had very little central leadership, or leadership that has tended to be harmful. Civil society involvement has been more or less total in Uganda, with tight integration between government and elements of civil society such as churches, nongovernmental organizations (NGOs), donors, business associations, labor associations, traditional authorities and traditional healers, schools, and community-based organizations.[11] In South Africa, this has not been the case. Although there is major involvement of civil society organizations, it is fragmentary, competitive, and quarrelsome. The relation between activist organizations concerned with AIDS and government has also been characterized by conflict and distrust. Political factors, however, do not entirely explain the different configurations of the trends or their directions.[12]

Cultural and social factors strongly influence the choice of sexual partners as well as the number of sexual contacts and their periodicity, and they determine the degree or level of social control that social groups such as family/clan, church, or peers might have on sexual behavior of their members. The effectiveness of these controls is often determined by still other factors, especially the presence or absence of the potential for coercive violence and the presence or absence of heritable fixed property that can be used to discipline sexual or other behavior by withholding inheritance or access to it.[13] It appears that coercive violence is not an effective means of sexual control. Use of controlled violence, from beatings to community-sanctioned murder, primarily occurs in strongly patriarchal societies,[14] such as rural Islamic villages from the Middle East to Pakistan and India where property-owning corporate kin groups exist and are strongly sanctioned by the community. Where violence does occur, sexual behavior is strongly associated with family honor, and families are corporate property-holding groupings with enduring systems of political conflict and alliances with other family property-holding corporations. In other words, sexual behavior is never the only thing at stake.

Such community-sanctioned coercion occurs to a very limited extent in Uganda and not at all in South Africa. Although there is a very high level of violence against women in South Africa, there is no indication that violence occurs as the result of community-sanctioned disciplining of women for shaming or bringing dishonor to families or to the community as the result of their sexual behavior. Shame and honor, as these concepts exist in, for instance, Mediterranean societies, are essentially absent in both Uganda and South Africa. By contrast, concepts of respect and jealousy, supported by witchcraft beliefs and networks of gossip and influence, are far more important. Almost universally in Uganda and South Africa, violence against women is locally attributed to jealousy, to drug or alcohol abuse, or to "people getting out of control." Except in the few cases in which supposed witches are punished, such violence is never sanctioned by families or communities.

One significant area of difference between the two countries is the fact that most Ugandans are closely tied to kin group, clan, or ethnic identities and these, in turn, are closely associated with property ownership. By contrast, most of the present South African land was alienated from black African ownership by the South African state, and few South Africans own any land outright as heritable property. Even white South Africans, who are more likely to have title to land and houses, generally have heavy debt burdens, and few transfer property through inheritance. Very few nonwhite people have any freehold-tenure land that can be inherited.[15]

The existence of heritable land in Uganda gives kin groups significant control over their members, particularly by senior, especially male, members over the junior members. It probably represents a significant system of social control over sexual behavior. Property is usually inherited, or otherwise transferred to juniors, only on the death of senior members of the family, clan, or lineage. Those who die from AIDS (or any other cause) cannot inherit property or pass it on to family or children. This seems to represent a powerful deterrent. Although it evidently does not limit the overall volume of sexual activity, it probably limits the range of persons with whom one can and does have sex.

In South Africa, on the other hand, family property is extremely limited for the vast majority. It is also rarely transferred as inheritance to junior generations. Although property transfer does occur, it is generally transferred at the time of marriage through the institution of bride-price, in which the husband's family gives a relatively significant amount of "cattle" (today, usually in the form of cash or other goods) to the bride's family. Other gifts are exchanged in the opposite direction as well, but the bulk of wealth is transferred from the groom's to the bride's family. This represents a horizontal exchange of wealth. The absence of fixed and real property-holding family corporations in South Africa means that kin have almost no control over other members of their group.

Bride-price is also customary in much of Uganda, but the property (cattle, money, and other goods) exchanged is exchanged by corporate kin groups. This explains the custom of wife sharing in western Uganda, for instance, because the bride-price is raised jointly by all members of the family, who then have joint sexual rights as a consequence. In South Africa, bride-price is raised and paid by the groom, possibly with help from his family, but they do not claim joint corporate rights. In Uganda, these patterns lead to clusters of sexual relations (joint family access to the new bride) and support the family property complex, while in South Africa, there is no family property complex, and bride-wealth is primarily the responsibility of the individual.

The history of Ugandan land tenure arrangements is centuries long, but since the early nineteenth century, the conquest of most of the southern part of this country by the centralized kingdom of Buganda (from which the country gets its name) has established and stabilized strong association between kin groups and specific lands, termed *mailo* (from the English term *mile*, the unit in which landholdings are measured).[16] Under the laws of the British protectorate, some precolonial landholding arrangements were preserved and only small amounts of urban lands were alienated to European or Asian (Indian) settlers. The small amount of land owned by settler groups (predominately Indian) or foreigners was commandeered under Idi Amin's government, although some of this has been returned since Museveni took power. In the main, land tenure arrangements dating back to the nineteenth century have endured until today. Most of the land is owned by corporate kin groups of one sort or another and all of it is heritable.

In South Africa, land tenure regimes allow very little scope for freehold title to land. Out of a total land area of 1.22 billion hectares, 86.2 million hectares (85.6 percent) are surveyed "farms," large tracts of land that are owned by one legal person.[17] Although the state owns some of this land, forty-six thousand private owners (0.1 percent of the population) own most of it.[18] The remaining 14.5 million hectares of agricultural land is predominately communal land in the old homelands, areas designated under apartheid (up to 1994) for exclusive settlement by black African people.[19] Private ownership in these areas is a rarity. Most of the nonagricultural land, comprising 21.6 million hectares, lies in nature reserves or state lands, or is owned by public works.[20] Overall, the state owns twenty-seven million hectares. Thus, there is very little scope for private ownership of real property.

As a result of all these differences in property ownership patterns and heritability, Ugandan and South African kinship structures and household formation, including levels of social control attached to them, are radically different.

SEXUAL NETWORKS AND FAMILY PROPERTY REGIMES

We can now explain the effect of different configurations of sexual networks on the dynamics of the HIV/AIDS epidemic in terms of different family property regimes. Depending on the kinds of choices people make about sexual partners, the sexual network can take on different shapes and cover different populations. For instance, if one highly sexually active person is having sex with ten people regularly (for example, a sugar daddy/mama), and each of his/her partners is having sex with two others, then we have a wheel-and-spoke-shaped network, where one person is linked to many people and those people are linked to fewer people. Several such interlinked networks can form a densely linked cluster with relatively few links outward. Alternatively, we might have large numbers of people in a population linked to two, three, or four people; all have multiple links to others through circles, chains, or filaments of sexual contact that ramify widely. This forms a randomized or small-world type of network, with many possible links between most people in the network.[21]

The clustered subnetwork will be relatively isolated from the rest of the population if none or only a few people have sex with people outside of that network. This network will be less efficient in transmitting HIV to a larger population, but highly efficient *within* the clusters if core people have the virus. On the other hand, the randomized small-world network will be highly efficient at transmitting the virus to *all* of the population, since there are many possible links across all possible participants in the network. For the small-world networks, it does not matter where the virus is first introduced, since it will spread to all parts of the network very efficiently.

This has implications for HIV/AIDS transmission. For clustered, lumpy networks, if the links between clusters are cut, HIV will be isolated within different subnetworks and will not be able to spread beyond that. A phase transition—as in Uganda—will occur in HIV incidence and prevalence when a tipping point is reached. If one or two critical links are eliminated—they stop having sex, start using condoms, stick to one partner, or die—then prevalence in the whole population will decrease very rapidly. For the small-world network, in contrast, if a few links are eliminated, there will be *no effect at all* on the entire network, since the network will function like the Internet—that is, even though some links go down, the network as a whole continues to function. In the case of HIV, so long as most people have multiple partners at regular intervals, the elimination of some people will have no effect on the efficiency of transmission through the entire network, since all persons are multiply linked to other parts of the network. Therefore, small (or even quite large) changes in sexual behavior will have little appreciable effect.

Uganda

It appears that Uganda's sexual networks were probably highly clustered with limited links between clusters. This is caused—or supported—by a number of factors that affect social differentiation.

First, Uganda has a relatively large degree of social differentiation in a relatively small population (twenty-three million people, as opposed to more than forty-five million in South Africa), with class and status differentials[22] that are founded partly on the hierarchy of the southern kingdoms, partly on wealth in land, and partly on other criteria such as position in government. The distinctions are deeply rooted in history, since the origins of the largest states of Rwanda, Bunyoro, and Buganda can be clearly traced back five centuries or more. These differences are both ethnic and political, since each kingdom was a distinct political entity in precolonial and colonial times. Many Ugandans continue to think of themselves as separate polities even today, especially since the restoration of their kings by Museveni. I was struck, for instance, by the fact that on the day I visited Rubaga Girls School, where I used to teach in the early 1970s, the flag of Buganda, the newly restored kingdom, was raised before and next to the Ugandan national flag. Rubaga is next to the first Roman Catholic cathedral in Uganda and adjacent to the old Lubiri, or king's palace. It lies at the heart of old Buganda. But each kingdom also has its own history of different tribes and languages, and they are ranked with respect to one another's history of conquest and incorporation. Inequalities exist both within and between these social divisions, as well as between virtually all individuals. Jacques Maquet termed this "the premise of inequality" in reference to this set of kingdoms and their political structures.[23] Another anthropologist writing about the oldest of these kingdoms, the Nyoro, noted that "ideas of superordination and subordination" were pervasive in social life, such that "every social relationship has . . . a hierarchical or 'unequal' aspect."[24] These authors were writing in the mid-twentieth century, when such broad generalizations were possible, but the essence of their observations rings true to anyone familiar with Uganda. This means that *within* these ethnic groups there are significant degrees of status difference that inhibit sexual contact across these barriers. They also inhibit sexual contact across the larger ethnic divisions.

Although the official national language in Uganda is English, there are significant ethnic and linguistic divisions, too. Ethnically, Uganda divides roughly into northern and southern halves. The southern half is dominated by the kingdom of Buganda, but includes three other kingdoms—Toro, Bunyoro, and Ankole—together with other tribes or ethnic groups such as the BaSoga, BaGisu, and BaChiga, which were politically organized with distinct historical identities but lacked kings in the precolonial period. All of the people in the southern half speak one or another language of the Bantu family of languages, with Luganda being the most widely spoken. Most of these are not mutually intelligible. In the north, people speak languages that are not related to the Bantu languages of the south, but rather to the Sudanic and Nilotic (languages of Sudan and the Nile valley) to the north of Uganda. These groups did not have kings and were not centrally organized into states as most of the people in the south were. The Madi, Alur, Lugbara, Langi, and Iteso in the central part of the north were primarily agriculturalists, while the Karimojong and Jie in the dry northeast relied on cattle herds and dry-land sorghum crops for subsistence. In most of Uganda's cities and towns, one language or ethnic group dominates, but none of them are ethnically or linguistically exclusive. In more rural areas, by far the majority of people live in monolingual communities. Linguistic differences, like political, ethnic, and status differences, also tend to create sexually endogamous groupings. One recent study, for instance, found that unmarried women and married men in multilingual communities were far more likely to engage in extramarital and multiple partnerships than those in monolingual communities.[25] Although this did not appear to hold true for married women or unmarried men, it does suggest, at least, that language differences structure the sexual network in specific ways.

Especially in the south, there were strong status differences among the political elites of the kingdom, and between the high-status cattle keepers (part of the larger Tutsi ethnic category) such as the BaHima (Museveni's ethnic group) and the BaIru (servants), who were agriculturalists. Other clearly differentiated status groups in the nineteenth century included fishermen, hunters, blacksmiths, bark-cloth workers, and so on. Important status distinctions are still made today based on the precolonial histories of clans associated with these pursuits, in addition to other, newer status differences based on profession, political party membership, and rural/urban distinctions, among others. Finally, all of these differences are crosscut by religious affiliation. The vast majority of Ugandans belong to one of three faith communities: the Roman Catholic, the Church of Uganda (Anglican Communion), and Islam. Evangelical Christians, primarily funded by Christian fundamentalists from the United States, have greatly increased their numbers in recent years, too. These distinctions, although not apparent everywhere, tend to divide the Ugandan population into relatively small endogamous (and sexually exclusive) groups based on economic, ethnic, and status factors. Most social interaction, especially ties of close friendship or sexual intimacy, tends to take place within these groups rather than across them.

The relatively high prevalence of polygyny is another factor that contributes to the clustered configuration of the Ugandan sexual networks. The Demographic and Health Survey of 2001 shows that 21.8 percent of all married women reported that their husbands have at least one other wife, while 10.4 percent reported two or more cowives.[26] The polygynous family is the simplest and clearest example of a hub-centered network or cluster. This consists of a husband married to several wives who each has her own household establishment and children. In fact, the wives may also have other lovers, and the husband is not necessarily faithful to his group of wives. The idea that one should be limited to even several wives seemed surprising to one Muslim man with whom I spoke in July 2003. "If I stayed with only the wives I have, how would I find another wife?" he asked. This pattern is relatively common. In some cases, informal or effective polyandry around a wealthy sugar mama such as a female professional or trader, or wife sharing, as attested in western Uganda among a group of brothers whose family wealth in cattle had been exchanged for a wife, were also practiced.

Clan or kin-group organizations are another factor that governs sexual access. Rules of kinship and marriage, and of rituals pertaining to life crises such as circumcision, death, and marriage both permit (or require) or forbid sex at different times. For instance, there is often a period of informal sexual license associated with large family funeral gatherings. Like any large gathering, these occasions also provide moments of sexual opportunity. There are often periods of sexual license during circumcision ceremonies in eastern Uganda. Wife inheritance is another instance in which sexual activity is regulated by rules of kinship and family/clan tradition. Traditionally, in most of the southern kingdoms (as in the Bantu-speaking areas of Africa), the surviving brother of a deceased man was expected to marry his brother's widow. If the deceased had died of AIDS, it is likely that the surviving widow was also HIV-positive, and this custom is believed to have led to increasing rates of infection. These practices appear to have changed radically in the early 1990s. It is very likely that these changes contributed to the sudden phase transition, or catastrophe event, that occurred in the HIV prevalence rates in 1992, as shown in chapter 2.

Most people in Uganda are linked through kin networks to heritable property, thus giving senior family members some degree of control over juniors. This pattern is based on the political structures of the old kingdoms in the south, and on the clan-based land tenure systems of the agricultural chiefdoms of the north. In the kingdom of Buganda, for instance, the clan chiefs, the *abataka,* held clan lands on behalf of

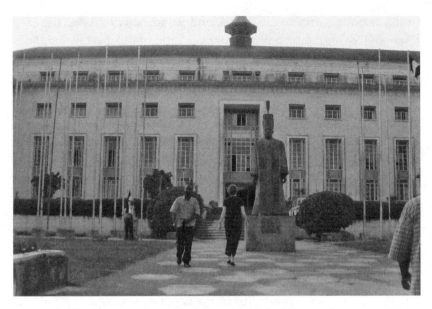

FIGURE 8. The Bunga, or Buganda king's council building, in Mmengo, where the *lukiiko* (king's council) is housed. Mmengo today is a suburb of Kampala, Uganda. (Photograph by R. Thornton)

the members of the clans. At the end of the nineteenth century, there were approximately fifty such clans in Buganda with clan landholdings. Their names and symbols (or totems) are memorialized today in the foyer of the Bunga, the seat of the Ganda king, or *kabaka,* and his council (see figure 8). For much of the history of the kingdom, the *abataka* competed with the hierarchy of the king's own men, who, as leaders of the army or providers of other services to the kingship, were also entitled to land, especially conquered lands. The king's men, then, constituted another group of landholders, who derived their position originally from the kingship during the expansion of the Ganda kingdom, but who became, with their descendants, holders of freehold-tenure land. The system of land tenure was confirmed and legalized by the installation of the British protectorate, and protected from expropriation by non-Ugandan settlers. Thus, the system of land tenure in Uganda is based on freehold tenure, originally by clan heads and elites, but now devolved to family units. Unlike South Africa's, Uganda's system of land tenure, and therefore of property and kinship, has been relatively stable for more than a century. Similar arrangements exist in Toro, Bunyoro, and Ankole, the other principal kingdoms of Uganda.

In the north, traditional local-level land tenure systems have remained largely unchanged due to the relative isolation of this part of the country. Because Ugandans own and inherit land, the moral pressure of families remains strong.

Since Uganda was never colonized, but remained a British protectorate from the late nineteenth century until independence, traditional systems of authority based on kingship and chiefship have been relatively stable over a period of centuries, and are strongly linked to systems of land tenure. As noted earlier, the systems of land tenure have also remained stable. "Most people's cultural patterns are constructed around land relations," notes Rebecca Mukyala-Mukiika, a Ugandan sociologist.[27] In 2003, for instance, the *kabaka* ceded the residence of the former *katikkiro,* or prime minister of Buganda, to the Uganda government to house the Joint Clinic Research Program, the leading HIV clinical research center in Uganda. Many Ganda people, especially royalists, objected to this because of the strong link between land and kingship. The move was justified by the *kabaka* as being in the national interest. This and other compromises and collaborations have enabled traditional systems of authority to become involved in AIDS prevention. Contemporary Uganda has—so far—successfully integrated these institutions into civil society and into the massive mobilization of civil society in response to AIDS.

Close cooperation has not always been the case, or even a possibility. After President Milton Obote, in collaboration with his military chief, Idi Amin Dada, abolished the kingships and all traditional leadership positions in 1967, resentment simmered, especially among the traditionalist Baganda of the Kabaka Yekka (Kabaka Only) Party, but also among other Ganda conservatives and in the smaller kingdoms. Responding in part to several strong social movements that demanded ethnic and communal rights which only the restoration of the kingships could provide, President Museveni restored all but one of these, Ankole, in 1993.[28] The 1995 constitution further entrenched the cultural rights of these kingdoms.[29] The Museveni government believed that because of the popular legitimacy of these kingships, they would be strong stabilizing agents, especially at the local level. This move was coupled with the implementation of a decentralization policy that shifted many of the functions of government to culturally homogeneous local councils and committees.

While I was conducting research in Uganda in 2003, it was clear to me that these local committees were effective and active. They helped to select a good cross section of their communities for interviews and focus groups on AIDS and HIV in the several cities we visited, including Kampala, Mbarara in the southwest, and Mbale in the southeast. It was also clear that people, especially in Kampala and Mmengo, the heart of the Ganda kingdom, were profoundly respectful of the king and the kingdom. At Rubaga Girls School, a Roman Catholic school where I had taught science in the late 1960s and early 1970s, the national flag of Uganda and the flag of the kingdom of Buganda flanked the diocese flag at a school function I attended. Local, cultural, and religious rights and identities were asserted even in the context of a Catholic school fête.[30] Traditional forms and idioms of Kiganda song, dance, speech, and ritual in the public performances featured strong HIV and AIDS messages. The parish priest and school pastor spoke forcefully in support of faithfulness in marriage and use of condoms, after asking blessings for both the nation and the kingdom of Buganda.

The majority of Ugandans are closely attached to their land for survival, subsistence, status, and prestige, among other reasons; this attachment also means that they do not travel widely. There is a low degree of physical mobility and travel except along trade corridors, and this is relatively highly structured since people travel only in limited and well-defined circuits, especially between urban areas and rural family landholdings, or for trade along a few major roadways. Paved highways connect the main urban centers, especially in the south, and an arterial route connects the border of Kenya with the northwest border of Tanzania, but it does not extend much beyond this even today. In the northern half, continuing violence and terrorist raids led by the Lord's Resistance Army drastically inhibit all but essential travel. The relatively high cost of gasoline, automobiles, and even public transportation also militates against large-scale mobility. My personal impression, both in the late 1960s and early 1970s, when my family lived there, and again in 2003, was that Ugandans in all parts of the country were exceptionally house-proud and dedicated to their homes, gardens, and farms. They did not stray far from these without good reason or very often. There are small markets within walking distance of everyone, and churches and schools are everywhere. Most people, then, typically do not travel much farther than they can easily walk.

Most people are strongly associated with some form of freehold-tenure land, and residence in rural villages has been stable, probably for centuries.[31] This stability—until it was disrupted during the period of political and social degeneration under Obote and Idi Amin between

1971 and 1986—may have allowed HIV to remain endemic in the population for many years, even generations or centuries, before breaking out of its isolated sexual networks and going global in the late 1970s. It has been suggested that a low-level endemic HIV infection may account for the low population densities in Buganda and the southern kingdoms, despite their obvious ecological advantages, and may account for the heavy toll taken by otherwise ordinary diseases in Buganda in the late nineteenth century.[32] The spread of HIV may well have been limited by the residential and social isolation of most Ugandans until very recently. This probably also helps to account for the sudden drop in HIV prevalence in 1992 and afterward, as social arrangements and routines began to settle down again following the years of disruption. In either case, the residential stability of people in the Ugandan landscape is likely to have created closed clusters of sexually active persons with few links to other clusters. This is a critical feature of the distinctive configuration of the Ugandan sexual network.

The configuration of social and sexual networks is also affected by the fact that only approximately 15 percent of Ugandans are urban,[33] compared with 58 percent of South Africans. The relatively low degree of urbanization is partly due to some twenty years of conflict, and collapsed infrastructure and scarcity of jobs in urban centers, but it was also the case before the period of social collapse. People have never had to move to cities for work or to survive because subsistence agriculture continued to work well and provided sustained livelihoods for all. Even when Ugandans choose to live in an urban area, they try to maintain continuing links to the rural areas and to clans and families that can provide them with farm produce and other amenities.

Other data on sexual and marital patterns lend support to the contention that Uganda's sexual networks differ markedly from those in South Africa. Uganda shows a relatively late age for onset of sexual activity, for instance, compared with a much earlier debut in South Africa. In Uganda, the median age at sexual debut for women increased from 16.5 years in 1989 to 17.3 in 2000–2001, and for men from 17.6 years in 1995 to 18.3 in 2000–2001.[34] According to Maria Wawer's research in Rakai, however, the median age at first sexual intercourse in the forty villages of Rakai where the study was based may have fallen from 17.1 to 16.2 years for men, and from 15.9 to 15.5 years for women.[35] Not all studies support these ranges for age at first sexual intercourse, however. A study conducted between February and April 2005 in Mayuge District of eastern Uganda, with 197 children ages

8–14 and 100 adult parents or guardians, led the investigators to the conclusion that 58 percent of these children had had sexual intercourse at least once (43 percent of boys and 57 percent of girls), mostly (70 percent) with others close in age.[36] But, despite some variation, the age at first sexual intercourse is apparently very close to the relatively early age at first formal marriages for the majority of the population. The median age at first marriage in Uganda was 17.7 years in 1969.[37] Other data show that 50 percent of 15- to 19-year-olds were already married in 1995, according to Department of Health Services (DHS) surveys.[38] Marriage does not necessarily exclude other sexual contact, of course, but it does set up formal means for control of sexual activity. These Uganda marital patterns differ strongly from the extraordinarily late age at first marriage in South Africa, if South Africans choose to marry at all.

Although we do not have details of the actual configuration of sexual networks, all of these factors suggest that sexual networks are normally highly clustered and often discrete, with few links between them and few long-distance or randomized links across the population as a whole.

South Africa

By contrast, it appears that South Africa has highly randomized, multiply interlinked networks in which the majority of sexually active people have sex with at least two others. There are many reasons for this.

Relative to Uganda and many other African countries, South Africa has a low degree of social differentiation by language, ethnicity, region, or class and status, and these factors have relatively little influence on choice of sexual partners. Virtually all South Africans today live in multiethnic, multilingual communities, even in rural areas. This is due, partly, to the exceptionally high mobility of people—men, women, and children alike. But even high mobility does not fully account for the mixed ethnic identities of South Africans. It appears to be deeply rooted historically. Any social arrangements that existed prior to 1820—the year that Shaka Zulu was murdered by his half brother, the Zulu kingdom fully established, and the first large group of British settlers established in the eastern Cape—were almost completely swept away across what is today the country of South Africa by warfare, large-scale migrations, shifting allegiances, and changing ethnic, territorial, and racial boundaries for the subsequent ninety years or so. In contrast to Uganda, whose ethnic and political identities are supported by histories and stable landholdings known for a half millennium into the past, there is no contemporary political identity in South Africa that is more than two centuries old, and most are younger than that. (The Bushmen/San and Khoekhoe, South Africa's first people, no longer exist as distinct ethnic groups and their descendants are now classified as colored in South Africa's racial vocabulary.)

Moreover, identities are only weakly associated with territory or land. There have been too many political and territorial redraftings of the landscape to permit such stable identities. The last wholesale redrawing of the South African map was as recent as 1996, when the four former provinces that had existed since the middle of the nineteenth century (Cape, Natal, Transvaal, and Free State) were divided into nine new ones. Change has been so pervasive and well accepted that the old territorial identities evoke little nostalgia and are almost entirely absent from conversation, and even from memory. At this level, territorial identity seems to have been flexible. The traumatic history of apartheid, most recently, but also of the Anglo-Boer War and other violent conflicts has perhaps contributed to South Africans' willingness to forget their differences, or perhaps has made it even more amazing that they should forget them. Because everyone learns at least two national languages in school, and most speak more in their daily lives, communication is rarely difficult. But, in any case, it is remarkable that few differences in language, ethnicity, class, or status have much impact on everyday social relations, including sexual relations, today.

This is likely to seem incredible to many who know South Africa as the land of apartheid, but the political system that remained in place for most of the second half of the twentieth century had a paradoxical effect. Although it was built on the premise of ethnic and racial differences and sought to strengthen them wherever possible, it evidently failed in this mission. Ideologies that developed during the struggle against apartheid included rejection of differences of all kinds, and political movements were inclusive of all ethnic, racial, and regional groups. In fact, in contrast to the Ugandan premise of inequality, South African political culture is premised on a deep commitment to equality, or even equivalence, within certain limits.[39] This is especially true for young black males, who assert their personal autonomy wherever possible and expect other men to do the same. Hierarchy is weakly developed in black South African traditional cultures because of this principle. This was strongly reinforced during the long struggle against apartheid, in which the political principle of equality was the ideological foundation of the struggle, but was probably an important cultural principle from at least the nineteenth century. In stark contrast to Uganda, where "every social relationship has . . . [an] 'unequal' aspect,"[40] in South Africa persons are held to be fundamentally equal. This principle of equality has tended to permit large-scale migration, especially of men (but also of women) because each head of household is believed to be effectively autonomous. This autonomy is both a goal for young men who seek to leave their parental homes, but also a condition that has permitted large numbers of people to seek their own fortune regardless of domestic arrangements or other social commitments. The result has been a highly mobile population that is constrained by few social barriers in the formation of social, economic, political—and sexual—networks of relationships.

The principle of equality or equivalence may also help to account for the distinctive marital patterns in South Africa. There is an extremely low prevalence of marriage (monogamous or polygamous). In 1995, for instance, 58 percent of women ages 15–49 reported that they had never married, and in 1999 this percentage had climbed to 60 percent.[41] A series of surveys of villages under the authority of a chief or traditional authority, which I conducted in 2000 with my students Joseph Nkuna and Kereng Kgotleng, supported these statistics. For instance, in Emjindini, a predominately Swazi-speaking tribal trust area with collective land tenure under Chief Kenneth Dlamini, 60 percent of all household heads interviewed (N = 335) were not married.[42] Similarly, in Mafefe, a SePedi-speaking village in Limpopo Province, 53 percent of household heads were not married, although the median number of children per household was three, and the absolute number of children ranged from zero to seventeen. In Mafikeng, a predominately SeTswana-speaking town in Northwest Province, 61 percent of all household heads interviewed were not married. The median number of children was three per household (range: 0–11, N = 306) in the Mafikeng sample. In Dan village, a predominately XiTsonga-speaking community near Tzaneen, Northern Province, 51 percent of heads of household were not married, with a similar number of children per household as in the other samples (median = 3, range 0–12, N = 345).

In short, the majority of childbearing couples, at least in these areas, are not married. Consequently, the number of sexual contacts outside of marriage is high, partly because of the low prevalence of marriage and partly due to the long window between age at sexual debut and age at marriage. This does not in itself lead to promiscuity, but it does largely eliminate the institution of marriage as a means of control. In fact, marriage is effectively delinked from childbearing. Although South Africa has the lowest fertility rate in Africa, births to adolescent unmarried women is high, though still lower than sub-Saharan Africa as a whole. More than 30 percent of nineteen-year-old girls are reported to have given birth at least once.[43] There is typically a long gap between the first child, borne in adolescence, and other children, which may be borne after marriage, however. Thus, marriage and childbirth are effectively independent of each other. When so few are married, the exhortation to be faithful (to a marital partner) makes as little practical sense to most South Africans as the idea of abstinence until marriage.

The low prevalence of marriage is itself probably a consequence of the fact that larger kinship units such as clan or kin-based organizations are virtually absent, and, where they exist, are small in size and exercise little control over the behavior (sexual or otherwise) of their members. In any case, there are no property-holding lineages or clans, and even larger family business units are rare, especially among black South Africans. On the other hand, the low rate of formal marriage and the late age at which marriages occur also mean that larger clans or kin-based organizations rarely form. It is probably not possible to say which is the cause and which the effect, but the result is that most people are born and grow up in households that contain an eclectic mix of close and distant kin, or nonkin (girl/boyfriends, parents of girl/boyfriends, etc.) who cooperate in domestic arrangements but do not constitute formal or genetic families. Occasionally, larger kin units are present, but they are relatively rare and do not form corporate or property-holding groupings. Inheritance of property, then, is also rare. Larger clans or kin organizations, where they exist, are generally informal and exist only for those who are more wealthy or who are linked to royal or elite lines of descent. For the vast majority, however, there are no superordinate groupings of kin, and no hierarchies of senior kin that might work to control sexual access or behavior. This pattern is pervasive in South Africa, but probably mostly limited to it. Patterns in Botswana, Lesotho, and Swaziland are different, although citizens of these countries travel frequently to or reside within South Africa for varying lengths of time.

Again, South Africa shows marked differences from Uganda with respect to systems of traditional authority. While Ugandans, especially in the areas of the old kingdoms—Nyoro, Toro, Ankole, and

Buganda—generally have affection for kingship and traditional author-ity and believe it exerts a positive moral influence, South Africans are widely ambivalent about their heritage of traditional authority.[44] Although the existence of chiefs and kings is guaranteed by the South African 1994 constitution, and their cultural rights entrenched, tradi-tional authorities have no political power. In South Africa, the majority of chiefs and kings were aligned with the apartheid government—often more by default than by choice—and were targets of resistance before 1992. This radically decreased their moral authority. In Uganda, since these institutions were abolished in 1967 and reestablished only after 1994, they were not contaminated by the period of state violence, corruption, and misrule during that period. They have consequently retained moral authority in the eyes of many Ugandans.[45] In the last decade there has been a resurgence of support for chiefship and king-ship in South Africa, but the system of traditional authority is still weak, and virtually impotent in the face of state authority. It exercises little control over behavior of any of its members/clients.[46]

South Africa has a high degree of physical mobility among men, women, and children. Most people travel at least some of the time to large parts of the rest of the country for work, for ritual events such as funerals, church celebrations, and pilgrimages, and for other reasons. Labor migration from rural areas—so-called labor reserves—to urban areas and mining compounds used to drive much of this migration, especially in the first three-quarters of the twentieth century, but mine employment has dropped dramatically since then, and most of the internal travel is now for other reasons. The overall extent of inter-nal travel is difficult to measure since transportation is not regulated and statistics on internal travel are not kept. There are some useful indicators, however. First, many people have automobiles or access to them. There are in total approximately 11 people per automobile in South Africa and around 6.4 persons per working vehicle of all kinds,[47] and 4.6 million adult South Africans (16.1 percent) own or use a car.[48] By contrast, there are more than 500 persons per passenger car in Uganda.[49] Road infrastructure in South Africa is also excellent: 20.3 percent of all roads in South Africa are paved, compared with 6.7 percent in Uganda. More important, South Africa has a finely reticulated road network that covers the entire country (1.2 million hectares).[50] This is not true of Uganda. Telecommunication coverage can indicate the degree of communication in a country, and could also be a proxy measure of physical mobility. Accordingly, there are 114 telephone land lines per thousand people in South Africa, compared with only three in Uganda, and 190 mobile phones per thousand people in South Africa, compared with eight in Uganda.[51] The high levels of mobile phone use appears to be a regional phenomenon, since all of the southern African countries rank in the top ten of fifty continental African countries with respect to mobile phone use. After South Africa, Botswana ranks second (123 per thousand persons), Namibia is third, Swaziland is fourth, and Zimbabwe and Lesotho are seventh and tenth, respectively. In sum, South Africa and southern Africa as a region have dense communication and transportation networks.

As we have seen, for the majority of the population in South Africa, freehold-tenure land is exceptionally scarce and land ownership is rare. This leads to the instability of residential groups in rural villages, as well as in townships, cities, and other residential areas, and to the instability of household constitution. Probably millions of people (the number is not known) have access to land in communal areas, but they do not *own* the land, except as members of communities that hold the land communally. They do not possess title deeds, and in most cases cannot because the land is not surveyed. Land in these areas is usually allocated by the chief or the headman, the traditional authorities in these areas. Although legislation has recently been introduced to make secure tenure possible in these areas, as of 2006 nothing had changed. Until the end of apartheid in 1992, black people in urban areas had to rent living accommodations, and rentals rarely included land. Although there was some freehold-tenure land in urban areas by the middle of the twentieth century, this was progressively decreased by apartheid legislation. Since 1994, this issue has been redressed. In the last decade, the government has provided 1.7 million housing units for low-income persons and has secured freehold tenure for 400,000 houses in urban areas. The majority of urban residents, however, do not have secure tenure in their housing, or they rent from others. Other rural people are resident on farms owned by the few large landowners, and thus do not have ownership rights to their property.

Relative to much of the rest of Africa, there is a high degree of urbanization in South Africa. The majority of the South African population lives in large urban centers—55–58 percent overall, with 92 percent of the white population, 98 percent of the Indian, and 84 percent of the colored populations living in urban areas. Approximately 45 percent of black Africans live in urban areas.[52] Because of the high levels of mobility, those who do not live in urban areas (especially black people) have relatively frequent contact with urban centers and with other close associates, kin, and sexual partners who live in urban centers. Although most people classified white, colored, or Indian (these categories are self-selected in the census and other statistical surveys) are urban, many do travel to rural areas or, especially, between urban areas.

As noted earlier, South Africa shows a pattern of early initiation of sexual activity and late marriage. The 1998 DHS survey reported a median age at first sexual intercourse as 17.8 years, but also reported that 37 percent of respondents were having sex by age 19, and 75 percent by age 24.[53] The median age at first marriage for African (black) men is 28.4 to 31.9, depending on how this is calculated (raw rates or singulate mean age at marriage). African women's median age at first marriage is 24 to 29.6 years, while the mean for South Africa as a whole lies between 25 and 30.8 years.[54] There is also a high prevalence of transactional sex and/or prostitution.

All of these factors tend to contribute to the formation of densely interconnected sexual networks, in which the majority of the sexually active population is multiply linked to all parts of the network, both near and far, and across most social categories. Race continues to divide the country's peoples and thus differentiates sexual networks into several different networks based on racial group, but there is little evidence to suggest that the shape of the sexual networks is significantly different in any of them. There are considerable—but so far unmeasured, and possibly unmeasurable—sexual links across all racial subpopulations. Differences that do exist are probably due to the differing density of contacts and their timing rather than to strong social differentials within each racial group. In other words, it appears that in South Africa there are strong cultural similarities with respect to sexual networking both across and within racial subgroups.

In Uganda, it is likely that the relatively rapid rise in HIV prevalence in the late 1980s and early 1990s was related primarily to the cross-linkage between otherwise isolated, clustered, or fractal networks. Perhaps this was due to the fourteen years of warfare and chaos that gripped the country from the coup d'état by Idi Amin in January 1971 and under his successors, Milton Obote and Tito Okello, until President Museveni reestablished orderly rule in January 1986. Ugandans see that period as a time of moral collapse, not just economic and political chaos.[55] According to this model, the increase in HIV prevalence was the result of social disorganization that linked previously separate communities (and sexual networks) to one another, and the later sudden decline in

HIV prevalence is due to the severance of links between these separate densely clustered networks. The rapid decline in prevalence was caused by changes in all of the ABC factors—increasing abstinence, being faithful to one partner and reducing the number of concurrent partners, and using condoms—and to the D (death) factor, particularly the death of persons who connected these networks, especially soldiers, truck drivers, sugar daddies (and sugar mamas), prostitutes, and traveling "businessmen" who ran smuggling and contraband operations during the period of instability and warfare.[56] Although these factors resulted in a rapid decline in prevalence overall, isolated pools of infection that did not cross-link to one another were maintained. For instance, among fishermen on Lake Kasenyi who had access to voluntary counseling and testing clinics, prevalence was 81 percent. Lakeshore villages on Lake Albert showed a 24 percent prevalence, compared with only 4 percent for neighboring inland villages.[57] Most fishing villages in Uganda are exceptionally isolated, accessible only by boat and, in dry weather, by footpath or track. Large local differences such as these can be caused only by limited linkages among these clusters or communities. These residual local pockets account for the fact that declining prevalence does not tend toward zero, as the power-law model shows (see chapter 2).

In a network of this configuration, so long as some (relatively few) people who provide significant linkages across densely intralinked clustered subnetworks no longer serve as transmission links (because they die, start using condoms, abstain, stick to one partner, or restrict their sexual activity to their own network), overall prevalence is likely to decline rapidly. This would explain both the rapid rise to a cusp in 1992 and the rapid decline afterward, which appears to reflect a sudden change of state in the social mass. It also helps to explain why HIV prevalence has decreased without significant declines in birth rates or overall declines in sexual activity, and why trends follow power laws rather than exponential growth curves more typical of ordinary demographic and epidemiological processes.

In South Africa, it is likely that the more typical growth curve, or exponential, rise in HIV prevalence, and the very high levels of HIV that are reached—up to 38.6 percent (95 percent confidence interval range = 30.0–48.1 percent) among black African women ages 25–29—is caused by the existence of a large and pervasive small-world network of sexual contact with relatively little segregation into clusters of subnetworks.[58] A network configured in this way presents little in the way of structural barriers to HIV transmission, and thus HIV infection is able to propagate freely, at first approximating an exponential model of free growth, then evolving to a linear trend suggestive of free diffusion of the virus. The spirit of freedom, including sexual freedom, and the new freedom of movement that accompanied the end of apartheid may have contributed to this. Long-term and enduring structures of kinship, domestic power relations, and property regimes are probably more significant causal factors, however.

CHANGING PREVALENCE:
A PROPERTY OF THE SOCIAL WHOLE

Since we lack specific empirical knowledge of these sexual networks, it appears that we can derive knowledge about them from different signatures that show up in HIV prevalence trends over time. This approach also suggests that the much-discussed link between poverty and AIDS may in fact be more closely related to—and complicated by—regimes and networks of property ownership, kinship and domestic power, rather than to absolute levels of economic prosperity alone. Indeed, there is no obvious relationship between HIV prevalence and wealth. Uganda, with its much lower HIV prevalence rate, is much poorer than South Africa. In South Africa, the AIDS deaths that have been most visible have been among the wealthy elites, even though the bulk of deaths have been among South Africa's far more numerous poor. Three of the poorest of the nine provinces—Limpopo, Northern Cape, and Eastern Cape—also have the lowest rates of HIV infection, and the wealthiest provinces—Gauteng and Western Cape—lie at opposite ends of the HIV prevalence spectrum. In other words, levels of wealth and poverty may be relevant to understanding the progress of the epidemic, but only insofar as specific forms of wealth—land, currency, and property—and the ways in which they are transacted determine the configuration of sexual networks.

We have shown that the configuration of these networks is determined by a complex set of *social* factors in addition to the individual *behavioral* factors. This suggests that intervention will be much more effective in situations where relatively isolated but still dense, nucleated, or highly clustered networks exist (such as in Uganda), since prevalence can be changed through the change in sexual behavior of relatively few people. It also suggests that population-wide interventions will be less effective than targeted interventions that aim to disrupt linkages between dense but relatively self-contained smaller networks. On the other hand, it also suggests that *all* interventions will be relatively less effective in multiply connected small-world networks (such as we find in South Africa), since elimination of even the majority of nodes will not affect the efficiency of HIV transmission in the overall network. Prevalence will probably continue to rise or remain relatively stable at high levels *despite* changes in sexual behavior of significant numbers of people. These networks function in many ways like the Internet, which was designed specifically to remain an active and efficient transmitter of information despite the elimination of some arbitrary number of specific nodes or links.

This may explain the apparent resistance of HIV prevalence to large-scale, costly interventions of all kinds in southern Africa. Thus, while small changes in sexual behavior can radically and rapidly reduce HIV transmission in minimally cross-linked clustered networks—such as those in Uganda—much greater population-wide behavior change is necessary in the interlinked networks such as those that seem to exist in South Africa.

In view of these differences, Low-Beer and Stoneburner asked in 2003, whether Uganda is unique in its apparent success in bringing down HIV prevalence, but warned in 2004 that "the Uganda evidence is still viewed with caution and confusion."[59] Is the pattern that we have seen in HIV trends in Uganda simply the consequence of unique historical processes that will never happen again in precisely this way? If not, can some factor or factors be isolated and exported to other countries, such as South Africa, where there is desperate need to find some intervention that works?

Although these questions are reasonable, they lead in the wrong direction. Changing HIV prevalence, as Caldwell and his colleagues suggested a decade after HIV was firmly identified, is strongly determined by the cultural and social roots of sexual networks.[60] The specific configuration of these networks determines what kinds and what quantity of behavior change (or death of HIV-infected persons) will have noticeable impacts on HIV prevalence over the population of sexually active people.

The search for one (or several) discrete and identifiable factors—such as abstinence or condom use—is, therefore, misdirected if the changing pattern of HIV prevalence is a property of the overall sexual network, a complex system whose properties are systemic and global rather than individual and local. Although people's motives, their assessment of risk, their behaviors, or even their deaths help to determine the configuration of sexual networks, according to this systemic perspective it does not matter how links (sexual contacts) are broken or formed; what is important is their density and timing. Changes in any or all of the ABC or D (death) factors may lead to change, but the *magnitude* of their effect will depend on the configuration of the social structures that underpin the sexual network and determine its characteristics.

Regardless of why or how links form or break, if the network configuration is still highly efficient at transmitting HIV, prevalence will continue to increase despite relatively large changes in any or all of the prevention factors. If the network is configured so that relatively smaller changes result in a reorganization of the overall network in a way that makes it more resistant to HIV transmission, then HIV prevalence will fall in a nonlinear way, probably according to a power law with an exponent approximating −0.5.

Historical factors are therefore relevant insofar as they can be related to the configuration of the sexual network. In Uganda, it is clear that a vast mobilization of all aspects of Ugandan civil society and government were involved in communicating the AIDS message and in helping to restructure Ugandan society. Clusters of high-density sexual links that existed around practices such as wife sharing, widow cleansing, and widow inheritance, and sexual license associated with nightclubs and with funerals, circumcision, and other rituals and festivals, were effectively stopped. Schools, churches, the army, all aspects of government at all levels, business and labor, traditional healers, and chiefs and kings, as well as NGOs and external donors, all worked together to bring about large-scale change at the national level. Changes in sexual behavior *and* mortality worked to restructure the sexual network. But without the high levels of social integration seen in the overall integrated response, it seems unlikely that changes in HIV mortality or behavior would have had the effect they did. Although Uganda found its own response through communication, education, and community mobilization programs,[61] the effect of this response was a fragmentation of a sexual network that was relatively easy to fragment. Unfortunately, it is probable that a similar level of integrated response in South Africa would have less effect because of the different configuration of the network.

These findings may also reflect differences between eastern African and southern African regions overall. In eastern Africa as a whole, median HIV prevalence decreased from 12.9 percent in 1997–1998 to 8.5 percent in 2002 in a way similar to Uganda's experience. In the southern African region as a whole, it increased from 21.3 percent in 1997–1998 to 23.8 percent in 2002.[62] It has long been assumed that the large regional differences between eastern, central, southern, and western Africa would eventually even out and diminish over time.[63] In fact, these marked differences have stabilized. In an article that surveys much of the evidence for these subregional differences in sub-Saharan Africa, Asamoah-Odei, Calleja, and Boerma call for greater attention "to the heterogeneity of the HIV/AIDS epidemic in subregions [eastern, western, central, and southern] and countries."[64]

Such regional differences suggest that the extent of sexual networks may indeed be regional. There are generally larger flows of population within these regions than between regions. There are widespread, though often subtle, cultural and social-structural similarities within regions. In southern Africa, the borders between South Africa, Lesotho, Swaziland, and Botswana are completely porous in all respects. This is increasingly the case, too, for southern Mozambique, Zimbabwe, and South Africa. Although the population flow is largely toward South Africa, cultural flows go both ways. There is probably less regional population flow in eastern Africa, partly because people are simply less mobile, but there are widespread linguistic, cultural, political, and social similarities and links there, as well. If trends in HIV prevalence can be related to the efficiency with which sexual networks transmit the virus, then this approach helps us to understand the heterogeneity of the epidemic at the national or even the regional level.

The focus on large-scale systemic processes of the sexual networks, contextualized in terms of the family social structures, domestic property regimes, and political systems, permits a move away from the current focus on individual behavior, risk assessment, and (supposed) rational action. This suggests, finally, that preventive interventions will have to pay more attention to the integration of all strategies at the national or even regional level to be effective. More than ABC or even D, what marks Uganda's experience and differentiates it from South Africa's is the degree of integration of prevention measures across all levels and divisions of society.

CHAPTER 4

The Tightening Chain

*Civil Society and Uganda's Response
to HIV/AIDS*

No one could see the link forming and stretching across the
country, a tightening chain that bound everybody together.
Doreen Baingana, Ugandan novelist, 2005

SYSTEM SYNERGIES

Uganda's approach converted the moralism of the ABC prevention
model (abstinence, being faithful, and using condoms) to the social ethic
of "zero grazing." This allowed for the mobilization of civil society,
and for the prevention of AIDS to be treated as a nation-building exercise. The synergies brought about by a comprehensive and integrated
response by government and civil society were largely responsible for
the change in HIV prevalence.

It first became apparent in 1996 that HIV prevalence in Uganda,
alone among African countries afflicted with HIV and AIDS, was
declining. Data from sentinel sites in antenatal clinics began to show
that a sustained reduction in HIV prevalence existed in many (but
not all) age groups and regions. This had begun to happen as early as
1989, but in aggregate, the decline was evident from 1992. The decline
continued strongly for five years, until 1997, and then began to level
out at around 8 percent overall, approximating the power-law curve.
This represented a huge reduction from levels of 30 percent registered
in western Uganda (Mbarara) and Kampala at the beginning of the
decade. By 2003, prevalence remained much lower, in aggregate, than
it had been ten years earlier, but by 2006 there were signs of message fatigue and HIV prevalence began to rise again.[1] The influence
of American policy, largely directed by Christian conservatives in the

83

United States, has also led to declining emphasis on condoms and increased emphasis on the ill-defined concept of abstinence.

The increases in HIV prevalence in 2006 were not significant enough to say definitively yet whether the earlier decline was permanent. Since the prevalence trend follows a power-law curve, reflecting the network of sexual contacts, further decline is likely to be very slow, if it occurs at all. Unlike other viral or bacterial epidemics, however, HIV prevalence is unlikely to trend toward zero in the near future. Indeed, a second rapid rise, paralleling the rise in the early 1980s, or even a reverse of the network phase transition or catastrophe event that seems to have occurred in 1992, is also a possibility. It is rarely possible to predict when a complex system like a sexual network (or stock prices or global climate, for that matter) might reach a tipping point and show dramatic and rapid shifts in direction and rate of change. It is also impossible to predict shifts in opinion and policy that are affected by political and religious regimes. "No one could see the link forming and stretching across the country," the Ugandan novelist Doreen Baingana tells us about the spreading epidemic.[2] These links are invisible until they are made apparent by experience of illness and death, and by careful analysis of the overall patterns and local manifestations.

What can be said, however, is that Uganda's success depended on what, over the years, has amounted to an extraordinary response by government and civil society to meet the crisis and to support appropriate changes in sexual behavior that would have an impact on HIV prevalence. More than the individual effects of behavior change—the ABCD of abstinence, being faithful, using condoms, and death—the synergies that developed between the configuration of the Ugandan sexual network and the degree of integration achieved in political, cultural, economic, social, and medical response is probably the real cause of its success. Because of the degree of integration of the response from civil society, business, and government it is also difficult to isolate any one factor. It was the total system that changed. Ugandan society changed in response to the HIV crisis, and the sexual network responded to this response. This combination created positive feedback that led to a tipping point at which HIV prevalence plunged to a much lower level. In other words, the two systems, one sexual and private, the other social and public, interacted synergistically to produce a change at the system level.

Apart from being an HIV/AIDS success story, Uganda's experience is a remarkable case study in political and social development. As AIDS became a tightening chain that bound everybody together, the common fear—always politically useful—was alloyed with hope for a new future. The government's integrated public response to AIDS became part of a highly successful nation-building program.

This was accomplished partly through the clear political direction provided by President Yoweri Museveni very early in the AIDS epidemic, but it is hardly due to him alone. Under Museveni, the government also delegated effective authority to competent and motivated leaders in the Ministry of Health and in churches, hospitals, and elsewhere, and then helped to provide resources to facilitate their activities. Major international donors provided most of the financial resources but very little of the actual implementation. Overwhelmingly, Ugandans themselves identified the problems, generated solutions, and integrated these into close-knit networks of mutual support that brought to bear the concerted action of society at large. Since this is relatively rare in Africa, or anywhere in the world for that matter, it remains all the more remarkable.

EXPLAINING THE UGANDAN SUCCESS STORY

The Ugandan success story, as it has been called, is both encouraging and puzzling. It is encouraging because Uganda's response shows that people—Africans in particular—can change their sexual behaviors sufficiently and in appropriate ways to meet the challenge of a mature generalized heterosexual epidemic. In South Africa, President Thabo Mbeki feared that Africans could be accused of being sexually undisciplined and promiscuous. The Ugandan story should have squashed this notion, but it seems that Mbeki did not pay attention to this aspect of the Ugandan experience. This has led to large amounts of donor funding flowing into South Africa for AIDS prevention programs, including millions from the U.S. President's Emergency Program for AIDS Relief (PEPFAR) announced by George W. Bush in 2003.[3] "The Bush Administration is basing its AIDS initiative on the success of Uganda, which has experienced the greatest decline in HIV prevalence of any country in the world," the conservative, Republican Party–aligned Heritage Foundation announced in a briefing paper. According to this policy document, "the best evidence suggests that the crucial factor was a national campaign to discourage risky sexual behaviors that contribute to the spread of the disease."[4] But the Bush administration also simplified and distorted this "evidence" and its message. The Heritage

Foundation policy document declares that "the White House correctly insists that U.S. AIDS policy be based on these lessons." Accordingly, the basis for U.S. government policy under the Bush presidency was the following:

- High-risk sexual behaviors can be discouraged and replaced by healthier lifestyles.

- Abstinence and marital fidelity appear to be the most important factors in preventing the spread of HIV/AIDS.

- Condoms do not play the primary role in reducing HIV/AIDS transmission.

- Religious organizations are crucial participants in the fight against AIDS.[5]

Although each of these "lessons" is true to a degree, taken as a group they do not begin to account for the complexity of the reality and, together, cannot be considered valid. This is especially true of the second point. Most of the evidence from Uganda shows that abstinence was, at best, a minor factor, and that marital fidelity is neither expected nor practiced by large numbers of people. Instead, the change in Uganda was a systemic change that involved synergies between behavioral and social changes, on the one hand, and changes in the configuration of the sexual network, on the other. To neglect this is to nullify the potential for success in other countries.

These simplifications are perhaps excusable, however, because the reasons for this change have been far from obvious. HIV is overwhelmingly a sexually transmitted infection that can be controlled only through limiting or stopping sexual contact among people, but changes in sexual behavior, though necessary, are not sufficient. It is also clear that Ugandans did not stop having sex. Uganda's birth rates did not fall during this period, and total fertility remains among the highest in Africa. Despite the fact that large numbers of people have died of AIDS, Uganda's population has continued to grow throughout this epidemic.

Behavior, especially sexual behavior, does not change easily or in isolation. Patterns of sexual behavior are generally quite stable. Thus, for sexual behavior to have changed there must have been larger social, cultural, political, and demographic factors that led to, motivated, and sustained these changes. Changes at the level of culture, social organization, politics, ecology, or demography are the distal causes. These distal "causers of causes" created an environment that both required change in personal sexual habits and practices (the proximate, or immediate, causes of the change in prevalence) and magnified their effect. In seeking reasons for the change in Uganda's prevalence rates, therefore, we can separate the more proximate from the more distal causes—that is, separate personal behavior changes from the social and ecological context of these changes.

In order to prevent or control sexual infections sexual contact must be limited or prevented, an approach summed up in the slogan "Abstain, be faithful to one partner, or use condoms" (ABC). The B factor has also come to include reduction in the number of sexual partners (from two or more to one). None of these interventions, however, proves to be effective in itself. Condoms may be used incorrectly or may fail. Few people are exclusively faithful to one other person throughout their sexual lives. And few people envision abandoning sex altogether. There are important temporal dimensions as well. When one begins sexual activity (and thus ends the implied abstinence of childhood) partly determines the age structure of HIV epidemics. When and how multiple sexual partners are encountered—within polygynous marriages, through casual sex (whether married or not), with commercial sex workers, and so forth—also has implications for the spread of HIV. The apparent simplicity of the ABC message, then, is an illusion.

How Behavior Changed

A great deal of research has shown that there was significant behavior change during the 1980s, that is, during the time when sexual behavior would have had to change if this were to account for the decline in prevalence beginning in 1992. It is clear, too, that behavior continued to change throughout the 1990s. No single change, however, can fully and unequivocally account for the change in prevalence: the change itself took place at a systemic level. Unfortunately, the uncertain impact of any or all *single* factors has made it possible for political and religious groups to assert their views using partial evidence, or by simplifying what is in fact a complex system.

The pamphlet titled *What happened in Uganda? Declining HIV prevalence, behavior change, and the national response,* published by the U.S. Agency for International Development (USAID),[6] led the way both in showing the overall decline in HIV prevalence and also in oversimplifying the context and complexity of that decline (see figure 9).

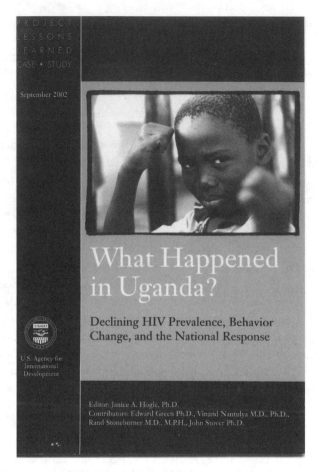

FIGURE 9. The USAID pamphlet that popularized the
ABC approach and gave oversimplified reasons for
HIV prevalence decline in Uganda.

This oversimplified picture cannot be empirically supported, despite
its appeal to policymakers. In its first sentence, the pamphlet states
that it "is not intended to provide a definitive explanation for Uganda's
AIDS prevention successes during the 1980s and 1990s," but it has
subsequently been taken to be sufficiently definitive to serve as a basis
for policy and to justify the allocation of fifteen billion dollars for additional programs

More detailed evidence shows that prevalence exhibits marked
regional, subregional, temporal, and cohort variation. In other words,
although HIV prevalence peaked overall in 1992 and then declined,

this was true only of the aggregate population. The reality is more complex. For instance, Whitworth and others, in a longitudinal study in the rural Masaka District from 1989 to 1999, show that no single age group or gender follows exactly the same trend shown in the USAID publication.[7] During this period, prevalence fell for females ages 13–19, 20–24, and 40–44, but increased for females ages 30–34 and 35–39 in the set of rural communities studied.[8] Peaks occur at different times, and trends are different for different age groups in this study. Similarly, the Ugandan data from antenatal clinic sentinel survey sites across Uganda show many different regional trends. For instance, prevalence began to decline in Jinja as early as 1990, whereas decline in Matany did not begin until 1994.

It is likely, therefore, that no single factor, or single behavior change factor, can account for the initiation of the decline and its continuation. Indeed, there are likely to be different causes for different age groups, regions, and genders. The initial decline, due—directly and indirectly—to mortality at first, was then sustained by significant and major behavior change in all ABC categories. Directly, mortality probably reduced prevalence since those who were HIV-positive died, reducing their proportion in the population. Indirectly, mortality also seems to have driven the behavior change, since many Ugandans watched close friends and family die in significant numbers during the late 1980s and early 1990s. Mortality, therefore, was also significant in the cultural environment as a motivator of behavior change.

The impact of AIDS mortality on sexual behavior change was probably greatly enhanced by a number of important cultural practices. First, most deaths occurred at home, and AIDS sufferers were cared for by their families. Second, Ugandans bury the dead within their living compounds. Graves of family members are often prominent features of the domestic space (see figure 10). Unlike people in many other countries, Ugandans generally do not use public or municipal cemeteries. When I visited the grave of our old family friend Kamondo and his family (see chapter 1), the importance of the visual and visceral impact of Ugandan burial practices on behavior change was brought home to me most forcefully. His parents were still alive, and they also remembered those days of thirty years ago, the time before AIDS, when Kamondo was still present in his family home, and as our families later got back in touch with each other over the Internet, his absence remained vividly present to all of us. Thus, mortality from AIDS had a daily visual impact as the living were forced to look at the graves of family members who had died

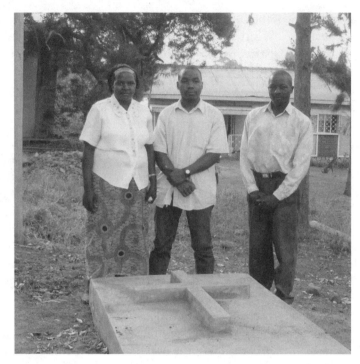

FIGURE 10. Kamondo's grave in the family homestead, with his
wife and two of his children. (Photograph by R. Thornton)

of AIDS. Finally, AIDS orphans are taken in and cared for by relatives
of the deceased in 99 percent of all cases. Death from AIDS thus placed
a very significant burden on the living.

Condoms may not have been a major factor in the initiation of
prevalence reduction in the population since they were not available in
large numbers before 1992, when the decline in prevalence had already
begun. They have been used increasingly from 1992 to the present,
however, and their use has probably contributed to the continuing
decline in prevalence.

Abstinence, similarly, cannot be isolated as causal. Although it
was consistently mentioned by all informants in focus groups and key
informant interviews, almost no one gave any concrete examples of
abstinence, and most expressed considerable skepticism about whether
abstinence was really possible. Appeals for abstinence could have
played a role only in delaying sexual debut among youths[9] and in the
abandonment of wife inheritance (since widows no longer automati-
cally entered into new sexual unions). Long-term abstinence was never

mentioned as desirable. Indeed, those who are entirely abstinent (the very young, the elderly, and priests and others practicing abstinence for religious reasons) are clearly not part of the sexual networks that transmit HIV and are irrelevant to the epidemiology of HIV. The number of abstinent people is probably insignificant in the total population, and the period of abstinence is small relative to an entire lifetime, and therefore abstinence is unlikely to have a statistically noticeable effect.

AIDS was not discussed in the popular press in Uganda until April 1985, and not discussed as a sexually transmitted disease caused by HIV until the following year. A mysterious disease known as *siliimu* or slim was, however, already a widespread rumor by 1985, though it was not yet connected with HIV or sexual transmission. There were only seven years between the first possible public knowledge of AIDS in Uganda and the beginning of the decline in prevalence. By the end of the 1980s, however, knowledge of AIDS was almost universal, and has remained so. The relationship between knowledge about HIV and AIDS and actual behavior change, however, remains as problematic in Uganda as elsewhere.

Uganda began a public debate about slim/AIDS in the media in 1985. The government of Tito Okello, who took power after the fall of Obote and before the Museveni government came to power, was the first to initiate steps to control the disease. Dr. Samuel Okware led the first initiatives. Although President Museveni was not the first either to discuss AIDS publicly or to make it a matter of public debate, his government moved swiftly after 1987 to develop a comprehensive response that eventually involved all parts of society.

President Museveni came to power in January 1986 and made a significant contribution to AIDS control programs with his early acknowledgment of the problem and the clarity of his messages about it. His primary contribution, however, was indirect. He enabled the growth of civil society and freedom of the press, and delegated authority to deal with AIDS to the Ministry of Health, where competent and motivated people began to design and implement highly effective responses after 1987.

Ugandans generally still believe in marriage, and marry early. The influence of Christianity and Islam cannot be doubted, but neither can these religions be credited with making a significant difference by themselves. The important role of faith-based communities was part of the synergistic integration of the many other forms of social organization in Uganda. Marriage and early age at marriage, however, do not necessarily mean that faithfulness to a single partner is the norm, or that numbers of partners are reduced as a consequence. Marriage, in fact, may be a kind of sexual license that heralds the debut of sexual access to many partners, especially for men, but also for women whose husbands are away or traveling. This was especially true in the period before the 1990s. A 1988 study of 15- to 24-year-old school-attending youths in Jinja found, for instance, that 75.6 percent of married males and 26.6 percent of the married females in the sample had more than one sexual partner.[10] Faithfulness in marriage seems to have increased, and practices such as wife sharing and widow inheritance were all but abandoned by the mid-1990s.

Churches and mosques were central in providing information, education, and communication (IEC) about AIDS and HIV, and in disseminating elements of the ABC message. This was facilitated by the fact that Ugandans overwhelmingly belong to three principal religions: the Roman Catholic Church, the Church of Uganda (Anglican), and Islam. Only a small percentage (1–2 percent in most surveys in the 1980s and early 1990s) belonged to other churches or to no faith, but this is changing rapidly with conversions to born-again and Pentecostal religious groups, which are largely backed by American supporters.[11] Unlike countries in southern Africa, in particular, Uganda seems to have almost no African syncretic or independent churches.

Approximately 25 percent of Ugandans are Muslim, and there appears to be good communication between Islamic and Christian leaders, and broad agreement on HIV/AIDS issues. The relative unity of religious organizations in Uganda and their early involvement in IEC interventions beginning in the 1980s are factors that greatly enhanced the effectiveness of campaigns promoting behavior change, especially delay of sexual debut, faithfulness in marriage, and partner reduction. Churches did not initially (in the 1980s and early to mid-1990s) support the use of condoms, but by the mid-1990s, Christian and Islamic leaders had agreed not to interfere in the promotion of condom use, and sometimes to encourage it. (Some ten years later, however, under pressure from religious fundamentalists and the U.S. government's PEPFAR program, many of the religious leaders had reversed their positions on condoms.)

One of the most striking factors in Uganda's approach to AIDS, however, has been the early and comprehensive inclusion of all parts of society in control programs. Uganda quickly implemented HIV monitoring at antenatal clinic sentinel sites, and developed educational programs that reached all schools. Government agencies and civil society organizations coordinated activities between government departments, universities and research institutes, hospitals, churches, labor and employer organizations, nongovernmental organizations, and other community-based organizations. By the late 1980s—still early in the epidemic—Uganda had developed a national strategy. By 1992, the government had created a national coordinating agency based in the Office of the President, and already-established AIDS control programs in all major ministries became responsible for implementation of education and control measures in their areas of concern. The governmental approach was distributed and decentralized. All levels of government, in all regions, districts, counties, and parishes, were involved. This approach has gradually incorporated virtually every size and type of organization in the struggle against AIDS. The intensive, directed, and focused participation by all aspects of society must be acknowledged as one of the most important factors in Uganda's success. This does not, however, fully explain the fact that Ugandans have responded to these myriad initiatives.

Within the context of major social mobilization, Uganda also led the way in voluntary counseling and testing for HIV. This began too late to explain the decline in HIV prevalence in the early 1990s, but has clearly been a major factor in sustaining a behavioral response in many individual Ugandans.

Ugandans in all walks life have clearly responded by changing their sexual behaviors, and all of the factors probably have been significant in reducing the number of sexual partners over the period of the epidemic, and this, in turn, has reshaped the sexual network at the systemic, national level. Thus, the Ugandan success story cannot easily be attributed to any single cause, or to any type or category of social actor. Personal decisions to change sexual behavior have been made in the context of nearly universal fear of the consequences of HIV, comprehensive social and cultural support for change, and integrated management of all institutional interventions.

The Validity of the Uganda Prevalence Curve

The USAID ABC study in 2003 was motivated by clear data that HIV prevalence in Uganda had begun to decline in 1992. This decline was impressive and demanded explanation—if it was real (see figure 11).

The data were obtained from sentinel survey sites at antenatal clinics

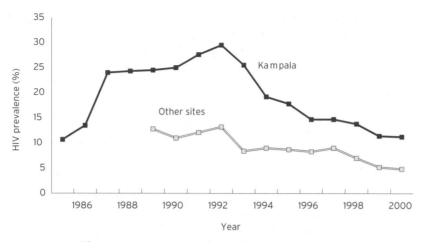

FIGURE 11. The "success story" graph: Median HIV prevalence among pregnant women in Uganda, 1986–2000, interpolated for one-year gaps in site
data. (Based on Hogle et al. 2002; data source: Ministry of Health, Uganda
2001)

in Kampala and six other sentinel sites at Rubaga Hospital (in Mmengo,
Kampala), Nsambya Hospital (Kampala), Jinja (Central District), Fort
Portal (Kabarole District in western Uganda), Mbarara (Mbarara
District, southwestern Uganda) and Gulu (Gulu District, northern
Uganda). The data were collected and summarized in a 2001 report of
the Ministry of Health.[12] HIV prevalence data for 15- to 19-year-old
pregnant women show a similar decline from 1991, from an average
around 30 percent in 1991 to around 5 percent in 2000. Prevalence
data for this age cohort are a good proxy measure for incidence because
people of this age will have presumably been infected only recently,
and will not have progressed to the point of AIDS illness and death.
Since similar trends exist in all of the antenatal clinic data, it appears
that most of the decline was due to the lower rate of new infections
(incidence) rather than to overall mortality. This, in turn, suggests that
these data are both valid and consistent. Several studies that examined prevalence and incidence over a ten-year period in southwestern
Uganda confirm this suspected declining trend for incidence.[13]

   This decline had become evident in 1996,[14] and continued to be
observed. It is summarized in the USAID's *What happened in Uganda?*
and in other documents.[15] These concluded, in the words of the
USAID's report, that the decline in HIV prevalence was largely due to
"a complex set of epidemiological, socio-cultural, political, and other

elements that likely affected the course of epidemic in Uganda,"[16] and that these were often absent in other countries where HIV prevalence has continued to rise.

Attributing Causes to the Statistical Decline in Prevalence

The causes of Uganda's decline in prevalence is not obvious, however. Emmanuel Sekatawa, of the Makerere University's Institute for Statistics and Applied Economics, told us in a 2003 interview that a new national prevalence study was in the advanced planning stages, but, although the study "will try to account for changes in prevalence, [there] is going to be a problem of attribution [of causes]. Evaluation and monitoring were not built into [any previous] programs." Dr. Sekatawa is as keen as others to account for the apparent decline but, as a statistician, he is extremely cautious about whether this is possible, given the available data. "We can't account for the decline," he said. "We don't know how much was due to condoms. We believe that all interventions contributed, but we can't specify which ones. [We] do not even know where condoms go when they come into country . . . urban or rural. [We] do not know what worked."[17] Dr. Sekatawa drew a graph of a decreasing exponential trend, asymptotic to a line above the x-axis, and asked, "What will bring it down lower?" He shrugged.

Nevertheless, several factors are likely to have been involved. The USAID report summarizes the "key elements . . . in roughly chronological order" that may have led to this decline:[18]

- · High-level political support with multisectoral response, which set the tone;
- · Decentralized planning and implementation for behavior change communication, which reached both the general population and key target groups;
- · Interventions that specifically addressed women and youths, stigma and discrimination;
- · Religious leaders and faith-based organizations, which have been active on the front lines of the response to the epidemic;
- · Africa's first confidential voluntary counseling and testing services;
- · Social marketing of condoms, which has played a key, but evidently not the major, role;

· Increased emphasis on programs to control and prevent sexually
  transmitted infections;

· A decrease in multiple sexual partnerships and networks, which
  appears to be the most important determinant of the reduction
  in the incidence of HIV infection in Uganda.

Other independent studies have produced strong support for the
reality of the decline in HIV incidence suggested by the prevalence statistics. For instance, the AIDS Control Programme (ACP) in Kabarole
District, funded by the German aid agency GTZ, was conducting sentinel surveillance in antenatal clinics every six months from 1991 to 1995
at three sites: Fort Portal, a semiurban roadside trading center, and a
rural community. These data were compared with population surveys
conducted in 1993, 1994, and 1995 to determine the representativeness
of the antenatal clinic data. Using these data, the researchers concluded
that trends seen in antenatal clinic data were in fact representative of
the whole community, especially in semiurban and rural communities.
For women ages 15–20 there was a constant decline in both HIV and
syphilis rates between 1991 and 1996, with declines from 30 percent
to 10 percent in Fort Portal, from 18 percent to 9 percent in the trading site, and from 10 percent to 5 percent in the rural site. Prevalence
of HIV infection among women ages 21–45 rose during this period,
however, though the rate appeared to be stable in the roadside trading
site and the rural community.[19] This study concluded that the ACP was
producing significant results, especially in the area of behavior change,
due to the combination of multiple factors including IEC campaigns;
care and counseling; sexually transmitted disease treatment; procurement, distribution, and training in the use of condoms; and training to
build organizational capacity. Although it appeared seven years before
the USAID report, this 1996 report came up with many of the same
explanations for the apparent decline that had only recently begun to
register clearly in the data.

In both these reports, and in Ministry of Health reports, the data
from the sentinel sites are usually generalized across the country as a
whole. Since the sentinel sites are mostly distributed across southern
Uganda, and since absolute numbers of respondents are not available
from the Ministry of Health,[20] it may be that these data cannot be
generalized and are not valid. The consistency of trends across most of
the sentinel sites, both across sites and across age cohorts within sites,
however, suggests very strongly that these data are valid and therefore

probably generalizable across the country. This of course masks potential hot spots of prevalence and incidence, and does not permit a disaggregation of descriptive statistics for different regions or risk groups. In other words, Uganda as a whole probably does indeed present a clear success story—but this does not mean that the problem is solved or that there are no significant populations in which HIV incidence and prevalence continue to increase.

Contextualizing the Data

The positive results in achieving lower HIV prevalence have been achieved with a tremendous amount of personal, and often selfless, dedication by large numbers of people at all levels of government, business, and civil society.

The countrywide HIV prevalence curve represents statistical summaries, and therefore does not show regional and age differences. The epidemic progressed rapidly across the landscape, and has progressed to older persons over time. For instance, the epidemic clearly began in the southwestern part of the country and spread rapidly eastward, and then to the north. Prevalence rates in the northeast are still much lower than elsewhere in the country. Matany, in the Moroto District in northeastern Uganda, reached a peak of 7.5 percent two years later than other sentinel sites in the south and central regions, and declined with the others to below 2 percent in 2001.[21] Antenatal clinic data for Nsambya, Rubaga (in Kampala, central region), Jinja (central), and Mbarara (western) all show higher prevalence rates from 1989 to 2001, while Tororo and Mbale in the eastern region show consistently lower rates. All exhibit the same trend, peaking at about the same time (except Matany) and falling to similar prevalence rates between 5 and 10 percent by 2001.

There is also an age factor: the epidemic is progressing into older age groups. Rates of decline have been highest in the youngest sampled age groups (15–19 and 20–24 years old), while prevalence is higher in older age groups (25–29, 30–34, and 35 and over). Declines in prevalence in older age groups are also generally slower, if they exist at all. The Mbale antenatal clinic data in the eastern part of the country even show an *increasing* prevalence trend for 25- to 29-year-olds, for instance.[22] A ten-year study of HIV prevalence in rural southwestern Uganda[23] shows a *decreasing* trend among male and female 20- to 24-year-olds beginning in 1989, when the study began. Prevalence in this age group decreased from 21.1 percent to 8.2 percent (p < 0.001) for females from 1989 to 1999, and from 7.7 percent to 2.2 percent for males. Prevalence *increased most rapidly,* however, for 30- to 34-year-old females (11.5 percent to 20 percent, p = 0.03) and slightly less rapidly for 35- to 39-year-old females (9 percent to 14.7 percent, p = 0.06). This increase for women in their thirties is at least partly due to a cohort effect, in which a bulge in prevalence for a particular cohort moves through age groups as the cohort ages. For men, however, the trend was in the opposite direction, with a decline from 19.5 percent to 16 percent for men 30–34 years old during this period. Only men ages 20–29 showed an increasing trend, but none of the trends in the male age groups were statistically significant. Prevalence also increased for 25- to 29-year-old females during the period, from 14.5 percent to 17 percent.

Overall, however, "seroprevalence in adults of all ages fell from 7.8 percent at the first survey round (1989/1990) to 6.4 percent at the tenth survey round (1998/99), a highly significant reduction (p < 0.0001)."[24] This is largely because of falling prevalence for males of all ages, and low and declining prevalence for females under 19 and over 40 years old. Overall, too, there is an aging trend in the population, with the median age of HIV-infected women rising from 26 to 30 years old, and for men from 32 to 35 years old.

None of these data[25] for any age group, male or female, show the pattern of the trend shown in the USAID publication *What happened in Uganda?*[26] Peaks occur at different times, and trends are different for different age groups and different for males than for females. Dr. Okware, a pioneer in the struggle against AIDS and the person responsible for the Ministry of Health surveillance reports, acknowledges that there are likely hot spots that are not sampled. The refugee camps in the north (where large numbers of people who fled from the depredations of the Lord's Resistance Army are likely to have higher than normal prevalence rates) and many rural areas were not sampled adequately or at all.[27] Thus, the geographic and temporal progress of the HIV virus may yet present some surprises. This does not negate the validity of the other data, which probably do represent a good part of the population adequately.

There is strong evidence in the interview and ethnographic data[28] that knowledge of HIV transmission and AIDS was disseminated as early as the second half of the 1980s and that this did indeed lead to changes in behavior, but this was a complex process, involving many nongovernmental actors in the broad-based civil society that began to emerge as early as January 1986, when Museveni came to power. Information about the modes of transmission of HIV, about the fact that it is incurable and leads inevitably to death, and about the prevalence of AIDS in the population was communicated person to person, in the press, and on the radio from the beginning of the Museveni government, and possibly even before, even in the last days of the second Obote regime. Knowledge emerged from many sources, with many different interpretations, during the early to mid-1980s, and seems to have pervaded the whole of Uganda (especially southern Uganda) very early in the epidemic. Today, there is virtually 100 percent awareness of the disease, its causes, and its prospects. This is not to say that there is consensus; there is not. Knowledge and direct experience, however, have penetrated all aspects of life in Uganda. They have led to significant changes in behavior through many channels, including modes of social organization, modes of governance, politics, business, and culture.

CHAPTER 5

AIDS in Uganda

Years of Chaos and Recovery

I think AIDS is now part of us.
   Namara Dinah, clinic sister
   and midwife, July 2003

FROM RUMOR TO DISEASE TO EPIDEMIC

Uganda is often associated in people's minds around the globe with Amin and AIDS. This is unfortunate, but the suffering that Uganda has gone through in the decades of the 1970s and 1980s seems to have given it the resolve and strength to defeat both the tyrant and the disease, and to arrive at the beginning of the twenty-first century as one of Africa's success stories. But in July 2003, as Amin[1] lay dying in exile in Saudi Arabia and debate went on about whether to allow him (dead or alive) back into the country, either to die or to be buried, fears were expressed that HIV/AIDS might come back, too, if vigilance was not exercised. During the height of Uganda's social chaos, when Amin was being driven from power by the Tanzanian army in 1979, AIDS had broken out into the general population from some isolated population(s) where it had clearly been endemic for some time. Some Ugandans had begun to recognize it and had given it the name "slim," or *siliimu*. Later they recognized that it was "now part of us." This recognition and the willingness to take ownership allowed the struggle against AIDS to be built into the nation-building process itself. Because Ugandans already had a "native category" (*siliimu*) for AIDS at the beginning of the 1980s, when the virus was finally identified in 1984 it could not be represented as a conspiracy or plot against Africans by the West (as it was in South Africa), and the virus was tackled quickly and honestly. This, more than anything else, may have saved many Ugandan lives.

Despite adversity, Uganda reestablished peace, good governance, and a strong civil society. This remarkable achievement is also closely related to, and partly responsible for, their achievement in meeting the AIDS crisis head-on and lowering HIV prevalence rates over a ten-year period. The Museveni government was open to partnerships with all segments and sectors of Ugandan society. It was aware of and paid attention to cultural practices and beliefs, and showed resolve and direction in its political leadership. These have been central factors in its approach to AIDS. But the political instability, warfare, pervasive violence, and rape that occurred in the era before the establishment of peace in Uganda in 1986 are also responsible, in part, for the problem itself. As important as good government has been, however, the response of thousands of churches, schools, nongovernmental organizations (NGOs), community-based organizations (CBOs), and other organizations of the broader civil society must be acknowledged. They have been supported by international donor agencies to great effect. These initiatives have been led by a number of extraordinary individuals, whose vision and dedication have also been exemplary. Ultimately, however, it is the ordinary Ugandan who had to change his or her behavior in profound and significant ways to bring about the AIDS success story in Uganda. These shifts in sexual behavior must be seen in light of what amounted to a complete reorganization of Ugandan society, cultural practices, and values. These changes were supported by organizations that mobilized resources and personnel to educate and motivate the Ugandan people. And, these, in turn, were supported fully and efficiently by international agencies such as the World Health Organization, the U.S. Agency for International Development (USAID), and many others.

The story of AIDS in Uganda is thus a complex web of causes, factors, motives, and action. Gaining strength over the last two decades of the twentieth century, this web resulted in a fully integrated, nationwide response on the part of all Ugandans and in all activities. Dr. Samuel Okware,[2] who led this response as the director of the National AIDS Control Programme in the Ugandan Ministry of Health, summed up the history in these words: "It started as a rumor. We discovered it was a disease. We found that it was an epidemic. We have finally accepted it as a tragedy."[3] Although he had originally coined this succinct summary of the history of AIDS in Uganda in 1993, he was still offering it—with good reason—as a concise summary of the AIDS epidemic in 2003. Dr Okware's four sentences express a historical unfolding. First, rumors of a new and mysterious killer eventually were confirmed with the diagnosis of a disease. The disease spread rapidly as its causative agent, HIV, infiltrated the entire country. Early recognition that this was an epidemic that could affect all parts of society led to mobilization of government resources, however. Extraordinary political commitment from the top levels of government to freedom in an open society led to the empowerment of civil society and to development of partnerships in dealing with the epidemic. The acceptance that this was a tragedy motivated people at all levels of society and from every village and town in what became one of the most coherent responses to a common threat ever mounted in Uganda, or perhaps Africa. Above all, *recognition* of the scope of the threat and refusal to deny its fearsome impact permitted effective responses to be mounted. *Acceptance* of the tragedy—like truth and reconciliation after a bitter struggle—both legitimated and motivated a major reshaping of individual behaviors, culture, and society.

TAKING SEX SERIOUSLY

In retrospect, and in the face of such an epidemic, Uganda's response may seem obvious. But recent history—and comparison with other countries—shows that many countries with problems of similar magnitude—or worse—have failed to mount anything like this level of response. Epidemics such as sleeping sickness (trypanosomiasis) in the 1940s in Uganda caused the deaths of an even larger share of the population.[4] Today, more people die of malaria than of AIDS. These epidemics did not result in the sort of total response that the struggle against AIDS has done.

Why? First, Ugandans take sex seriously. People in Uganda constantly confess to loving sex, and sexual networks are part of the social fabric. Customs and rituals in many ethnic groups prescribe sexual contact as part of the performance of duty. Ugandans value fertility greatly, and praise people with many children. Despite AIDS, fertility has not decreased. Indeed, many Ugandans say that life without sex is scarcely worth living.

Daily newspapers are full of how-to advice on sex and a tales of sexual intrigue, sexual styles, sexual adventures, love, and betrayal. Today, there is almost no topic related to sex that is not discussed in the popular press, both in English and in indigenous languages. There are a number of popular newspapers, such as *Red Pepper,* that are simply about sex. Although they do not contain explicitly pornographic nude photographs, they come as close as they can without full nudity. They are sold openly on the streets for slightly more than the cost of a daily newspaper.

The Luganda-language daily *Bukedde* mixes articles about sex and sexuality, which constitute about 25 percent of its column inches, with other stories about Ganda life and culture. The issue for 5 July 2003, for instance, includes stories about the personal lives of Catholic bishops, sex games, and the restored Ganda kingship. The leading front page spread is about transfer by the Ganda king *(kabaka)* of the former residence of the kingdom's prime minister *(katikkiro)* to the state for use by the Joint Clinic Research Programme, which provides research services on HIV/AIDS. A front-page feature line introduces an article about a popular party game in which women sit in chairs in a row, in short skirts or with their legs uncovered, while each man, blindfolded, feels their thighs and tries to guess which one is his wife. Another front-page item is a story about women who beat up their husbands/men, with six full-color photos.[5] On page 12 is a special section, called "Ssenga" after the tradition of having an older woman teach young women "how to please their husbands." This contains short items, such as a man's story of how he can be aroused only by prostitutes, and a full page of wedding pictures. There are also articles on *Big Brother Africa,* featuring the Ugandan participant, Gaetano, and his reality-TV romance with a South African woman. The mix is also enlivened by full stories about a Ganda cardinal welcoming newly ordained Catholic deacons in the Lubiri, the king's palace.

All of this was explained to me as I sat eating and drinking—and reading *Bukedde*—with the school board of a Catholic girls school and the parish priest, Father Kalomba, in Rubaga, the heart of Ganda culture and the center of the kingdom. Father Kalomba had just finished a speech to the schoolgirls and their parents about the need to control sexuality and to use condoms when abstinence failed. There could be no doubt that sexuality was part and parcel of Ganda life and identity, reflected in the newspaper in which Catholicism, marriage, sex games, and the politics of HIV/AIDS were all blended together. Although this is no different from the content of glossy Western women's and men's magazines, such as *Cosmopolitan* and *Maxim,* that are available in Uganda, *Bukedde* is a popular family daily newspaper aimed at Ganda traditionalists and Catholics. Many articles emphasized the value of marriage, tradition, and Roman Catholicism, and there could be no doubt about the importance of sex and sexuality in daily life.

A second reason for Uganda's high-level response to AIDS is that sexual networks of lovers, wives, and husbands are fundamental to the social order. Many people we interviewed insisted that this fundamental social fact has not changed. They felt that the worst aspect of the HIV epidemic was the limitations that it had put on sex. Dr. Okware spoke to us of his wish to "make the world safe for sex again."[6] All the Ugandans we interviewed admitted, however, that many aspects of this sexual culture have permanently changed for the better. Numbers of partners and therefore the size and reach of networks of sexual contacts have decreased, they asserted. Cultural practices that involve penetrative sex such as cleansing rites after death and circumcision, together with wife inheritance and wife sharing among brothers, have all but stopped. "We have changed our culture absolutely, but what do we put in its place? ... This culture had to change, but we do not want to lose everything," said Nakanyike Musisi, the head of the Uganda AIDS Commission and the director of the Makerere Institute of Social Research, pointing—somewhat ironically—to the pervasive influence of American popular culture that threatened to overwhelm Ugandan media.[7]

Third, Uganda was determined and able to mount an early and effective response to HIV/AIDS after the country's vast political and physical devastation over the previous fifteen years. This response to HIV/AIDS was led by President Yoweri Museveni, supported by a number of exceptionally capable medical doctors, initially including Dr. Samuel Okware, Dr. John Rwomushana,[8] and Dr. Kihumuro Apuuli,[9] among others. Later, the struggle was joined by many of the leading ministries of government and by the major hospitals and their staffs, including government hospitals such as Mulago in Kampala and mission hospitals such as Lacor in Gulu and Rubaga in Kampala.

POLITICAL COMMITMENT AND SOCIAL MOBILIZATION

Political commitment from the top was critical but probably not sufficient to explain the effectiveness of Uganda's response. It could not have happened without a strong sense of commitment from virtually every organization of civil society, and from individuals across the country. Why and how did this happen?

There are a number of factors that seem relevant. Uganda has a high level of literacy and there are good schools throughout the country. Although there are many local languages, English is the national language and it is widely and well spoken throughout Uganda. These factors made it possible to communicate effectively and quickly with the approximately twenty-four million inhabitants of the country.

In the south, especially, Uganda has a heritage of hierarchical political organization stemming from the history of early kingdoms dating from the sixteenth century. President Museveni, soon after taking power, quickly organized the country into a hierarchy of districts, counties, parishes, and villages not unlike Napoleon's thorough reorganization of France after the Revolution. Uganda was never a colony, so its political order was maintained—though transformed—during its sixty or so years as a protectorate of Britain. Museveni was able to draw on these traditions.

Religious communities are also well integrated and less fragmented than in many other African countries. The majority of Ugandans are Roman Catholic or Anglican (Church of Uganda). Islam has been firmly established in Uganda since the late nineteenth century, and is also a fundamental part of Ugandan culture. Approximately 25 percent of Ugandans are Muslim.[10] There are very few independent or African syncretic sects in Uganda. Because of this lack of fragmentation, the churches and Islamic communities were able to act in an integrated fashion to reach the large majority of Ugandans.

Finally, the determination to repair the country after the ravages of civil war, the "liberation" by Tanzania (which attacked Uganda in 1979 in order to reinstall the corrupt previous president Milton Obote), and the mismanagement of government throughout the 1970s and first half of the 1980s gave Ugandans a sense of purpose. AIDS stood in the way of redevelopment of the country and had to be countered if these goals were to be achieved. The struggle against AIDS was coupled with a political and economic agenda of reconstruction and development, and this enlisted the support of the entire country.

Ugandan history since the mid-1980s, then, has been a story of sex, death, and transcendence of adversity.

THE FIRST DECADE OF AIDS IN UGANDA

Amin came to power in a coup d'état early in 1972, driving President Obote into exile in Tanzania. Famous for his own sexual exploits and many wives, Amin's rule ushered in a period of economic chaos and decline, as well as untrammeled brutality and rape. Many of our research informants agreed that the prevalence of rape during this period (1972–1986), and during the wars that punctuated the political process, led to greatly increased HIV prevalence. "Sex is a very important part of war . . . rape, and so on," said Emmanuel Sekatawa, a statistician at the Institute for Statistics and Applied Economics. "[It is used to] demonstrate conquest or something. Unfortunately, it [also] increases HIV."[11] Everyone in the focus group discussions (FGD) we conducted, especially women, agreed that they had lived in fear of rape under Amin and Obote. "During Amin's time, life was so bad. Amin's soldiers used to take people [away] in a car boot [to rape them]. I was one. People lived in fear,"[12] said one woman from western Uganda. Men agreed. A man from northern Uganda commented, "Soldiers are injectors of AIDS because they don't ask."[13] "They take you by force," echoed his friend. Another man from western Uganda said, "Between 1979 and 1986 men would freely rape women. . . . It would only become a problem when the rapist was caught in the act. In such a case he would only be fined."[14] Soldiers were especially guilty of this behavior, and rape by soldiers became virtually "normal."

War, however, also seems to have curtailed ordinary sexual activities and opportunities for many. Mrs. Governor Goretti, a community counselor in Kikyenkye, a village about thirty kilometers north of Mbarara, said that rape was commonplace during this period, but "people did not have time to have [normal] sexual relationship as a result of war. People were more concerned about their security and for their children." Soldiers, however, "had multiple partners because they were mobile and everywhere they went they had partners." Mrs. Goretti distinguished clearly between the disruption of normal sexuality, in marriage and in bars and other places of entertainment, and rape during the wars and misrule of Amin and Obote. "People did not have sex so much because they were in confusion," she said. "It was the time Museveni was fighting Obote's government. This gave no opportunity for people to engage in sexual intercourse."[15] Shortages of everything and curfews imposed by government seem to have brought to a close a period of relatively free, uncoerced sexual expression in the late 1960s and 1970s as bars and clubs closed their doors. Instead, women came to expect rape by soldiers as almost a normal part of their lives. Men who could afford to also sought sex outside the home, but most just struggled to survive and stayed close to home.

When Tanzanian and Ugandan forces attacked Amin's regime in

1979, the Tanzanian soldiers were also accused of rape, but many young women welcomed the cash brought by the soldiers. Older women in Igorora village, Mbarara District, western Uganda—an area that has been in the path of several military campaigns—made a distinction between the relatively well behaved Tanzanian soldiers, who often married the girls from the region (and took them back to Tanzania), and Amin's troops, who simply raped at the point of a gun.

> *Respondent C:* The *Bakombozi* [Tanzanian soldiers, literally "liberators"] were not raping girls; this was the good thing about them.
>
> *Respondent A:* It was Amin's group that used to rape women.
>
> *Respondent B:* Aren't *Bakombozi* the same as Amin's soldiers?
>
> *Respondent C:* No, the *Bakombozi* are from Tanzania and were different from Amin's soldiers. Those of Amin would use force. Like the way we are here [a group of women sitting and talking], if they came, they would cock their guns and if we went to the bush they would follow us and rape us.[16]

This was a period of mayhem and disarray. Mulago Hospital, the principal hospital in Kampala, was looted by Amin's troops as they fled, while Amin's government workers looted the Ministry of Health on their way out.[17] Five major hospitals had been destroyed during the fighting.[18] Cash and goods were exchanged for sex, but many respondents who mentioned it commented that there was considerable prestige associated with going out with a soldier. They had money and power. After the defeat of Amin, the Tanzanian government returned Milton Obote to rule after elections that were widely believed to have been heavily rigged in favor of Obote's party, the Uganda People's Congress. Obote's second period of rule, known as Obote II, proved to be at least as brutal and corrupt as that of Amin. Both Amin and Obote were from the northern half of Uganda and were resented by the people of the south, whose culture and languages were considerably different. Despite this, there was a great sense of relief when Amin was deposed, expressed in sexual license. A group of middle-aged professional women in eastern Uganda described it as follows:

> *Respondent 1:* After the fall of Amin there was a lot of excitement. Originally people were like prisoners, so thereafter they felt free. There was a lot of socializing, drinking, and people had many sexual partners. Schoolgirls had sexual affairs with the *Bakombozi*. Some schoolgirls got married to them. Some schoolgirls had sugar daddies.

Respondent 2: Our people integrated a lot with Bakombozi; they became girlfriends and boyfriends and produced children with those people.

Respondent 3: Almost every woman was involved with the Bakombozi. They seemed to have money and yet people were very poor. Schoolgirls, married and unmarried women, got sexually involved with the Bakombozi.[19]

In the early 1980s, a resistance movement, composed mainly of people from the southern kingdoms and led by Museveni, broke away from the army and began a four-year-long war against Obote II. This was also the time that AIDS was first recognized in southwestern Uganda. Museveni's National Resistance Army (NRA) was initially based in southwestern Uganda, where AIDS, or *siliimu*, was already endemic. From there, they moved to an area known as the Luwero Triangle, north of Kampala. In July 1985, another army general, Tito Okello, overthrew the Obote II regime. Okello's grasp of power, however, was short-lived. The NRA made a final push to topple this regime in early January, taking Kampala on 25 January 1986.

On 29 January 1986, Museveni was declared president. He immediately promulgated the Ten-Point Plan, which promoted institutions of civil society, the rule of law, human rights, and political freedoms, together with ambitious plans for development based on a mixed economy relatively free from government control. Even more important, these promises were kept, and in the peace that followed, tens of thousands of new businesses, NGOs, CBOs, and other organizations sprang up across the countryside. USAID, among a few other donors, had resumed support for Uganda in 1980 after the return of Obote, primarily in the areas of agriculture, medical relief, and medical training. USAID had suspended aid to Uganda during Amin's rule and again briefly after Okello's coup. With the installation of Museveni's government, international aid began to flow into Uganda once again to help restore the war-torn social and economic infrastructure.

During the 1980s, Ugandans remember that, apart from rape, sexuality was rampant. According to a large number of informants, both men and women had many sexual partners. In the early 1980s, having multiple partners was a cultural ideal. It was acceptable and very common in Uganda for men to have many wives. According to Cissy Kiyo Mutuluuza, deputy director for clinical research at Kampala's primary AIDS research center, "This was happening all the time. That started to change with HIV. We also had wife inheritance and girls getting married very young, especially if poor or if not going to school. They get married to older men."[20]

Many believed that the value placed on having multiple partners was a consequence of the severe economic hardships experienced by many, with what wealth there was concentrated in the hands of a few, mainly male, businessmen (especially traders and smugglers), military and government personnel, and land or property owners. Young girls with few prospects were often willing to have sex with these men for money or other forms of support for themselves and their families. This was a consequence of poverty but was not entirely coercive. A group of relatively poor women from the Kampala suburb of Kifumbira, for instance, was asked if girls in the mid-1980s could choose to abstain from sex. They all agreed, "Not when he has showed you *omutwaro* [a ten-thousand-shilling note, worth about five U.S. dollars in 2003]."[21] Sexuality was often seen as a legitimate commodity, a tradable value or service that could be exchanged for other goods and services.

> When Museveni came in, if you can remember, he used young soldiers— the *kadogos* [small ones/boys] who came with money. Obviously, they would also come and move around with their guns freely in discos and interact with people. Afterward a lay [nonmilitary] person seeing a *kadogo* with money, especially women, would be forced to go with him. Women were forced due to poverty. So they earned their living from the *kadogos*. The *kadogos* were also excited about having sex with these elder women, now they could pull out whatever [money] the women could demand.[22]

During the previous regime, soldiers were feared greatly, but Museveni's army attempted to create an atmosphere of trust and acceptance of soldiers—what many people referred to as the "demystification of the gun." Most people saw this as a return to normality, and even "sexual behavior normalized."[23] For women in one of the discussion groups in Mbale, this implied, "Somebody would go where he was supposed to go. A girl would go with a boy, not necessarily a man with money, social life became confined within the age groups. There was a lot of freedom of association."[24] But they also agreed that this freedom under the new government meant, for many, sexual license as well. One woman in eastern Uganda explained, "Let me give you an example, for a young lady like I was. I was confined in the village [in the early 1980s], so when Museveni came in I got freedom of moving from Mbale to Kampala, and there I met people I had never seen, those who do not look like people in the village. They had a lot of money. So

I was caught up in a trap."[25] She made it clear that this trap was the lure of sexuality, "sugar daddies," good food, fashionable clothes, and the city life of night spots, bars, and the sex that went with this.

> When Museveni took over power, the situation was that people were really happy of the government and were assured of peace, and then the soldiers had to move in the villages freely and there were some parties organized. . . . When they heard that Museveni had taken over the leadership, and especially when they arrived in Mbale here, there were so many ceremonies being organized such as the kadodi dancing; discos were organized even in rural areas . . . everywhere. Soldiers had to leave the barracks and they were just moving, interacting with people freely in communities, telling them, "Don't fear, we have come to rescue you."[26]

Upon Museveni's ascendancy, then, sex also became part of the general rejoicing. "It was the rejoicing part of it that resulted in women interacting and finally moving out with kadogos because of the poverty and the kadogos were the source of money. As they rejoiced, the women got money from the kadogos in exchange for sex."[27] The period of rejoicing lasted for a couple of years and was associated in many people's minds with the realization that AIDS was a serious threat, and that many people were dying. In Museveni's own camp, it quickly became clear that HIV had infected many in his top echelon of officers.

> In 1986 when they went to Cuba, early 1987, they had captured power early January 1986, a high percentage were tested in late 1986 and 18 percent were positive and none were sick.[28]

> Those ones started dying in 1995, 1996. That cohort, maybe they had not got the disease while in the bush but maybe it was part of the celebration of 1986. So we heard one story. So when he [Museveni] came from meeting Castro, that is when he called everybody and started campaigning.[29]

Even before Museveni's presidency, however, AIDS had begun to raise alarms. The first AIDS case in Uganda was identified in 1982, almost as soon as the syndrome was identified in the United States among homosexuals and intravenous drug users.[30] Medical practitioners in San Francisco and New York City began to note the emergence of previously rare infections and cancers in men in 1979 and 1980. Pneumonia caused by *Pneumocystis carinii,* a bacterial infection that usually occurs in birds, and Kaposi's sarcoma, a type of previously very rare skin cancer that produces black or dark-colored nodules on the skin, seemed to be occurring together and in greater numbers. The Centers for Disease Control, in Atlanta, Georgia, published the first notice of this emerging phenomenon on 5 June 1981 in *Morbidity and Mortality Weekly Report,* and a second notice the following month. Reported cases of the new diseases and their apparent connection to homosexual men began to attract increasing attention. By then, it was becoming clear to Ugandans, especially those who were resident around the shores of Lake Victoria in Masaka and Rakai districts that what they had already begun to call *siliimu* was increasing rapidly, with more and more people dying of the disease. In the early 1980s, too, a group of infections and diseases that was now being identified as a syndrome began to appear elsewhere in the world. Dr. Anne Bayley reported cases of Kaposi's sarcoma in Zambia.[31] Soon cases were identified in most European countries, in Brazil and Mexico, and in other African countries, such as Rwanda and Zaire (now the Democratic Republic of the Congo). Isolated instances appeared even in Australia and New Zealand. By 1982, AIDS was beginning to be recognized as a global phenomenon with serious potential for epidemic spread.

In fact, AIDS was already spreading rapidly in the increasingly international male homosexual community, which had developed its own sexual culture that permitted and often encouraged frequent change of sexual partners. For example, Gaetan Dugas, a gay male flight attendant from Quebec, Canada, today has the distinction of being known as patient zero. Gaetan Dugas had apparently infected at least 40 of the 248 men who were showing symptoms of AIDS by the middle of 1982.[32] Mr. Dugas himself estimated that he had sex with at least 250 men a year. In his travels as a flight attendant, he may have spread the virus to the far corners of the world. It is likely, too, that he had been infected in the 1970s, because his Kaposi's sarcoma was already well advanced by 1982.[33] He was hardly the only one, however.

Seventeen confirmed AIDS cases were reported to the Uganda Ministry of Health in 1983, but this considerably underestimated the impact of the disease in Rakai District along the shores of Lake Victoria and on the Tanzanian border, where it had begun to hit hard.[34] By this time it was known widely as "slim," because people with the disease lost weight precipitously through loss of appetite, gastrointestinal infections, and diarrhea. A group of Runyankole and Rukiga speakers (western Uganda groups) in Kampala told us that it was first called *omunywengye* in their language. "I know *omunywengye* very well because I had an in-law who had that disease; he lost weight and his mother-in-law used to put banana leaves under his bottom to trap the watery diarrhea. That was in [the 1980s]. They said it was *omunywengye,* and

then he died."[35] There were other names for it as well, such as rough
cast (after the rough cement plaster applied to brick and cement walls),
or *mukenenya*, meaning someone who was reduced in size or drying
up (*ziridde*).[36] As AIDS reached the northern parts of Uganda, it was
called *etawoi* (wildcat) or *oridi* (something that squeezes you down,
squashes you) in Ateso, a language spoken in northern Uganda around
Lira and Kitgum.[37] A number of Acholi men commented,

> There is still not a name for AIDS in local languages.

> No one can exactly explain why [there is no African name]. People were
> calling it slim, *asein* in Ateso, meaning you have lost weight until you are
> like this [showing a squeezing motion with his hands].

> It was called slim by that time [early] 1980s. No other new names.

> In some places, in local languages like Acholi, [it is called] *acui* [meaning]
> "you just become thin."[38]

In Luganda and other Bantu languages in the southern part of
Uganda, the term "AIDS" is still not used in information, education,
and communication campaigns; *siliimu* (in Luganda) or *akakooko ka
siliimu*[39] (chronic disease of slim, in Runyankole) are used instead.
The KiSwahili word, *ukimwi*, coined in the late 1980s by the Swahili
Language Institute at the University of Dar es Salaam, is not used in
Uganda.[40]

Ed Hooper, a journalist whose 1990 book *Slim* was one of the
first extensive reports on the disease, asked a local health assistant,
Jimmy Ssemambo, "When was the first time that you came across
Slim?" Jimmy responded, "During 1982, when I was just posted here,
I visited a place called Lukuny on the lake; there I happened to come
across a case, which I at first suspected to be TB . . . it was a woman."
According to Hooper, the health assistant realized that her ailment
had been slim two years later "when a large number of people died in
Gwanda, another parish here."[41] Several FGD respondents claimed that
it must have been present even earlier. One said,

> I remember back then, around 1979, coming to 1980, I had a sister who
> died of the same symptoms; up to now we can recall how she died. So I
> think the thing began a long time ago. But people are believing they were
> being bewitched. That is when it started. The symptoms [were] the same

as the things we are seeing today. You can imagine that this is what she might have died of.[42]

Another recalled,

Me, I learned of it in 1980 when I lost my mother. They called it AIDS. She was a medical superintendent. After the burial they said this disease has just come called AIDS. People were doubting. Some say she was bewitched.[43]

Another remarked,

I remember that when my father was working in Nsambya [army] barracks, I used to see how people were having sex. I knew Okware, who went with the banning [i.e., exile] of his father in London. When he explained how his father died in London, he was black, thin. That was in 1980.[44]

And another commented,

[That was] when we discovered it was a killer disease from America. Historically, they say it started a long time ago, but no one was yet experiencing it. One from our family, in the late [1970s], the man died, but no one knew the cause. So they gave the woman to another. The whole family got down [died].[45]

Although AIDS was first suspected in Uganda in 1982 or 1983,[46] numbers of our informants, recalling their own family histories, believed that people had died of slim even earlier than that. Dr. Anthony Lwegaba, the district medical officer for Rakai District, first reported a local epidemic around Kyotera town in Rakai to the Ministry of Health in November 1984. He speculated that the newly identified syndrome "may not be new in Africa" and may even have originated there.[47] A cancer specialist, Charles Olweny, published a report in a medical textbook in 1984 citing AIDS as a possible explanation for Kaposi's sarcoma, which was being seen in Rakai District and at Mulago Hospital in Kampala.[48] The HIV-1 virus was first isolated in 1983, and blood testing became possible. Wilson Carswell, an expatriate surgeon at Mulago, sent blood samples of patients suffering from Kaposi's sarcoma to Britain for testing. All proved to have HTLV-3 (later called HIV-1). A team including Dr. Carswell, with Ugandans David Serwadda, Nelson Sewankambo, and Roy Mugwera, visited Rakai and Masaka to do further tests. They found that patients with slim were infected with HTLV-3, and they speculated that it was transmitted by sexual contact. They published their results in 1987.[49] By then, several other

articles about AIDS had appeared in the international medical literature.[50] Publications come out months or years after the discovery they
announce, however. Although it is difficult to fix a precise date on
the definitive identification of AIDS as a disease caused by HIV (or
HTLV-3, as it was called then), it appears to have occurred in late 1984
or early 1985.

It is clear, then, that HIV was already well established in the Ugandan
population in the 1970s, if not earlier, and that it had already begun to
travel the world. Ugandans in the villages around Lake Victoria, where
it first emerged as an epidemic, had already identified it and named
it in their languages. Numbers of people told me that by 1980 people
were already dying of the disease, but they told me this in retrospect in
2003. Nevertheless, the deaths of their kin—mothers, sisters, fathers,
as in the stories cited earlier—were not remembered as just any deaths,
but as deaths of a certain type. The classification and causes of death
were not yet known by medical science; these were Ugandan terms for
Ugandan knowledge.

Ugandans thus created an indigenous category for the disease by
naming it and recognizing it as a feature of their own family histories
and community problems. Indeed, HIV was already endemic in southwestern Uganda, especially in Rakai and Masaka districts, and in the
cities of the Buganda heartland, Jinja and Kampala. The fact that it had
already entered the cultural consciousness, oral history, and vocabulary of the people in this region meant that it was also already part of
their ideas about health, illness, disease, and death—that is, part of
their medical culture. Because it was an indigenous category *before* it
came to be identified by Western medical practitioners and scientists,
Ugandans seem to have been much more willing than South Africans to
accept the consequences of the emerging epidemic. They seem to have
taken ownership of it promptly, and this, as much as anything else, is
probably responsible for their ability to deal with it more effectively
than any other country we have so far seen.

CHAPTER 6

Siliimu as Native Category

AIDS as Local Knowledge in Uganda

THE BEGINNING OF DEBATE AND KNOWLEDGE

One of the most important aspects of AIDS in Uganda was the fact that Ugandans seem never to have believed that it came from some distant place to afflict them. They did not invent conspiracy stories. Even in the early years when people in southwestern Uganda were casting around for explanations of the rising epidemic, stories began to circulate that it had been brought in by Tanzanian soldiers who overthrew the regime of Idi Amin, but these were local people who spoke similar languages, not distant foreigners. The disease was stigmatizing, and many people had difficulty talking about it, especially at first, but the level of stigmatization never reached the ferocity that has been observed in South Africa. The fact that Ugandans accepted the reality of the disease made it easier for them to deal with its consequences and to tackle the challenges of preventing its spread. By the time AIDS was first formally recognized by biomedical professionals, Ugandans already had a conceptualization of the disease, including a native category and names for it in local languages. By 1984, when HIV was identified as the cause of AIDS, and the label "AIDS" had been assigned to the syndrome, Ugandans were already able to talk about it. And they did talk about it. In the regions where it first emerged, they already knew its potential for devastation.

Although it was locally known and discussed in Rakai and Masaka

districts, where people were most heavily infected and affected, the
first discussion of the disease appeared in the indigenous language
press. *Munno* (Your Friend), which is Uganda's oldest continuously
published newspaper, began in the late nineteenth century as a Roman
Catholic newspaper. By the beginning of the twentieth century, it was
hosting extensive debates about Ganda history, culture, politics, religion, and society affairs. Apolo Kagwa, then the prime minister of
the Kingdom of Buganda, often led these debates, and he published a
number of books that grew from seeds first published in the pages of
Munno. These included *Mpisa za Buganda* (Customs of the Buganda)[1]
and *Ekitabo Kye Basekabaka be Buganda* (Kings of Buganda).[2] *Munno*
had a century-long history as a forum for educated opinion and debate
in the indigenous language of Luganda when the debate about AIDS
began. On page 1, *Munno* published Uganda's first news item on the
disease on 13 April 1985, noting that *siriimu* was a "new disease":

> A new disease named SIRIIMU (slim) was rumored to be present in
> Rakai and Masaka district last year (1984) and it has been confirmed
> by experts that it exists, but the mode of transmission and the cure is yet
> to be known. *Munno* was the first to report on the details of this disease
> in a public meeting held in the District of Rakai, which was attended by
> the minister of local government, Mr. Laurence Kalule Settala. Residents
> worry about this new disease SIRIMU [*stet*]. The minister confirmed that
> a report about the disease was sent by the medical officer to the ministry
> of health headquarters in Entebbe, and that details of the study by the
> ministry are still being awaited.[3]

This article, in Luganda, is probably the first mention of *siriimu* in
the Ugandan public media. It was reported in English for the first time
five months later, on 13 September, in *The Weekly Topic*, a Kampala
newspaper.[4] The first article does not mention HIV (or HTLV-3, as
it was then called) or any other causal agent, and simply calls it "a
disease." Notably, the article says that there is no cure, although the
way in which it was transmitted was not yet known.

The written version of the name had not yet been fully standard-
ized. It appears in this article both as *sirimu* and as *siriimu*. In an
article of 1 June 1985, it appears as *siliimu*. The spelling of the name
fluctuates between the *r* and *l* spelling for the next couple of years,
with one instance of *ssiliimu* (30 June 1987). In the phonology of the
Luganda language, there is no phonemic distinction between an *l* and
r (like English spoken by a Chinese, in which *rice* and *lice* may be
indistinguishable) although the double constants (geminated or long

consonants) in *ssiliimu* are semantically significant. Thus, *siliimu* and *siriimu* sound like the same word (carry the same meaning) to Luganda speakers, but *ssiliimu* and *siliimu* sound as though they could be different words, that is, carry different meanings. By 1987, *siliimu* (a single or short initial /s/ and a long second vowel /ii/) had became standard.

Thus, there may have been some variation in pronunciation of the word. This suggests that the word may not have been a simple borrowing of the English word *slim* into Luganda. If it were, editors would have represented it with an *l* in all cases, recognizing its English origin. In fact, however, the English word could be a borrowing into Ugandan English of the Luganda *si(r/l)iimu* linguistic form. In this case, it would suggest that the disease had been endemic in Rakai and Masaka, perhaps limited to the exceptionally isolated lakeshore villages, for long enough to have acquired a name that was fully of local origin, linguistically indigenous. The folk etymology of the English term has it that AIDS makes people slim, but this may be a post hoc rationalization, since other symptoms, notably coughing from pneumonia and tuberculosis secondary infections, thrush and sores on mucus membranes, fever, Kaposi's sarcoma, extreme diarrhea, and dementia may be much more noticeable in many cases than wasting and "slimming." In any case, whatever the spelling, pronunciation, or etymology, it is clear that there was no ambiguity in meaning. None of the *Munno* articles use alternative words for *siliimu* such as the English acronym AIDS, the French acronym SIDA (introduced into some early reports and pamphlets from Rwanda and Zaire/Congo), or the KiSwahili acronym *ukimwi*. The relative stability and consistency of usage from the very first articles shows clearly that the term was already established in (at least) the regional Luganda of Rakai and Masaka, and was in common use (including in the other related languages in southwestern Uganda) by the mid-1980s at least. AIDS was, in all probability, already an indigenous category—that is, a well-known syndrome with recognized characteristics and a distinctive name—before the other terms for the disease emerged.

The *Munno* article mentioned a number of doctors who were involved in research on this new disease. It mentioned Professor B. G. Kirya of the microbiology department at Makerere University; Dr. Samuel Okware, assistant director of medical services/public health, of the Ministry of Health; Dr. Brew Graves, a program coordinator for the World Health Organization (WHO); Doctors J. M. Jagwe, E. Kigonya, J. Womukuta, and J. W. Carswell of Mulago Hospital; Dr. J. Wamukota of Makerere

Medical School; and Dr. Serwadda of the Uganda Cancer Institute. Many of these people subsequently became leaders of the research and mobilization initiatives against AIDS, especially Dr. Okware, who was put in charge of integrating the response, and Dr. Serwadda, who became one of the leading researchers in the field.

With personnel already engaged in what were then the early days of recognition and dawning awareness of the threat, and with the knowledge and name of the disease itself already part of the local culture and popular medical knowledge, it is clear that Uganda had begun to respond to the threat even before Museveni came to power, and only eighteen months for so after the first identification of the virus in the laboratory.

In back pages of the same 13 April issue, *Munno* published a more detailed report, *Bakakensa balaze ensi we batuuse ku ndwadde ya 'Siriimu'* ("Experts release their first report on 'siriimu' to the country"), with reports from the medical team that had been sent to investigate. The report is worth quoting at length because it indicates what was and was not known in 1985.

> In the recent past, there has been talk about a new disease now dubbed "Slim" [English, in Luganda original] in Rakai. This disease starts with fever, and then diarrhea that doesn't stop with currently available medication. The patient now becomes very thin: this disease has been named after "slimming," losing weight. The Ministry of Health got information about the disease early this year and promptly sent a group of professionals to this area from Mulago Hospital and Medical School. The aim was to examine patients in the area and see how the disease spreads, and how it can be cured. The team discovered that the "Slim" [English, in Luganda original] patients had a lot of other common major diseases such as tuberculosis and cancer. It was easy to call these patients Slim sufferers because all these diseases lead to severe weight loss [slimming]. Diarrhea and typhoid was also found to be prevalent in the area and it was easy to confuse this with Slim. After separating all the people with these diseases, the remainder of these patients may now be said to have Slim. Those who are said to have "slim" are now being vigorously tested in Mulago and other hospitals, and a treatment regime has been formulated. Despite the fact that the cause of the disease has not been identified and studies are still being conducted, the known facts are as follows. Those who have the disease are the traders and smugglers of goods from the neighboring countries. It made people think that this disease is like a sexually transmitted disease, although there is inconclusive evidence; however, it is known that it affects men and women. People should not think that they got this disease through sexual acts. Therefore, anyone who gets a fever and starts having diarrhea and a rash should go to the nearest hospital for expert

medical diagnosis. The patient might actually have a common disease that is easy to treat. Ugandan medical professionals have known how to treat the most of these common diseases. No evidence has yet shown that the disease can spread easily, so there is no need to isolate these patients. Doctors are ready to treat all the infected despite the fact that the origin of the disease, and how it spreads are yet to be known. There must be a cause that has to be identified. Some diseases are known to spread through the use of unsterilized needles. . . . The Ministry of Health has already contacted experts in foreign countries to find the cause of the disease and how it is spread. It should be known that this is not the first new disease called *Onyon-Nyong*. Within the next two years, it spread throughout the country and created a lot of fear. But with cooperation from patients and medical experts, the cause of that disease [*Onyon-Nyong*] was found. This disease was quickly brought under control with everyone's cooperation. The ministry is confident that with cooperation from patients and local and foreign medical experts, this disease will be defeated.

Appearing in April 1985 in Luganda, this article predated by six months the first announcement of "Slim disease: A new disease in Uganda," which appeared in the international medical journal *The Lancet* in October.[5] A year later, the AIDS virus was also reported to be present among prostitutes in Nairobi, Kenya.[6] The *Lancet* article called it the "new disease . . . known locally as slim disease," and identified it with the virus that had recently been discovered.

It is strongly associated with HTLV-III infection (63 out of 71 patients) and affects females nearly as frequently as males. The clinical features are similar to those of enteropathic acquired immunodeficiency syndrome as seen in neighbouring Zaire. However, the syndrome is rarely associated with Kaposi's sarcoma (KS), although KS is endemic in this area of Uganda. Slim disease occurs predominantly in the heterosexually promiscuous population and there is no clear evidence to implicate other possible means of transmission, such as by insect vectors or re-used injection needles. The site and timing of the first reported cases suggest that the disease arose in Tanzania.[7]

The article that appeared in *The Lancet* and the report that had appeared earlier in *Munno* show remarkable similarities. It is likely that the editors or reporters of *Munno* had been briefed by the team of doctors and researchers from Mulago Hospital (the main government hospital in Kampala) and elsewhere. The single striking difference is that the *Munno* article is ambiguous about whether it is sexually transmitted, while the medical article specifically links it to "heterosexually promiscuous" people. This aspect continued to be debated in the pages of *Munno* for some years to come. Both articles, however, suggest that the disease came from Tanzania (the *Munno* article says "neighboring countries," but this clearly means Tanzania).

The debate about *siliimu*/slim, then, had already begun during the final months of intensive civil war during the last days of the Obote II regime (that is, the second period of Obote's rule) and during Tito Okello's short-lived regime, and before Museveni's guerrillas stormed Kampala in January 1986. When Museveni came to power, knowledge of the disease was already widespread, at least in the southern part of Uganda where Luganda and English were the primary languages.

The fear of *siliimu* had also already begun to spread. A reader's letter in *Munno* on 6 June 1985 offered some speculation on the causes of slim. It claimed that the disease was caused by drinking a new local brew called *kayinja* that contained salt and tea leaves.[8] A reader replied to this letter, saying that *kayinja,* an alcoholic drink, was not to blame. He noted that the government was calling for assistance in meeting the threat of the new epidemic.[9] Another reader replied on 20 June, saying that he agreed that *kayinja* did not cause AIDS. He said that since both he and the previous writer came from Rakai, they both knew that slim came from having multiple sex partners.[10] As this public correspondence shows, slim was already known in 1985 and was being discussed in the newspapers and other public media. At least one reader already knew that it was sexually transmitted. On 17 February 1986, weeks after Museveni's army had marched into Kampala signaling the end of the civil war, *Munno* reported that AIDS was "causing chaos" and that "panic broke loose in Rakai District." The reporter said that the most "influential people economically, socially, and politically who are contributing to the country's development are succumbing to the disease."[11]

> The disease . . . has caused havoc in the district and people are so con-
> fused that they do not know what to do anymore. Many have vacated the
> district in the hope of evading the disease . . . but ended up spreading it
> elsewhere. They blamed the government for neglecting them, and there's
> no cure that has been found yet. People say they are fed up of burying
> people on a daily basis, and those who are spreading it rapidly around
> are the rich ones because they have money. One of our reporters who
> visited the area witnessed dozens of dead bodies lined up for burial all
> over the villages, and the residents said plenty are still on their deathbeds
> waiting for their time to come. They said dozens of patients had flooded
> hospitals and hospital staff couldn't figure out where to start and stop.
> They resorted to simply looking at them with nothing to do since they
> couldn't figure out what disease it was and how to treat it.[12]

This article makes the first public link between AIDS as a "rich man's" disease in Uganda and the threat that it posed to the development and reconstruction of Uganda. These insights in a Luganda newspaper did not appear in the academic and medical literature until some time later. It shows the sophistication of the debate that had already emerged in Uganda around the time of Museveni's ascendancy. Throughout the rest of year, *Munno* carried articles that documented the beginnings of an integrated response from the grass roots and government. A letter to the editor in April 1986, for instance, urged intensive cooperation in fighting the scourge.

> Dear editor: I kindly urge you to pass on my request to those in the Ministry of Health to set up programs and print articles in newspapers informing us about AIDS. Dear editor, I think the rate at which the disease is spreading won't leave anyone alive. It's incurable. Since it's now been discovered that the disease is so rife in Rakai, let's not close off the area like animals in a game park or in a zoo. . . . The reason in writing to you is because it seems that plenty of people in Uganda have died as a result of the deadly disease, not forgetting the United States as well, where it is said to have originated from. . . . By the way, what causes it and how do you tell one is suffering from the disease? It is more speculation or a rumor without a headline and an end, because many are saying that we should sip dog soup and so on and so forth [as cures]. Everyone seems to come up with their own story. So I'm requesting the Ministry of Health to gather traditional healers, medicine men, and scientific medical researchers and pharmacists to try all sorts of drugs and medicines to try and end this deadly disease.[13]

The writer was urging the nation to take an integrated approach that would bring together traditional healers with medical researchers, government departments, doctors, and others in developing a response.

The next day, *Munno* reported that not only AIDS but also the reporting of AIDS were sources of agitation. People were demanding clear leadership from the government and the facts about the disease from the professionals.[14] Typical of such debate, they accused the journalists of rumor mongering and using scare tactics to sell newspapers. According to *Munno,* people thought that the rural areas were being unfairly picked out as centers of infection: "[People said that people] also die of other, weaker diseases, not just from AIDS. They further said that in Kampala, AIDS is killing plenty of people as well, but these newspapers have not published articles such as those being published about Lyatonde [a popular truck stop and night club area in western Uganda]."[15] According to the *Munno* reporter, people had told him that the fear and confusion being created by journalists might itself be responsible for AIDS symptoms: "If people continue to listen to the rumors being spread about AIDS, then they will get depressed, and end up growing thin or even dying."[16]

Munno continued to report on the developing response, however. Donations for AIDS treatment and research were coming in from Germany and the United Nations (7 May 1986), and new equipment for testing for HIV had arrived from the United States and was being set up at Nsambya Hospital in Kampala.[17] Government ministers and National Resistance Movement (NRM) spokesmen were making use of these responses to begin to rebuild the nation after the depredations of the previous regimes. Entrenching themselves as the new government, they went out of their way to speak about AIDS and, according to *Munno* and *New Vision* (the government newspaper), were giving scientifically informed and appropriate messages about the disease at all their public rallies. There were a number of other new developments as well. In September 1986, *Munno* reported that AZT, a new AIDS drug, had just arrived in Uganda for use and further testing. "During [AZT drug] trials," *Munno* reported, "145 people were given the drug, of which only one person has died so far. The drug before AZT called 'placebo' was also tested on 137 patients, of which 16 died."[18] Despite the confusion about the role and nature of placebos in large-scale drug testing, the article also reported that AZT would soon be available in pharmacies.

The reporting shows that even as early as its first months, the new government had begun to integrate the struggle against AIDS into the struggle for nation building. This included the usual demonization of other countries when it was reported that the United Kingdom and other European countries were refusing to permit Ugandans to enter because of AIDS.[19] When, in October, a formal government-sponsored AIDS campaign was announced, *Munno* reported that "the deputy minister of health, James Batwala, has urged all Ugandans to join the campaign and fight AIDS together. . . . The call was made yesterday at an occasion when he was naming the council members of the national AIDS prevention council, which will be responsible for fighting AIDS in the country. The occasion was held at the city hall in Kampala."[20] The Ministry of Health's campaign against AIDS required all Ugandans to get involved in the struggle against the disease. The message was more than just a public health warning: Ugandans were told that AIDS was threatening to hinder development and reconstruction of the country.

The beginnings of a public debate concerning AIDS in Luganda had developed while Museveni and his Resistance Army were still in the bush, during their final push into Kampala, and it continued into the early days of the new regime. In November 1985, however, the Okello government had directed the Ministry of Health to prepare plans to deal with AIDS. These plans were preserved under the new regime and implementation began. Dr. Samuel Okware was given the brief to begin negotiation with donors for assistance. When Museveni and the NRM arrived, the new minister of health under Museveni, Dr. Ruhakana-Rugunda, appointed Dr. Okware as chair of an AIDS surveillance subcommittee, with Roy Mugwera and Wilson Carswell as the other members. By September 1986, the committee had begun to organize education campaigns, provide condoms, and provide for screening of blood donors.

Munno publicized the deaths of many people in Rakai District, and reported that the Rev. Emmanuel Lubega, of Masaka, among many other religious leaders who were quoted during these years, shared his concern and sympathy with all those who were suffering from *siriimu*. He urged people to return to God to be saved from the disease.[21] By May, the efforts of the AIDS committee under Dr. Okware's chairmanship had evidently begun to pay off, whether by God's grace or through hard work, or a combination of the two. By this time, too, *Munno* had stopped using quotation marks around the term *siriimu*. This typographical nuance suggests how fully AIDS had become part of the language and of public debate. In other words, meaning and knowledge were leading to action, and action continued to create meaningful reasons to join the struggle for both the task of nation building and an effective response to AIDS. These two goals gradually began to merge.

The AIDS threat was consistently linked to economic and social development. Of equal significance was the fact that all Ugandans were being called on to get involved. The campaign was not to be merely a government initiative, but was an invitation, if not a demand, for Ugandan citizens to respond to the epidemic. This foreshadowed Uganda's success in organizing institutions of civil society to become involved. Eventually, organizations that dealt with AIDS in one way or another began to mushroom around Uganda. Although the government had provided the conditions for the growth of civil society in this way, it is also clear that the public press, and in particular the vernacular language press, had led the way to a significant degree.

There were many popular explanations for the epidemic at first. Many people told us that at first some thought *siliimu* to be the result of witchcraft. The fishing villages along the southwestern coast of Lake Victoria had become major entrepôts for a vast smuggling trade from Tanzania that had grown up during the Amin and Obote II regimes. For most Ugandans, this trade provided many of the necessities of life such as soap, tea, sugar, matches, and oil. Boats brought the goods across the lake from Tanzania in order to avoid roadblocks. With money available, these fishing villages were also well known as places for sex and drunkenness. Virtually every focus group in our research related the same story, evidently widely circulated, that Tanzanians had been cheated by Ugandan smugglers, who had used witchcraft to avenge their loss. One interviewee recalled, "There was a lot of denial. There was a belief in witchcraft. It started around Lake Victoria. There was a lot of smuggling after the war. For example, traders brought in cigarettes. Some transactions were not very smooth. Thus, some people thought it was punishment for this."[22]

Based on notes from the time, Edward Hooper quotes a Ugandan journalist (who later died of AIDS) as saying: "People are quite sure that some cases can be caused by wizardry and sorcery. Some Ugandan traders go to Tanzania, get things on credit, come and sell, but they don't take back the money. So the Tanzanians end up using sorcery. They are supposed to have *mayembe* [horns] that can be sent to someone to kill him."[23] Tanzanians were not the only ones who were blamed for witchcraft in this period, even as late as 1989, according to one focus group informant. "Our neighbor died around that time . . . actually 1989. They said he had stolen fish from Masaka [Uganda] and the owner of the fish had bewitched him. That is why he could not be cured. They even took him to Congo and Nairobi for treatment but he died."[24] As many other focus group participants pointed out, the wasting away, the blackness of the skin, and its rough texture all pointed to a supernatural disease, in their view, which had previously been associated with witchcraft. It was now associated with AIDS.

AIDS was also attributed to a range of other causes. "It came in the name of 'slim,' affiliated to witchcraft, sharing razor blades, saliva, and the like," said one man.[25] One focus group in Mbale associated AIDS with the arrival of a white South African who worked for a construction company doing work in Mbale.

> In 1986, that is when a certain *muzungu* [white person] from South Africa came to work with Wade Adams in Mbale. They came to know later that he was among those people living with HIV/AIDS and was immune to

the disease. . . . He migrated from South Africa, came to Kenya and then
to Mbale in Uganda, and in Mbale, where he was working Wade Adams
Construction Company. . . . That is when it was discovered that he was
using each and every female he would come across and it was discovered
that he had HIV/AIDS. And he was intentionally doing it to infect each
and every body.[26]

At that time, most African countries were enforcing sanctions against
apartheid South Africa and it is therefore unlikely that the person mentioned was carrying a South African passport. There was considerable
movement of exiles out of South Africa into eastern Africa, however,
and some of these may indeed have found English-speaking Uganda a
congenial country. At this time, the first cases of HIV infection were
noted in South Africa, too, suggesting that there was at least some flow
of people between the two regions. In 1986, thirty-four cases had been
recorded in South Africa, and by the end of the decade there were 184
known instances.[27]

Stories such as this one about people who knew that they were HIV-
positive and deliberately infected as many people as they could were
common. This story is unusual only in that it features a white South
African as the culprit. There were also stories about people who kept
lists of people whom they had deliberately infected. When these lists
were found, they often featured the names of all the leading politicians
and businessmen (or businesswomen) of the community, according to
Ugandans interviewed in 2003.

A focus group in Mbale agreed that people in that area (eastern
Uganda) initially associated AIDS with famine or with new food crops.
"When there is war, people don't go to the fields (gardens) and at this
time, people had shortage of food. When they saw some people becoming thin, they associated it with lack of food and with witchcraft. It
was not [at first recognized] as HIV/AIDS because of these situations.
It was regarded as a result of famine and witchcraft and new varieties
of food available at a time used to eradicate famine."[28]

Other suspicions centered on the heavy field artillery that had been
used by the Tanzanian forces when they attacked Uganda through
Rakai District in 1979. These guns were called *saba saba* (seven seven).[29]
Numbers of people mentioned that the smoke from these guns, or some
lingering effect from them, had caused the disease. Whether or not it
was caused by *saba saba,* many people agreed that the disease had
been brought by the Tanzanian invasion and that the soldiers were to
blame. Since soldiers were often involved in sex, either coerced or vol-

untary, with local women, once the heterosexual transmission of HIV was confirmed, this view held credence for many people, especially in southwestern Uganda, where most of the fighting was concentrated.

Even Museveni and his soldiers, or *Bakombozi,* were blamed by some. A man from northern Uganda claimed, "When Museveni first came he was not popular. There was that belief that he had brought the disease . . . [and] his fighters who had sex with apes and monkeys [in the bush]."[30] A woman from Mbale in eastern Uganda said much the same thing: "In the community, . . . we used to say that, since before we did not have such a disease, then through the wars these people brought us the disease, since in the bush they lacked women so they must have had sex with chimpanzees, which resemble human beings. So up to today people think it was the *Bakombozi* who brought AIDS."[31]

Thus, slim was attributed initially to a number of causes. In order to develop effective interventions, these stories had to be discredited. For the most part, it appears that virtually everyone readily accepted the truth, once it was made known through the media that AIDS was sexually transmitted and lethal. Indeed, common sense had already led many people to this conclusion, since it was often people with money and a large number of sexual partners who sickened and died first. Information, education, and communication interventions, when they came, found most people ready to accept the facts.

THE SPREAD OF SLIM/*SILIIMU*

HIV spread very rapidly across Uganda from the southwest toward the east and north. By January 1985, the first case in the north was confirmed at Lacor Hospital, three kilometers outside Gulu town.[32] A study in the West Nile District in northwestern Uganda, published in 1986, however, found no evidence of HIV infection in that part of the country.[33] It is likely that cases had existed even earlier. Dr. Pietro Corti, the medical superintendent of the Lacor mission hospital, said,

> We started to realise more than two years ago [1980–1982] that we had cases of young men and women having diarrhoea, being sick, having lung disease, sometimes suspected of TB, sometimes other things—that they were not reacting to any treatment, but going downhill slowly, slowly. We felt very uneasy about these cases, and then we learnt more about AIDS in other places like Kampala. . . . The impression is that, as far as numbers are concerned, we are a bit behind Kampala, but not very far behind. I would say every six to ten months we more or less reach the level of Kampala people.[34]

Dr. Corti confirmed that AIDS had firmly taken hold in the north as well, and expressed the belief that "the wars have been one of the main elements in spreading AIDS in Uganda—I don't think there is any doubt—because exactly the same thing happened to all the other venereal diseases."[35] Focus group data and key informant interviews conducted during my research in 2003 suggested the same thing, but this was in addition to considerable evidence of promiscuity, early sexual debut, and multipartnering in all parts of Uganda. The final battles of the NRM insurrection against the Obote/Okello regime were fought in 1985, with suspension of many services, including health services, throughout Uganda. The U.S. Agency for International Development suspended financial support to Uganda for six months or so during that year, until the NRM finally set up a new government in Kampala.

Gradually, Ugandans learned of the nature of this new disease. Speaking in 2003, a woman in a suburb of Mbarara in western Uganda explained how the truth had dawned on her even in the earliest years of the growing epidemic: "In 1983, a woman died and when we went for her burial, a doctor who had treated her told us about her illness. He said she had not been bewitched, that they had tried blood transfusion in Nairobi, had given her the best treatment in Mulago [Government Hospital, Kampala], but she died. She had lost all the hair on her body. He explained that she had died of a disease called AIDS. He told us what each letter in this word stood for. Since 1983, we started burying AIDS victims."[36] The speaker must have been in error about the exact date (1983), but she was speaking to us about her earliest knowledge of the disease. Knowledge of AIDS seems to have spread more slowly than the disease itself, but at least by the end of the 1980s, it was no longer attributed to witchcraft or other causes. It came to be understood as a heterosexually transmitted disease that had no cure.

Public knowledge about AIDS was fostered tremendously, too, by poster campaigns that were direct and to the point. One poster from the late 1980s urged Ugandans to consider the needs of their families and to "behave responsibly" (see figure 12). Another poster of about the same time, with the message "love carefully," did not pull its punches about the consequences of failing to do so. Against a backdrop of skulls and an emaciated man clearly dying of slim, the poster emphasized that a significant change in behavior was necessary "to avoid AIDS, the Global Worry." The "love carefully" poster became well known across Uganda, and the slogans of these posters were still remembered by people we interviewed in 2003.

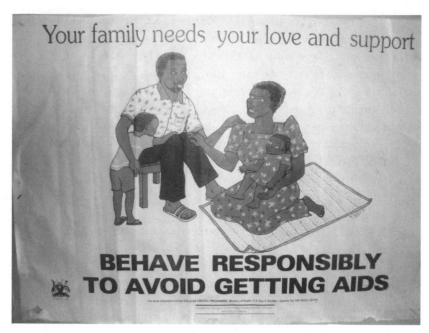

FIGURE 12. "Behave Responsibly to Avoid Getting AIDS" poster, circa 1989.
This poster was displayed in the Uganda AIDS Commission offices in Mmengo,
Uganda, in 2003. (Photograph by R. Thornton)

These posters were widely distributed to clinics and other public
venues and most Ugandans would have seen them. The early posters,
however, seem to have been mostly, if not entirely, in English. Since the
messages were simple, and the pictures clear and to the point, most
Ugandans would have been able to read them, as all Ugandans are
required to study English in school from the primary level on.

Munno continued to publish articles on AIDS, as did *New Vision*,
which had been set up by Museveni as the government-approved
English-language newspaper. At the beginning of 1989, *Munno* carried a report that indicated the extent of popular and government collaboration and cooperation in developing a response to the threat. On
23 January, for instance, a leading article carried the headline: "The
gospel of AIDS is spread countrywide." It reported:

> A campaign to fight AIDS, which has affected more than 180 countries
> worldwide, has been taken up and it aims at spreading awareness coun-
> trywide. The task has been handed to political mobilizers countrywide
> who were first taught skills about the disease. The skills training is taking

place at Lweza Training Conference Center on Entebbe Road [a main road between Kampala and Entebbe, the administrative capital on the coast of Lake Victoria to the south]. . . . The political mobilizers were picked from all districts across the country, though some will arrive later. The minister of state for health, the Honorable Ronald Bata, opened the conference. He said that, right now, everybody knows about the disease, which has become the major cause of death countrywide and has claimed a lot of lives. He said that right now, all we need to do is to educate the masses about how they can avoid getting the disease and also to urge those already infected not to spread it, and be looked after with love.[37]

By this time, the scope of global HIV infection was beginning to be understood. The WHO drafted a global strategy for prevention and control of AIDS, which was approved by the World Health Assembly meeting in Venice in May 1987 and by the United Nations General Assembly in October 1987.[38] Uganda was party to these resolutions and began to apply them as quickly as possible. By October 1985, the AIDS Control Programme (ACP) was established in the Ministry of Health under the leadership of Dr. Samuel Okware. Its functions included epidemiological surveillance; protecting the safety of the blood supply; provision of information, education, and communication; provision of patient care and counseling; and control of sexually transmitted infections. In addition, the National Committee for the Prevention of AIDS was established to oversee the implementation of the ACP.[39] During the 1986 World Health Assembly in Geneva, the minister of health of the recently established NRM government announced the presence, and admitted the severity, of HIV/AIDS in Uganda.[40] He explained that Uganda had begun to take significant steps toward controlling the disease.

Thus, a popular response to *siliimu*/slim that had begun in the final days of the Obote II and Okello regime during 1985 quite quickly led to an integrated government response. Efforts to stem the tide of AIDS were folded together with efforts to build a new Uganda. Well before the full future impact of the disease could be known or even glimpsed, the Ugandan government and people had begun to respond effectively and with determination to the threat. The fact that ordinary Ugandans had already recognized and accepted the threat was a significant contributing factor.

CHAPTER 7

The Indigenization of AIDS

Governance and the Political Response in Uganda

GOVERNMENT RESPONSE

By 1988, HIV prevalence was beginning to skyrocket. At the Kampala antenatal clinic surveillance sites, HIV infections had increased by approximately 150 percent since 1985, when figures were first recorded. This turned out to be the period of the steepest rise in HIV prevalence. The government response, still located primarily in the Ministry of Health (MoH) through the AIDS Control Programme (ACP), was supported by a significant response on the part of civil society. For instance, the Ugandan Women's Effort to Support Orphans was founded and chaired by the first lady, Janet Museveni, with funding from international donors.[1] According to focus group discussion participants in July 2003, President Yoweri Museveni had also begun to tour the country making speeches about HIV/AIDS and urging people in schools and churches, and at funerals for AIDS victims, to be aware of the dangers of promiscuity and to limit their number of sexual partners. Dr. Dorothy Balaba, currently head of the Traditional and Modern Health Practitioners Together against AIDS and Other Diseases (THETA), recalls:

> I think it was the late 1980s. . . . When I was in high school we had a youth conference where the president addressed all the school-going children in 1988. We went to a conference center in an urban setting and talked about HIV. The president himself in person came and addressed

us. [There was seating for] 2,000. . . . One of the big places where most of the urban schools had a talk by the president. Our school was invited. We were at Gayaza High. He was talking about abstinence, . . . condoms, . . . well, really "ABC." Mostly on abstinence.[2]

During 1987 and 1988, a national seroprevalence survey showed an overall prevalence of 6–9 percent.[3] The U.S. Agency for International Development (USAID) began to import subsidized condoms and to oversee their distribution. The government of Uganda began to recognize at this time, too, that AIDS was no longer simply a health matter, and began consultation and discussion on an approach that would bring all levels of government, government-supported institutions such as schools and clinics, and organs of civil society including nongovernmental organizations (NGOs), faith-based organizations (FBOs), and community-based organizations (CBOs) into a nationally integrated response to AIDS. This eventually resulted in the "multisectoral approach" to AIDS control in the early 1990s, but discussions in the late 1980s represented a significant departure from the position that AIDS was primarily a medical matter. President Museveni, together with the leaders of the health care system, began to make it clear that AIDS affected all parts and all levels of Ugandan society.[4] According to Emmanuel Sekatawa, a leader in the development of the National Strategic Framework for HIV/AIDS, "There was recognition that there are many problems with AIDS that are not medical and that go beyond the health sector. For example, all the orphans have implications for inheritance. Thus, AIDS goes beyond the sexual." In response to this recognition, he said, "We brought people together to decide how to build a world without AIDS. Then we went to the nation. [We] arrived at consensus about vision, mission, and objectives. . . . This helped each individual sector see their role in the fight against AIDS. They could clearly see their role. Even churches could see what they could contribute; people believe in them. It allowed us to articulate various dimensions of AIDS, the biomedical, etc."[5]

Although not recognized at the time—or even now—Dr. Sekatawa was explaining the process that led away from mere medicalization of AIDS, and the narrow focus on behavior to an indigenous understanding rooted in local cultural forms and knowledge. Issues such as the effect of orphanhood on inheritance of property, and the role of churches, could be integrated with the biomedical without succumbing to the hegemony of the biomedical worldview and technicism driven by USAID, the World Health Organization (WHO), and other large agencies.

The ACP was established in the Ministry of Defence[6] in 1987–1988 in response to a warning from Cuba's Fidel Castro that large numbers of the Ugandan National Resistance Army (later the Ugandan National Defence Force) personnel who had been sent to Cuba for training were HIV-positive. Cuba refused to admit them, since Cuba had instituted a strict policy of quarantine of all HIV-infected people. The AIDS Support Organisation (TASO), was started in a small shed on the grounds of Mulago Hospital by HIV-positive people who wished to become involved in and to promote care of people living with AIDS (PLWAs). This small initiative grew rapidly from its origins at Mulago. USAID began to support training for peer educators and counselors involved in rapidly growing information, education, and communication (IEC) efforts, and funded care and support initiatives (such as TASO), sexually transmitted disease (STD) management, and grants to NGOs and to the National Resistance Army. TASO was first given USAID funding in 1988 with funding continuing to the present (2008). Ten years later, TASO had cared for at least 50,000 clients and their families and trained hundreds of AIDS counselors in Uganda and elsewhere in Africa. Their programs greatly helped to reduce the stigma associated with AIDS, and thus lowered levels of resistance to IEC programs and of discrimination against those who suffered from AIDS. USAID also continued to provide food relief and support for children who had been orphaned by the death of one or both parents from AIDS. The WHO began to provide large funding to support the ACP in the MoH for IEC, epidemiology, surveillance, patient care, and STD control.[7] By 1988, business became involved with the initiation of the AIDS in the Workplace project by the Federation of Uganda Employers.

These shifts in policy resulted in the near-total involvement of all government, business, labor, religious, educational, and other civil society institutions and organizations. This was significant, but it could not have happened if Uganda had not developed its own indigenous understanding of the disease.

Dr. Dorothy Balaba discounted the earlier contributions of the MoH, however. "They were not doing much. They were responsible for the adverts, and the TV, but it was not until they created the Uganda AIDS Commission [that things started to happen]. Then all the ministries had to become involved. It was created in the office of the president, but every ministry was represented. Every ministry became active. Before that it was seen as a health problem only under the Ministry of Health."[8]

Medical interventions, research, and public health initiatives were not neglected. In 1988, several large-scale research projects that were designed to study the epidemiology of HIV and the natural progression of AIDS in communities were begun. The Rakai Project, a joint effort of Makerere University, the Uganda Virus Research Institute, MoH, Columbia University, and Johns Hopkins University, began its study in Rakai District along the western shores of Lake Victoria, where the virus had first been identified and where deaths from AIDS were rapidly increasing. The German international aid organization GTZ, together with the Ugandan MoH, initiated the Basic Health Services Project in Kabarole and Bundibugyo districts (in the far western region of Uganda) and by 1991 had added a comprehensive AIDS control project including IEC/behavior change; care and counseling; STD treatment; condom education, procurement, and distribution; and programs that sought to reduce the personal and social impact of HIV/AIDS through training and capacity building.[9] Research to study maternal and pediatric HIV infection was developed through a cooperative program with Makerere University, Mulago Hospital, the Uganda MoH, and Case Western Reserve University. USAID, in conjunction with the government of Uganda and the WHO, began to supply larger numbers of condoms to the Maternal and Child Health Division of the MoH and provided $1.5 million in funding to the ACP overall.[10]

By the end of 1988, 7,249 AIDS cases had been officially reported to the MoH,[11] but this figure probably grossly underestimated the true death rate from AIDS. A review of the ACP recommended considerable increase in activities, especially at district and community levels, and the preparation of district-level plans that would include all governmental and political structures in the fight against AIDS.

THE SECOND DECADE OF AIDS IN UGANDA

Recognizing the scope of the problem and the efforts that were being made to respond to it, the Centers for Disease Control (CDC), in Atlanta, Georgia, sent Dr. Elizabeth Marum to lead the combined USAID/CDC response to AIDS. Research programs were discovering by 1989 that there was already an extremely high level of awareness of AIDS and HIV across the entire spectrum of the Ugandan population. The Swedish International Development Cooperation Agency began at this time to support further IEC programs together with an emphasis on care and support of HIV-positive people and those suffering from AIDS.

USAID expanded its Family Health Services (family planning services) programs and extended greater support for assistance to orphans and funding for two private-sector AIDS projects. It also funded Save the Children, an NGO based in the United Kingdom, to work with the Department of Child Care and Protection in the Ministry of Gender, Labour, and Social Development. By 1991, it was estimated that 1.2 million children had lost at least one parent, and 250,000 to 300,000 had lost both parents. The principle focus of USAID then was family planning, AIDS prevention, and orphans.[12] USAID funding reached its highest level since funding had been stopped in 1979 after the fall of Idi Amin's regime and the beginning of Milton Obote's second presidency (Obote II). The government of Uganda, with support from USAID, developed a policy on care and support of orphans that emphasized community and home-based care for orphans, rather than seeking to institutionalize them.

All of these efforts by donor agencies, public health services of the government, and civil society organizations led to better integration of a nationally coordinated response in Uganda. In February 1990, AIDS information centers (AICs) began to be set up around the country, especially in the south, to provide voluntary counseling and testing (VCT) for HIV.[13] By the end of 1998, around a half million clients had visited VCT centers, and the numbers continued to grow rapidly.

The year 1992 was pivotal in Uganda's AIDS epidemic. Although it could not have been known at the time, this was the year in which HIV prevalence peaked at nearly 30 percent in Kampala (based on antenatal clinic data for Kampala sentinel sites at Rubaga and Nsambya hospitals). At that time, it was still far from clear what the future trend of HIV prevalence would be in Uganda, and there was little agreement on the actual situation. The February 1993 foundation document for the new Multisectoral AIDS Control Approach (MACA) said, for instance, that "there is evidence that possibly about 10% [not 30 percent!] of the adult population could be already infected by HIV." The document noted that the "current estimate for doubling rates of the disease is about eight to twelve months."[14] The prevalence peak was experienced at different times in different parts of the country, with Jinja peaking in 1989, Lacor Hospital (near Gulu in the north) in 1993, and Matany (in the northeast) in 1994.[15] There were also wide disparities in regional prevalence. Seroprevalence in Rakai District varied from 1 percent in some rural villages to 33 percent in trading centers.[16] The national seroprevalence survey of 1988 also indicated considerable variability, from "as high as 50% and as low as 6%."[17] This variability was the result of the "lumpiness" of the sexual network that was transmitting HIV across the country. This clustering of HIV infection in specific parts of the sexual network introduced instability into the network dynamic, which led to the beginning of the collapse of HIV prevalence.

The Uganda AIDS Commission (UAC) was founded by an act of Parliament in 1992. Its primary goals and guiding principles had been under discussion during the previous four years. The critical document, "AIDS control in Uganda: The multi-sectoral approach,"[18] was published in February 1993, but its objectives were already being implemented in 1992. It called for the MACA to be implemented in all parts of central government, district government, CBOs, and NGOs, among others. The UAC would coordinate these activities. MACA was immediately adopted with the goals of (1) reducing the spread of HIV; (2) mitigating the health and socioeconomic effects; (3) strengthening national capacity to respond to the epidemic; (4) establishing a national information database on HIV/AIDS; and (5) strengthening the national capacity to undertake research.[19] This was strongly supported by international donor agencies, who had also been involved in the drafting of the plan. The United Nations Development Programme (UNDP) funded community-level IEC, care, and support projects and poverty alleviation.[20] USAID increased its funding of AIDS community education activities and supported IEC programs in churches and mosques.

In July 1993, Uganda presented its plan to the Summit of African leaders at the Organization of African Unity meetings in Dakar. It emphasized the commitment to an agenda for action including political commitment, multisectoral action to prevent transmission, care for PLWAs, support for AIDS research, support for multisectoral planning and action, and prioritizing AIDS as a target for external funding. Unfortunately, Uganda seems to have been among the very few countries that took this agenda to heart.

THE MULTISECTORAL APPROACH TO AIDS

The founding of the UAC was a major step in the coordination of the government's response to AIDS, but it was fraught with intricate political maneuvering in its early stages. The controversy revolved primarily around the question of whether the AIDS problem, and hence the nature of the response, was primarily medical (and therefore should be controlled by medical doctors based in the MoH) or was a more generalized social, political, and economic problem (and therefore required broad-based social, political, and economic responses developed and controlled by social scientists and political structures). By contrast, South Africans never resolved these kinds of disputes, and never managed to create and effective center in government to manage the epidemic. Eventually, in Uganda, an effective compromise was reached, which permitted inputs from both medical and social science. A similar compromise has so far eluded South Africa. The Ugandan MACA document noted,

> Because the coordination was being done by the Health Sector, the epidemic continued to be addressed almost exclusively as a health problem. Consequently, there was generally inadequate response and participation by other organisations in the public and private sectors, who felt that AIDS prevention and control was not their responsibility. It was later realised that the impact of the epidemic went beyond the domain of health and cut across all aspects of individual, family, community, and national life. Government therefore decided on an alternative approach towards AIDS control. A multi-sectoral AIDS control strategy was opted for.[21]

This proved to be the right choice: the Ugandan multisectoral approach has been highly effective in shaping communication strategies, developing condom distribution plans, creating organizational structures, and, ultimately, changing behaviors in ways that led to lower incidence and the decline in HIV prevalence.

The idea for the UAC began to be discussed in the period from 1988 to 1991, with the MACA framework being developed beginning in July 1991.[22] It involved a broad grouping of social scientists, medical scientists, and doctors, together with specialists in agriculture, statistics, development, and other fields, and the managers of AIDS control programs in government and the private sector. According to a number of people interviewed, the first plan developed by Uganda was presented to the WHO and the World Bank for funding. The WHO, in particular, was said to have rejected the first plan, claiming that the HIV problem was largely medical and therefore should be managed by medical specialists. Several consultants brought in by the World Bank and the WHO to advise on the plan called instead for a multisectoral approach, that is, an approach that would seek to coordinate responses and interventions from government, NGOs, FBOs, CBOs, and other informal organizations that were beginning to be acutely aware that AIDS now affected virtually every aspect of life. Finally, with assistance from the CDC, a comprehensive and successful plan was put together that would ultimately fund the UAC.

The UAC secretariat was set up and began immediately to develop plans for the multisectoral approach that would eventually lead to the establishment of formally appointed AIDS response contact personnel, called focal persons, in all ministries, and coordinate the activities of the now large and growing number of organizations in civil society, including Christian and Muslim FBOs, trade unions, the Federation of Uganda Employers, schools, NGOs, and CBOs across the country. In practice, however, most of the activity in the 1990s and up to the present is still located in the southern part of Uganda due to the security situation in the north. Only the lower tier of towns north of the Nile–Mt. Elgon line that roughly bisects Uganda, such as Gulu, Apac, and Lira, have received adequate attention.

The UAC immediately ran into political difficulties because of its location within the Office of the President. The ACP had already been established in the MoH in 1986. As the first government-initiated and funded formal response to AIDS, the ACP believed that it should continue to take the lead in shaping the response from government. The UAC was criticized as being too political, too policy-oriented, and too diffuse in its direction since it included many people from fields other than medicine. The ACP, by contrast, was controlled by medical specialists and led by Dr. Kihumuro Apuuli, a medical doctor. Eventually, Dr. Apuuli was appointed by President Museveni to the directorship of the UAC. From this position, Dr. Apuuli was able to coordinate the ACP within the UAC. This new framework resolved the political problems concerning which organizational unit or which type of educational specializations would control the government response. It was an astute move and had significant benefits. By contrast, as late as the end of 2006, national AIDS policy in South Africa was still directed from the president's office, with the deputy president in charge. This has critically exacerbated the political conflict over AIDS in South Africa.

The organizational location of the UAC in the Office of the President, rather than in a ministry, gave it the power it needed to implement and coordinate policy. The national policy on AIDS articulated by the MACA planning document stressed: "All Ugandans have individual and collective responsibility to be actively involved in AIDS control activities in a coordinated way at the various administrative and political levels down to the grassroots level. The fight against AIDS is not only directed at the prevention of the spread of HIV but also addresses the active response to, and management of, all perceived consequences of the epidemic." [23] The inclusiveness of this policy is extraordinary and powerfully enabling. It directs attention to both individual responsibility and to collective efforts and points out that effective AIDS control should not limit itself to prevention alone, but address both real and perceived consequences while managing the response administratively and politically. Moreover, the document envisions a fully coordinated and total response: "The process of preventing HIV infection, and controlling its consequences by various organisations and individuals in the country should be comprehensive, and sensitive to all aspects of the epidemic and emphasise capacity building for sustainable activities among sectors and individual organisations." [24]

This policy was predicated on the belief that "the current trend of the disease will not change much" [25] and conceptualized the response as a process rather than as mere administrative structures. It focused on a number of key political principles that had already been articulated by the Museveni government:

- strengthening the role of women in development;
- decentralization of planning and service administration;
- promotion of self-reliance and community empowerment;
- development of close partnerships between government and NGOs and CBOs;
- continued strategic political will and support for AIDS control;
- a demand for positive public response to AIDS that would include rapid and substantial behavior change;
- increasing allocation of resources for HIV prevention at all levels of government and response to the effects of the epidemic; and
- mobilization and sensitization of the public on the impact of AIDS.

These were the keystones of Uganda's multisectoral AIDS approach, but they also constituted major moves in the direction of national reconstruction more generally. The ACP became part and parcel of the process of political reform that was being led by the new government. In practice, this policy had already been in effect for some time; MACA represented the formulation and articulation of what was actually happening on the ground. It was a uniquely Ugandan initiative, and it noted that although "international support and assistance" were welcome, it "will not unduly influence national priority interventions."[26] It was built on a number of the principles of Museveni's Ten-Point Program of the National Resistance Movement, which called for, among other things, the restoration of democracy, the restoration of security of person and property, the consolidation of national unity and elimination of all forms of sectarianism, building an independent, integrated, and self-sustaining national economy, and restoration and improvement of social services.[27] Significantly, MACA was not just a government initiative or plan. It called for behavior change on the part of individuals and families, and tied the struggle against AIDS to an overall development strategy and to strengthening of democracy, personal security, and human rights. It broadened the base of AIDS prevention strategies to include all parts and all levels of society. It explicitly sought to empower women and to build institutions of civil society. Moreover, it articulated a belief and a means for all of these components to work together.

Although MACA was exceptionally comprehensive, it does not mention what has come to be called the ABC approach. Instead, it calls for behavior change across the spectrum of sexual practices. It notes that several demographic and social factors require attention, including

- early initiation of sexual activity (noting that 75 percent of both male and female children have had sex by age 17);[28]
- migration and mobility (noting that there is rapid urbanization in what has been an overwhelmingly rural population, with "breakdown of traditional moral instruction");
- a "knowledge versus moral and behavioral change gap" (noting that Ugandans are already overwhelmingly aware of HIV and AIDS but, despite this, "change of sexual partners is often rapid and sexual intercourse outside of regular relationships is frequent," with "dispersed and interlinking networks of sexual contacts");
- economic survival strategies linked to sexual risk (noting the effects of war, rape, disruption of family structures, poverty, illiteracy, and "increased use of sexual activity by women as an economic survival strategy");
- biological factors including STDs and blood-borne risks; and

· cultural practices, including language and communication
issues, gender relations, and alcohol use.

MACA insisted that all of these issues had to be addressed in order
to control the HIV/AIDS epidemic, and that "a multiplicity of behavior
options have to be encouraged."[29]

The MACA document is particularly explicit in calling for change
in cultural practices, and details these in several sections. It notes, for
instance, that "certain sociocultural practices have contributed to the
rapid and sustained spread of HIV/AIDS. For example, inheritance of
widows is quite common, scarification for treatment using a common
instrument, uvulectomy,[30] tooth extraction, circumcisions, tattooing.
Overnight parties with open access to alcohol and sexual laxity are a
regular occurrence at last funeral rites in some areas of the country."[31]
Under the heading "Cultural Practices," the MACA document also
highlights the plight of women in Uganda as particularly burdened by
care of AIDS patients, more likely to be infected, and often culturally
disempowered.[32]

While Uganda's policy integrated AIDS control measures into the
national reconstruction program and political reform, it was also revo-
lutionary in its straightforward discussion of cultural practices and
the complex role that sexual practices played within systems of kinship, religious and ritual life, gender, language and communication
practices, migration, and mobility. It was, in effect, a manifesto for
revolution.

AIDS AND CULTURAL PRACTICES

Here, Uganda stands out among other African governments in *specifically naming and describing* African cultural practices that lead to risk,
thus integrating the struggle against AIDS into local cultural forms
and practices. Focus group discussions universally mentioned these
practices, among others, as major contributors to HIV risk. Elsewhere
in Africa, and even in the past in Uganda, cultural practices having to
do with sexuality were rarely talked about, and certainly not openly
criticized.

It was also exceptional in seeking to empower and promote positive
traditional African cultural practices such as those of traditional healers (traditional medical practitioners), including traditional surgeons
(who perform circumcisions, uvulectomies, and tooth extractions),[33]

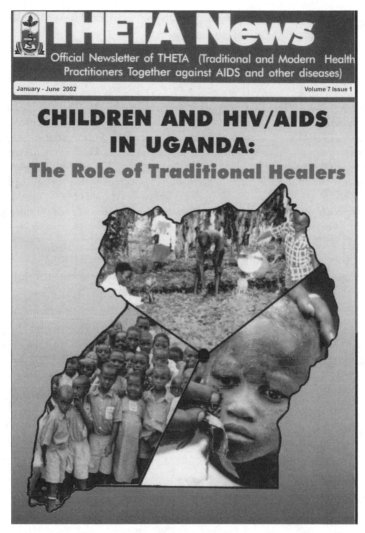

FIGURE 13. *Theta News,* official newsletter of the Traditional and Modern Health Practitioners Together against AIDS and Other Diseases (THETA).

traditional birth attendants, and syncretic practitioners who use herbal treatments, often in conjunction with biomedical treatments. The MACA document states, "The Commission will collaborate with all these groups which are essentially concerned with *body healing* [emphasis in original]," adding further that "spiritual and physical diviners will also be educated and guided." This policy led to the foundation by

TASO and Médecins sans Frontières, in 1992, of THETA, initially as a research initiative.[34] Dr. Balaba explained,

> The HIV epidemic was a mystery. People were dying, it must have looked like a god was unhappy somewhere. So people went to traditional healers. It started off as research. We wanted to know what they had to offer. So we started with research; this involved over 500 clients. We were looking at herpes zoster. We provided clients with herbs, comparing [their use and effectiveness] to a control standard. What we found out is that these were effective against herpes zoster, chronic diarrhea, and comparing against Western treatment. That success is what prompted us to start a program. We realized that traditional healers were respected. When they talked to people, people believed in them. We tried to see if they could communicate. We found out that they were natural counselors. We found out that they were good counselors.[35]

Dr. John Rwomushana, current UAC director for AIDS research and policy, told me that he had supported the inclusion of traditional healers in the MACA plan since this was a central institution of African culture. He acknowledged that there had been resistance from others, especially other medical doctors.[36] Dr. Rwomushana served as the first chairman of THETA. Today, THETA publishes a newsletter three times a year (see figure 13) and is involved with intensive training of traditional health care practitioners throughout Uganda.[37]

The MACA strategy for behavior change was similarly comprehensive. It called for sustainable behavior change and risk reduction through the following measures:

- Creating and sustaining peer and community behavioral support resources groups;
- Improving access to HIV testing and individual counseling;
- Improving access to STD diagnosis and treatment facilities through training for health workers and healers plus improved testing and treatment guidelines;
- Improving provision of condoms by improving procurement, storage, and distribution systems;
- Providing IEC in various formats for presentation in community meetings;
- Providing health care and condom dispensing sites near job locations; and
- Developing and promoting guidelines on family housing at work

locations, linked with adequate support and work opportunities for spouses to keep families together.[38]

As thorough as the MACA document is, however, nowhere does it mention the ABC program that has recently been associated with Uganda's approach to controlling the spread of HIV. Instead, it seeks to embed activities aimed at the control of HIV in a broad social framework.

Of course, the multisectoral approach, as such, was not meant to address specific behavioral interventions. If anything, it emphasizes condoms, changing cultural practices, and control programs embedded in government ministries and other organizations. (One is tempted to call it the CCC approach.) This approach has guided virtually everything that Uganda has done in combating AIDS throughout the 1990s and up to the present. The emphasis on a total sociopolitical integration, and the attempt to change behavior through programs that are embedded in the larger social, cultural, and political fabric of Ugandan life, gives the MACA an especially African character. It subordinates the emphasis on the individual—a characteristically Western approach—to the social and the cultural context. In particular, Uganda has been exceptional in the development of support programs for PLWAs through TASO and in the rollout of VCT.

The UAC, through MACA and the implementation of the National Operational Plan, has also sought to continuously monitor its progress. Developments through the middle of the decade reflect this. Condom imports and distribution rose swiftly after 1992. An estimated twelve million condoms were sold and/or distributed in 1993[39] as USAID and other organizations expanded reproductive health services. There are few reliable data on total numbers of condoms distributed in Uganda, but a compilation of figures from multiple sources shows that the number available greatly increased only after 1992 (see figure 14). Contrary to a widespread belief—propagated by President George W. Bush and the Heritage Foundation, a conservative research institute—that condoms played little or no role in Uganda's decline in HIV prevalence,[40] millions of condoms were in fact distributed in Uganda beginning in the mid-1980s. USAID began to import condoms in 1985, even before the Museveni administration took control of the government and while fighting continued. The International Planned Parenthood Foundation began distribution in 1989, and the United Nations Population Fund and the WHO joined the effort a

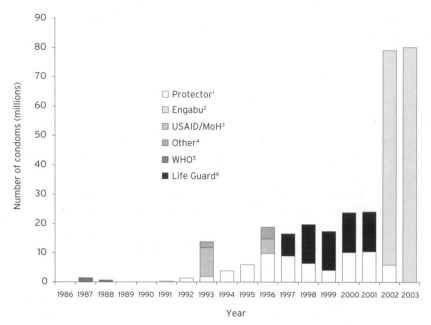

[1]Data from "Protector sales from launch date," provided by Twebese Rukandema, Commercial Marketing Services, Kampala.
[2]Data from Ministry of Health, Uganda 2002a. Apparently, these figures are projections.
[3]Kagimu and Marum 1996: 14.
[4]Kagimu and Marum 1996: 14.
[5]*New Vision*, 20 February 1987. The article states that 1.4 million were available, and 600,000 "on the way" (for 1988?).
[6]Data interpolated from Hogle et al. 2002, "Number of social marketed condoms sold in Uganda." Source: Deloitte Touche Tohmatsu, Commercial Marketing Services, Uganda Report 2001.

FIGURE 14. Partial compilation of total condom imports and local distribution in Uganda, 1987–2003.

year or two later, pushing condom availability from these sources alone to more than ten million a year. USAID's shipments continued to increase into the mid-1990s before beginning to fall, but many organizations provided large numbers of condoms through the rest of the 1990s, including the German development bank Kreditanstalt für Wiederaufbau (Reconstruction Credit Institute), the United Kingdom's Department for International Development, Population Services International, Marie Stopes International, Pathfinder International, and others.[41] In addition, the Ugandan government itself sourced, manufactured, and distributed condoms through the MoH, and later through the brand names Protector, Lifeguard, and Engabu (meaning "protector" or "shield" in Luganda). Precise numbers have been difficult to ascertain, but estimates are given in figure 14. International donors stepped in to help the overall program as well. The UNDP funded AIDS control programs in at least eleven ministries, including the Ministries of Gender, Education, Agriculture, Internal Affairs (Police and Prisons), Justice, Finance, Public Service, and Local Government. The Danish International Development Agency assisted with funds for TASO, which was also funded by USAID. The World Bank supported blood screening for the National Blood Bank, and provided seventy-five million dollars in loans for the implementation of a sexually transmitted infections program. In order to evaluate the effectiveness of this program, the collaborative Rakai Project began a five-year study to examine the effect of modified mass treatment of STDs on the incidence and prevalence of STDs and HIV infection. Other donors included CARE, World Learning, CONCERN, AMREF, and World Vision.[42] The first United Nations Program on HIV/AIDS (UNAIDS) country program adviser was posted to Uganda in 1996.[43]

By the end of 1995, Uganda had organized and hosted the International Conference on AIDS and STDs in Africa. At this conference Uganda first announced what appeared to be an observed decline in HIV prevalence. By then, 48,312 cases of AIDS had been officially reported,[44] but the true number was estimated to be around 340,000.[45]

Numbers of new statutes were passed by the Ugandan Parliament to discourage discrimination based on HIV status and to provide additional support for AIDS and HIV interventions. The Children's Statute of 1996, for instance, encouraged community care with financial support of families who care for orphans. As a result of this, as few as 1 percent of all orphans are housed in public institutions.

SUCCESS ACKNOWLEDGED

During 1996–1997, a comprehensive review of AIDS control programs was conducted by the UAC, ministry-based AIDS control programs, UNAIDS, and representatives of NGOs.[46] It found, for instance, that overall knowledge of HIV/AIDS in Uganda was extremely high, and that many strategies for risk reduction and behavior change had been implemented. Cultural practices involving multiple sexual partners were effectively discouraged throughout the country. Approximately 300,000 were reported to have benefited from VCT provided by

AICs,[47] in addition to other benefits provided by Uganda's strategy. The report noted,

> Virtually every component of the WHO-recommended Global Strategy for responding to the AIDS epidemic has been implemented in Uganda, including intensive education campaigns, condom education and distribution, voluntary HIV testing and counselling, STD treatment and control, and the provision of safe blood supply. Programs to provide long term supportive care and terminal care for persons living with AIDS have been implemented in many areas, and counselling has become available in many areas. Persons living with AIDS have formed associations both to provide mutual support and to educate communities about HIV prevention. Numerous efforts have been developed to reduce the social and economic impact of the epidemic on individuals, families, communities and the society at large. Uganda's efforts to control and respond to the AIDS epidemic have been greatly enhanced by strong political leadership and will at every level. There have also been commendable efforts to mobilise and unify the response to the epidemic at the external, national, district and community level including the establishment of the multi-sectoral Uganda AIDS Commission, line Ministry AIDS Control Programmes, and District AIDS Coordinating Committees.[48]

In addition to the huge success of these programs based on the multisectoral approach, there were a number of significant developments in biomedical treatment. For instance, SOMARC, the USAID-funded social marketing project, developed drug kits for treatment of sexually transmitted infections, especially in men with urethral discharge.[49] Uganda began to participate in a study designed to examine the effectiveness of Nevirapine, an antiretroviral drug (ARV), on mother-to-child transmission of HIV.[50] The government of Uganda established the Drug Access Initiative, which advocated for reduced prices on ARVs and supported the infrastructure to administer them, while the U.S. National Institutes of Health began providing research grants to American scientists to study the HIV epidemic and to test and identify effective treatments.[51]

Following the glowing review it received for its programs, Uganda began to develop the new National Strategic Framework for HIV/AIDS. In particular, it further integrated AIDS control programs into national development goals. AIDS activities became part of the Poverty Eradication Action Plan. At the same time, the Local Government Act of 1997 reorganized and decentralized government services, with financial and administrative devolution of education, medical and health services, social development activities, and management of remedial

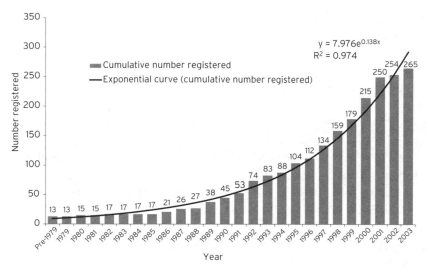

FIGURE 15. Cumulative growth of Ugandan NGOs, CBOs, and FBOs dealing wholly or in part with HIV and AIDS (by date of registration to provide HIV/AIDS services). Data from files in the offices of the Uganda Network of AIDS Services Organisation, Nakulabye, Kampala.

welfare programs and welfare programs for children and the elderly to the district level. Since all of these services and agencies involved an AIDS component, this meant that control over AIDS programs was also devolved to a level closer to the community. The effect of these interventions, and their overall effectiveness can be inferred from the average national prevalence among adults which fell from 18.5 percent in 1995, to 14.7 percent in 1997, 9.5 percent in 1998, and 8.3 percent at the end of 1999. In 2001, Uganda received an additional fifty million dollars in loans from the World Bank to secure and support all AIDS activities in all sectors at the national, district, and community levels.[52]

Notwithstanding the effectiveness of Uganda's response, cumulative AIDS deaths had mounted to 947,552 by the end of 2001,[53] and there were approximately 1,050,055[54] PLWAs out of a total population of twenty-four million (4 percent), while even more HIV-positive people had yet to manifest symptoms.[55] Clearly, even though the incidence and prevalence had dropped, Uganda was still left with a major challenge.

Remarkably, Uganda seemed ready to deal with this challenge. The growth of agencies and institutions in civil society that had been enabled and empowered by the Ugandan approach was exponential. A sample of local organizations, NGOs, CBOs, and FBOs that dealt wholly or in part with HIV or AIDS showed tremendous growth during the 1990s and through 2003. Figure 15 shows this remarkable development. The fact that this curve is almost perfectly exponential ($R^2 = 0.9749$), rather than linear, suggests that each of these civil society organizations was responsible for the establishment of others. In effect, the creation of such organizations has been organic, with each one reproducing itself several times over. The MACA policy and the overall encouragement of the development of a civil society response by government and by international donor funding have spawned numerous spinoff organizations, as the goals and tasks of each organization grew and specialized. For instance, TASO and Médecins sans Frontières created THETA. This sort of organic process has been at work since the late 1980s, resulting in an exponential growth in HIV/AIDS-related organizations. This has greatly enhanced the ability of government to cope with the HIV/AIDS problem in Uganda. Significantly, many of these organizations are also involved in economic development projects of all kinds. They represent a tremendous growth of democratic ideals and grassroots involvement.

Uganda, then, has not only been successful in decreasing HIV prevalence throughout the country, but has leveraged its response to HIV/AIDS into an effective and pervasive commitment to economic growth and social empowerment. The establishment of the UAC successfully managed political conflict by placing control of the AIDS programs in the hands of independent administrators, most of whom were highly qualified professionals rather than politicians. Although government response was probably not effective in lowering HIV levels directly, especially in clusters of high-density sexual networks, it probably did have the effect of helping to eliminate some of the contacts across these clusters, and thus bringing about the collapse of the network, which did result in rapid HIV declines overall. Although prevalence remained high in many areas and locations, the transmission of HIV across the country as a whole was disrupted through the integrated efforts of government and civil society. By building the struggle against AIDS into the program of nation building, Uganda succeeded in "owning" the epidemic. Although the disease was endemic, it also became *indigenous*.

CHAPTER 8

South Africa's Struggle

The Omission and Commission
of Truth about AIDS

A nation, previously divided by race, now threatens to be
destabilised by gender inequality, violence, and disease. A
truly African solution would be to set up an HIV truth and
reconciliation commission, where under strong health policy
and scientific leadership, everyone could come together and
reach a consensus on how best to draw a line under past
misguided views and to move forward with convincing
strategies. Only then can South Africa's leaders give hope
to future generations.

Editorial in *The Lancet*, 20 May 2006

TO APPEAR LIKE NORMAL ILLNESS

In 1987, the president of Zambia, Kenneth Kaunda, announced that
his son, Gwebe, had died of AIDS.[1] "It does not need my son's death
to appeal to the international community to treat the question of AIDS
as a world problem," the senior Kaunda said.[2] The epidemic that had
begun in northern central Africa was rapidly making its way south. In
that year, there were approximately fifty-one cases of AIDS known in
South Africa.[3] Eighteen years later, Nelson Mandela's son, Makgatho
Mandela, died on 6 January 2005. Two of Africa's best known and
greatest former presidents had lost their sons to AIDS. In the interven-
ing years, HIV prevalence in South Africa had skyrocketed from near
zero to an estimated 5.5 million people living with HIV at the end of
2004,[4] while perhaps 1.5 million had already died[5] by the time Nelson
Mandela lost his son.

Mandela, who had made efforts to "normalize" the image of AIDS
in South Africa, and who had campaigned for AIDS to be recognized

and treated like any other disease, said at his son's funeral, "Let us give publicity to HIV/AIDS and not hide it, because [that is] the only way to make it appear like a normal illness."[6] It was exceptionally important for Nelson Mandela to say this, but he should not have had to say it at all. Half a decade into the new millennium, South Africa had by far the worst HIV epidemic in the world, and yet there was still debate about how to deal with it. The principal question was whether it could be considered normal and, more than this, normal in whose terms?

Of course, it was normal if this is taken to mean common. Black South Africans are aware of the terrible toll that AIDS is taking because of the number of funerals they have to attend. When someone dies, almost everyone who knew the deceased is expected to attend the funeral. All family and relatives, friends, colleagues, fellow church members, coworkers, and any one else who has had more than casual contact with the deceased and who hears about the funeral in time will try to attend. Nearly everyone appreciates the tremendous strain that this has put on resources. With the rise in deaths, municipalities are running out of room in cemeteries, while families and households grieve, collapse, and sink further into poverty. In this, AIDS is now normal.

Mandela's words are more complex than this: he says that South Africans must do what they can to make AIDS *appear* like a normal illness. In fact, it still does not even appear as an illness to many South Africans, who continue to deny its existence, especially as a cause of death. In announcing the death of a colleague at the national South African Broadcasting Corporation (SABC), the news reader noted that one of the network's weather announcers had died of "AIDS-related illness" on 15 June 2006. This was a departure from the way deaths from AIDS had been announced previously. People were said to die "after an illness." The indirect reference to an undefined illness, however, had already come to signify death from AIDS. In this way, it was as normal as the hidden network of sexual relations that drove it: everyone knew it was there, but no one would admit to the fact. AIDS was becoming normalized as a missing presence. It did not *appear*.

Mandela's successor, Thabo Mbeki, has fought mightily against accepting this reality. At the other end of the political spectrum, people in rural villages, and especially traditional healers, debate whether AIDS is curable, and some claim to cure it. The essence of the debate is whether the ancestors knew about AIDS. If they did, then traditional medicine ought to be able to cure it because it is an African disease among Africans; if the ancestors did not, then traditional medicine cannot cure it and we must die. The struggle against AIDS, then, depends on a peculiar image of its nature and origins, an image that is deeply embedded in South African cultural imagination. South Africans ask themselves, "Is AIDS ours, African—from us and within us—or is it foreign, un-African, from without rather than from within?" This is not unusual in South Africa today. South Africans, for instance, typically blame the worst aspects of crime on people they call "Africans," that is, immigrants from Africa north of the South African border. For South Africans, especially black South Africans, what they call "Africa" is a dangerous and foreign place. The deep ambiguities of reference to what is "ours," that is "African" or "South African," or to what comes from outside versus what comes from inside, create significant barriers to acceptance.

Uganda had already made this determination years before the virus was discovered, described by science, and named. It had its own name for it, and recognized it as its own problem, for which Ugandans must come up with a solution. There were, of course, many who helped to find solutions, but Uganda's ownership of the problem facilitated its response. South Africa, especially its leadership, has not accepted this burden of possession, for the most part, and so still wanders through a nightmare of uncertainty. This "denialism," as it has come to be called in South Africa, has characterized the response to AIDS almost from the start. [7]

In the late 1980s, HIV was still scarcely noticeable in South Africa. There were a few discussions of it in the newspapers, but these all pointed fingers at Africa north of the South African border. It was implied that HIV would not affect South Africa. Indeed, in the dying days of apartheid, some thought HIV might be a good thing, as it would result in the deaths of black Africans. Although this attitude was not expressed in the public press, so far as I am aware, it was expressed at dinner parties and garden gatherings. SABC, the state-owned and sole broadcaster in South Africa, ran a few stories on the new disease that had been reported in Uganda and had been identified in migrant mine workers, especially from Malawi. The contracts for these workers were subsequently canceled. Dr. Willie van Niekerk, the minister of health and population development, proclaimed in 1988, "Promiscuity is the greatest danger, whether one likes it or not," in reference to homosexuals and foreign black mine workers. Dr. Marius Barnard, the shadow minister for health in the parliamentary opposition, the Progressive

Federal Party, suggested that HIV/AIDS "carriers" should be isolated as they were in Cuba.

Most people had other things on their minds, however. South Africa was in the midst of rising violence in the townships as bomb blasts and protest actions gradually gathered in force and urgency. 1985 was a watershed year in which violent events by both police and resistance movements became, if not commonplace, at least alarming. In that year, South African churches, led by Bishop Desmond Tutu, began to campaign steadily and forcefully for change. Armed police patrols began moving through South African townships, and several groups of protesters and innocent people were killed. In an attempt to reassert control over the rising violence, the prime minister, P. W. Botha, offered to release Mandela if he agreed to forswear violence. Mandela refused to do so and remained in prison, and Botha declared a state of emergency. It was to last for the remainder of the decade, until F. W. de Klerk succeeded a tired and confused Botha as prime minister in August 1989.

The events of the last half of the 1980s made it clear to everyone that the end of apartheid was merely a matter of time. It came sooner than most expected, and without major bloodshed. In February 1990, soon after taking office, de Klerk effectively declared the end of apartheid by announcing that he was lifting the ban on the political parties that had led the resistance to the apartheid government, including the African National Congress (ANC) and the South African Communist Party. He began to release political prisoners and acknowledged the end of the apartheid regime. He announced, too, that Nelson Mandela would be released, and Mandela finally walked free on 11 February 1990. Prime Minister de Klerk led his party to the negotiating table with the ANC, together with all of the other parties from the left and right. Fifteen years later, the remainder of the National Party (NP), the old party of apartheid, quietly folded itself into the triumphant ANC, which after two democratic elections commanded two-thirds of the vote.

By the end of 1991, the first formal negotiations aimed at founding a new government were begun, but ended in failure because of the continuing violence in South African townships. The negotiations were called the Convention for a Democratic South Africa (CODESA). On 20 December of that year, Mandela spoke to the constitutional assembly, saying, "Today will be indelibly imprinted in the history of our country. . . . [T]oday will mark the commencement of the transition from Apartheid to democracy. . . . History will judge us extremely harshly if we fail to turn the opportunity, which it now presents to us [to the] common good. The risks of further pain and affliction arising from violence, homelessness, unemployment, of gutter education, are immense. . . . The price of CODESA's failure will be far too great."[8]

Eventually, through a successful series of negotiations, a new constitution was written and the first full-franchise democratic elections were held in South Africa in April 1994. On 10 May of that year, Nelson Mandela became the first president of what was soon to be called, informally but proudly, the New South Africa, or the "new dispensation." As Mandela's CODESA speech suggests, the burden of the past was far too great to give equal attention to the reform of government and all of its aspects, to the ending of violence that had by this time become pervasive and increasingly arbitrary and aimless, and to everything else that must be done. It was imperative that the moves toward a new government not fail. Everything else rested on this. The efforts were successful, of course, but the rising tide of HIV was lost from sight.

Efforts to control AIDS, however, were beginning by 1990, when the first survey of antenatal clinics shows that 0.7–0.8 percent of pregnant women attending the clinics tested positive for HIV.[9] The survey provoked little notice in the press, but the Department of Health has continued to conduct surveys annually since that time. It was not until 1992, however, that the first significant efforts were made by government to address the problem. When it did, these efforts were heavily burdened with a political legacy and ideological agenda that did nothing but divide and fragment efforts from the beginning.[10] By now, much has been written on AIDS in South Africa.[11] This chapter offers, in particular, a synoptic view of cultural meanings and contrasting political discourses around AIDS that have affected the relationship between the South African people and their government and civil society.

THE SHAPE OF THE SOUTH AFRICAN RESPONSE

HIV crept into South Africa just as political power was being smoothly transferred from the old party of apartheid, the Afrikaans-dominated NP, to the predominantly black ANC. The shape of the response to AIDS was already being formed even as South Africa was negotiating the transition. Although the impact of any serious efforts to combat

AIDS would not be felt in South Africa until sometime toward the end of the decade, two pivotal developments seem to have begun to direct those efforts. The first development was the formation of the National AIDS Committee of South Africa (NACOSA), the founding of the AIDS Law Project (ALP), and the organization of the AIDS Consortium, all in 1992. These three organizations determined that the approach to AIDS in South Africa would have much in common with the approach that was taken in the United States, especially that which developed around gay organizations in California and New York. They also adopted the struggle tactics that had been developed during the decades of active political struggle against apartheid. These organizations gave birth later to the Treatment Action Campaign (TAC), an organization built around demands for treatment rather than prevention. TAC used the media and strong confrontational political tactics in direct struggle with government, while ALP provided support for challenging the government in court.

The second development was the founding of Soul City, an "edutainment" organization that proposed to use entertainment to educate the public about HIV and AIDS and other health and development issues. The Soul City program was based in the Institute for Health and Development Communication, a nongovernmental organization (NGO) with international and South African government funding. This was followed by the establishment of LoveLife, an organization that used mass advertising—billboards, glossy publications, and road shows—as a means to educate people about HIV. This initiative helped to channel funds and government attention toward mass media as the principal means for communicating their message. From the start, South Africa's strategy has been highly political, centralized, and based in expensive high-tech mass media. Echoing the rhetoric of the struggle against apartheid (or "the Struggle," as it is known in South Africa), Nelson Mandela called the efforts to halt the epidemic "the new struggle."[12] Prevention messages have been indirect, often obscurely so, and explicit sex education has been consistently resisted. Discussion of AIDS in the media routinely places it in a political rather than sociocultural context.

These approaches contrasted strongly with Uganda's approach, which emphasized communication strategies based in small organizations, schools, businesses, churches, and community theater using popular but indigenous music. It was highly decentralized, nonpolitical (President Museveni had banned political parties and had decentralized government), and it emphasized medical-technical approaches to both prevention and treatment. Prevention messages were sexually explicit, with widespread use of direct and explicit sex education in schools reinforced with significant media support and educational materials. While the president of Uganda offered encouragement and direction, he generally delegated to technically competent individuals the responsibility for carrying out these programs. He did not so much lead the way as get out of the way of implementation by others. By contrast, the first president of the New South Africa, Nelson Mandela, paid little attention to AIDS during his presidency, and his successor, Mbeki, often obstructed effective prevention and treatment, preferring instead to direct an alternative course of action that appeared to have little scientific validity. His personal authority was pervasive in government and little happened without his direct, personal assent.

The two directions that the South African approach took—human rights and mass media—have had some contradictory results: one tending to entrench attitudes toward secrecy and privacy, the other encouraging openness and freedom of expression around HIV status. The focus on human rights has entrenched an attitude against personal disclosure of HIV status and against mandatory testing in appropriate circumstances. Contact tracing has been discouraged, as have explicit messages and sex education.[13] Research has often been hampered by bureaucratic insistence on complex ethical research protocols based on those used in invasive medical procedures and drug testing. It has given legal force to many people's desire for privacy, but has also discouraged voluntary testing, even with counseling. Although this emphasis on privacy is not a bad thing in itself, it has tended to counter the other major direction in South African policy development, the effort to get people to "talk about it"—one of the slogans used by the Soul City programs and by LoveLife, South Africa's largest mass AIDS education NGO. The overwhelming move to public media, including prime-time entertainment, has emphasized the importance of speaking out and talking about sex, especially among youths, and between youths and their parents.

These two tendencies, though in some senses opposed to each other, have achieved an accommodation, and have come to define the South African response to AIDS. The emphasis on human rights enshrined in the new South African constitution and defended strongly by the courts also permitted effective challenges to the resistance from the Mbeki government.

AIDS and Human Rights

The convening in October 1992 of NACOSA was the first step in South Africa toward addressing the HIV/AIDS problem.[14] NACOSA received considerable funding from the European Union, which had been funding AIDS programs in South Africa since 1987.[15] Its name and political constitution reflected those of CODESA, which was struggling with the challenges of political change. This was the year that HIV prevalence in Uganda began to plummet while it was just beginning its steepest rise in South Africa. Elements of the NACOSA plan were good: it was, at least, a start. It aimed to generate a unified national plan that would direct a coordinated response. The conference was attended by 442 delegates, but the emphasis fell on what, in retrospect, seem to be indirect concerns: racial inequalities, human rights, and poverty. Instead of stressing an aggressive and integrated medical and epidemiological attack through research, prevention, and palliative care, as Uganda had done, the conference pointed to the poverty of many South Africans and asserted that improvement in living standards was the key to prevention. Objectively, all but the poorest and most marginalized of South Africa's poor were not as poor as most Ugandans at the time, and they had access to generally better health facilities.

Even in the early 1990s, however, South Africa was still loath to compare itself to any other African country. All South African parties to the political conflicts of the twentieth century sought comparison with the developed world, especially Europe and North America, and with the other English-speaking Commonwealth countries of the south, that is, India, Australia, and New Zealand. Comparison with other African countries, where political violence, poverty, injustice, and exclusion based on ethnic identity and race were often worse than in South Africa, was held to be odious because it tended to weaken the moral force of resistance to apartheid. This made political sense, but blinded most people to obvious comparisons with the rest of Africa. South Africans in general and the South African government in particular rarely looked to the north for ideas or solutions to problems. This was a tragic omission. Even though South Africans were in general much wealthier than most people to the north, it was in South Africa that HIV prevalence has reached its highest mark on the continent. To the north, countries were poorer, but their response to HIV was often superior to South Africa's.

The political-economic focus of NACOSA was consistent with the broader political environment of the transition to democracy, and seems to have taken this opportunity to address grievances rather than to address the problem. Race was also a significant issue, with black and white delegates each believing that the other side was responsible. Blacks believed that AIDS was still primarily a disease of white homosexual men or other Africans, and therefore not a problem for black South Africans. Some white South Africans saw AIDS as a problem with the pattern of black sexuality and family life arising from the disruptions of migrant labor and apartheid laws that resulted in the breakup of black families who were not allowed by apartheid laws to live together near their places of work. Even though HIV prevalence was already highest in Natal, a predominately Zulu province in South Africa, the Inkatha Freedom Party that primarily represented a Zulu constituency did not attend the conference.[16] This highly politicized and adversarial approach—as opposed to a dispassionate public health or technical one as exemplified in Uganda—continues to underlie much of the South African response. It was revitalized by the second president of the New South Africa, Mbeki, in his campaign against exorbitant costs of antiretroviral (ARV) medications from the large pharmaceutical manufacturers.

It was clear by this time that Uganda's response to AIDS was exemplary, even if it was not yet certain that HIV prevalence was falling. The plan that emerged from NACOSA strongly reflected elements of South Africa's political transition by placing greater emphasis on human rights and rights to confidentiality[17] than on more practical concerns. It attempted to assert national central control over provinces that had already begun to develop fairly effective local responses, especially in the Western Cape (where prevalence was still low) and in Natal (where prevalence had already increased to a level higher than that in Uganda at its peak). HIV prevalence was found to be as high as 13 percent among males who attended a sexually transmitted infection clinic in Johannesburg, and 18.7 percent among females at the same clinic.[18] A national AIDS coordinating committee was subsequently set up, and at a workshop in September 1993 attended by forty people, the coordinating committee drew up a document that encouraged grassroots involvement in fighting AIDS, and required that the legacy of apartheid be recognized as a contributory factor to the spread of AIDS in South Africa.[19]

NACOSA's invocation of grassroots involvement—an important political strategy in the struggle against apartheid, and a South Africa political buzzword that appears in virtually every speech even a decade and a half later—was meant to channel the political strength of the masses against the new threat. But, unlike in Uganda, where significant political commitment and infrastructure was mobilized to do just that, in South Africa the words remained just words. There was no political commitment to mobilize the masses and the fabled grassroots energy failed to materialize. At that moment, there was still too much work to be done to wind up the apartheid regime, and later on many of the political activists had either received comfortable employment in government, or subsided into bitter unemployment.

An HIV and AIDS Charter was drawn up in 1992 by several political activists including Edwin Cameron, Edward Swanson, and Mahendra Chetty. [20] This charter[21] was modeled, both in structure and in wording, on the Freedom Charter[22] written by Nelson Mandela and other ANC activists, which had guided the ANC's struggle since its adoption in Kliptown in June 1955. Since both Cameron and Mandela were lawyers, both charters used the formal language of legal documents. And, since Cameron and the other drafters of the AIDS Charter were gay males, they also felt a sense of political disenfranchisement. Cameron and others also set up, in 1992, the AIDS Consortium to coordinate NGOs and other organizations that were beginning to organize around the issue. Originally based at the Centre for Applied Legal Studies at the University of the Witwatersrand in Johannesburg, it moved out in 1998 to become independent, and in 2006 had more than one thousand organizations affiliated with it. The AIDS Charter provided an orienting doctrine and legitimating charter for many of these organizations, while the informal networked structure of the AIDS Consortium and its affiliates mirrored the structure of the organization of the mass democratic movement during the 1980s in the last days of apartheid. The AIDS Charter clearly framed HIV and AIDS as political issues that required struggle to overcome. It also set the agenda for confrontational legal challenge as one of the bases for this contest.

The struggle against AIDS, then, merged medical and political issues seamlessly, drawing on both American and South African experiences of racism and homophobia. Ironically, it seemed to suppress widespread political mobilization against AIDS because the era of mass mobilization had passed—or was by now, most hoped, passé—or because the other pressing political issues simply overwhelmed it. In any case, what emerged as HIV tightened its grasp on South Africa was nothing like the Ugandan response.

The AIDS Charter closely parallels the Freedom Charter in many respects. The AIDS Charter, noting the threat of discrimination against people with HIV infections, "sets out those basic rights which all citizens enjoy or should enjoy and which should not be denied to persons affected by HIV or AIDS as well as certain duties." Responding to the expulsion of HIV-positive foreign mine workers from South Africa by the previous government, the charter declared that no restrictions should be placed on any person's freedom of movement, just as the ANC's Freedom Charter demanded, "Freedom of movement shall be guaranteed to all who work on the land." In response to suggestions that people with HIV should be isolated or quarantined, the AIDS Charter stated, "segregation, isolation or quarantine of persons in prisons, schools, hospitals or elsewhere merely on the grounds of AIDS or HIV is unacceptable." The Freedom Charter declared, "All people shall have the right to live where they choose." In line with the Freedom Charter's demand for equal and free education for all regardless of race, the AIDS Charter declared that "all persons have the right to proper education and full information about HIV and AIDS." In these and in many other respects—health care, security, education, employment, housing, gender, provision of justice, and so on—the AIDS Charter treated HIV-positive people in political terms and demanded their freedom. In short, the AIDS Charter aligned itself strongly with the ANC and the freedom movement in general by asserting an identity between people who had been discriminated against and disenfranchised for reasons of race with those whom they feared would be further discriminated against by reason of their HIV status or sexuality and sexual preferences. This was hardly an unreasonable fear since some infected individuals had already been killed and others thrown out of their homes or denied employment. The fears were valid and the mode of their expression familiar and commonplace, but their consequences were partly unforeseen.

The AIDS Charter helped to entrench the politicized understanding of AIDS in the country. Although fully consistent with the human rights–based approach of most NGOs and left or liberal organizations, it prevented the possibility that AIDS might be seen as a disease like any other, as Mandela pleaded that it might on the death of his own son fifty years after the adoption of the Freedom Charter. AIDS now had a political identity that other diseases did not have, and this effectively prevented mandatory tracing of sexual contacts, which had become routine for syphilis, for instance.[23] As openly gay men, the authors of the AIDS Charter were fully aware that this was the approach taken by gay men in the United States when AIDS was first discovered among them. They saw themselves as double victims of discrimination and stigma by virtue of their sexuality and their HIV status. In the midst of a struggle for the human rights of homosexuals in the United States, this politicization made sense; in Africa, faced with a generalized heterosexual epidemic whose proportions vastly exceeded that of the American gay community, it was, perhaps, less appropriate. In any case, it made explicit a right not to divulge HIV status to anyone, not even a current lover. This is embedded in the South African political consciousness.

Eventually, however, this approach appeared to be counterproductive. In 2002 in *The Lancet,* De Cock, Mbori-Ngacha, and Marum identified what they called "HIV exceptionalism."[24] They argued that an approach modeled on Euro-American human rights issues and demands for privacy (unless the individual actively chooses to "come out" and publicly declare his or her own HIV status) was not helpful in Africa where universal "know your status" campaigns should be the norm and routine testing for HIV in all public facilities should become mandatory. The provision of social justice through treatment and accurate identification of HIV infections was more important than narrow legalistic interpretations of human rights, they maintained. The power of this argument grew, and Edwin Cameron, now a High Court judge, reversed his position on the right to nondisclosure of HIV status as a human right in August of 2006, arguing—by this time with many others—that the provision for privacy and nondisclosure of HIV status prevented AIDS from being viewed as a normal illness. The crucial difference was that by 2006, unlike the situation in 1992, AIDS was now treatable and could be considered a chronic disease. He recommended that routine tests be carried out for HIV wherever possible, and that reporting to responsible monitoring agencies be made mandatory. The South African government, however, has failed to act on these suggestions.

AIDS NGOs and support organizations in South Africa explicitly adopted the style and often the substance of the underground anti-apartheid movement of the 1980s. Surprisingly, the new government colluded in this by acting toward HIV-positive people and those with AIDS in a way that was in many ways like the way the apartheid state had acted with respect to black people. People living with AIDS and organizations that supported and represented them became political actors, while the state maneuvered to thwart them.

The tendency to central control by the national Department of Health was already clearly present in the NACOSA plan. Indeed, two members of the eight-person drafting committee became ministers of health — Dlamini-Zuma and then Tshabalala-Msimang — and both resisted effective intervention to slow the progress of HIV.[25] At a time when Uganda was moving to decentralize AIDS control programs, and thus to shift responsibility to the local level and to the many parts of Ugandan civil society, government, and economic institutions, the new South African government, like the old, continued to hold closely the secrets and mechanisms of state power. South Africa was still suffering from academic boycotts and cultural sanctions. Though these had ceased by then to be useful, they continued to hinder the flow of new research on AIDS into South Africa. The go-it-alone attitude that had come with sanctions busting during apartheid lingered on to isolate the developing South African AIDS response from the rest of the world. The political bickering continued to foster isolation even after May 1994, when the new government was finally installed.

The new government, however, immediately set about trying to implement the recommendations of NACOSA, and external agencies began to join in with increasing foreign aid. Still divided about the causes of AIDS, the bulk of the effort was placed on information, education, and communication strategies, and on reforming the government health care system so that it would permit health care access to the rural poor and to black people more effectively than it had done in the past.

Nkosazana Dlamini-Zuma, a former ANC activist, was made the first minister of health under Nelson Mandela. She was the person ultimately responsible for the government's AIDS program implementation. Before her marriage to Jacob Zuma, Nkosazana Dlamini had qualified as a medical doctor in 1978 at the University of Bristol, after going into exile in Britain as the result of her political activities in South Africa with the then-banned ANC. She was active in ANC politics in Britain while working as a doctor in two British hospitals before returning to southern Africa. She was medical officer in the Pediatrics Department of the government hospital in Swaziland from 1980 to 1985, where she met and then married Jacob Zuma, who later became deputy president and then president of the ANC in 2007. She subsequently divorced him. She then left southern Africa again and became involved in exile in ANC politics overseas. On her return to South Africa in 1991 with many other exiles, she secured a post as a research scientist with the

Medical Research Council in Durban. She served as a member of the
steering committee of the national AIDS coordinating committee, and
was chairman of the ANC Women's League in the southern Natal
region, among other activities. Her biography is typical of many of the
current ANC elite, who are often connected not only by their political
relations and shared experiences in exile and in the resistance to apartheid, but also by a dense set of marriage and sexual links.

Dlamini-Zuma was well qualified for the new post and well connected with the ANC elites, and she had practical experience as a
medical doctor. It has therefore been a source of great puzzlement why
she and her successor as minister of health, Dr. Manto Tshabalala-
Msimang, should have been so contrary and reactionary in leading
government AIDS interventions and programs. As minister of health,
Dlamini-Zuma was a central player in efforts to get the large international pharmaceutical companies to reduce the price of drugs used to
treat AIDS and other tropical diseases, especially tuberculosis. Ironically, she then refused to allow government hospitals to dispense the
antiretroviral drug AZT, and prevented the use of Nevirapine in government hospitals for prevention of mother-to-child transmission of
HIV until she was forced to do so by a court order. Her major legacy
in public health legislation was the passage of the Tobacco Products
Control Bill in 1999, which effectively prevented smoking in all public
places. Effective government-driven AIDS programs languished while
smokers were cleared out of pubs, government buildings, and other
establishments. Under Dlamini-Zuma's leadership, the South African
Department of Health also went off in a number of other strange directions. Several of these were extraordinary scandals that did little to
advance the cause of AIDS prevention and undermined the credibility
of the South African government's ability to manage an AIDS prevention program.

The Sarafina II Scandal

One of Dlamini-Zuma's first efforts as minister of health was to commission an extraordinarily expensive musical entertainment. In 1994,
the European Union had granted the South African Department of
Health eleven million ecus for AIDS prevention programs.[26] During
June 1995 the Department of Health decided that a play or musical
that presented the message in the form of popular entertainment would
be a useful way to proceed. Mbongeni Ngema, a well-known producer

of South African musicals was hand picked to produce it. Ngema's previous hit musical, *Sarafina*, featured high-energy Zulu song and dance with a weak story line about political struggle. It had been a great success in New York and London around the time of Nelson Mandela's release from prison. With the eyes of the world focused on South Africa, this play had highlighted South African cultural achievements and had presented the struggle against apartheid in a highly positive light. A film version was the first South African production to be screened at the Cannes Film Festival. It was perhaps not surprising that the Minister of Health would have thought that musical theater might be an appropriate medium in which to promote a new HIV and AIDS prevention program. Intentional or not, the idea for basing an AIDS prevention message on an antiapartheid film fused the South African politics of struggle with the public health problem of AIDS. This might have been effective had it not run so rapidly off the rails during the financial free-for-all that developed around the newly powerful ANC elite as it took over the state and its resources.

According to the subsequent report of the Office of the Public Protector, Ngema gave an initial estimate of eight hundred thousand rand for the development of an AIDS prevention play. The Health Department then formulated a plan to develop a touring play that would be culturally sensitive and that would tour all of South Africa for twelve months. According to the Office of the Public Prosecutor, the terms of the tender were as follows:

> To supply a detailed script/framework and costing of the production.
>
> The theatre production must consist of a play and music around the theme of HIV/AIDS awareness and prevention in South Africa. The play must be culturally sensitive to all people in South Africa. The company must have the capacity and infrastructure to tour the production countrywide for 12 months. The most important aspect of this play is the complete quality in all respects of the production. It must therefore be stressed that the highest quality must be obtained in the production and not the least cost.
>
> The opening of the play must take place on the first of December 1995. Consultation with the National HIV/AIDS and STD Programmes is essential.
>
> The company must be committed not only to the prevention of HIV/ AIDS and STD in South Africa, but the overall development of all its people.[27]

Ignoring the usual bidding procedures, the government AIDS Directorate invited bids from only three entertainment companies, and two companies presented bids. One of them was Mbongeni Ngema's Committed Artists Theatre Company. The short time scale, political qualifications, and other specifics clearly favored Ngema, who already had *Sarafina I* in production. Ngema's tender of fourteen million rand for the production of *Sarafina II* was accepted over the tender of six hundred thousand rand from the other company. Predictably, *Sarafina II* was a slightly remodeled version of the earlier international hit musical, with the same cast and story. It was first performed on World AIDS Day, 1 December 1995. The opening was attended by the European Community ambassador, Erwan Fouéré.

Clearly, European Community funds were misused in this project, and an investigation was immediately launched. The affair soon escalated to the level of international scandal. The play itself was never seen again, and the contract was withdrawn. The Office of the Public Protector was requested by the principal opposition party, the Democratic Party, to investigate, and the report of the public protector, Selby Baqwa, was submitted to Parliament in May 1996. Baqwa's principle finding was simply that normal tender procedures had been ignored. Later that year, it was reported that an anonymous donor had come forward with 10.5 million rand to pay for *Sarafina II* so that the European Union funds could be returned. Since the donor did not wish to be identified, there were fears that this involved some measure of influence buying or other corruption, or that there was no such donor and the funds were actually coming from ANC party sources or from elsewhere in the government budget. The minister of health declared that because they could no longer ensure the anonymity of the donor, the offer had been retracted.[28] In any case, nothing more was heard of the recycled play, whose message about AIDS was weak in any case. It was not until 1998 that a special investigative unit pursued criminal charges against Ngema and managed to recover some of the government funds that had been spent on his play, most of which had been used to buy automobiles and to build an expensive house in Durban. By April 1999, Ngema had declared bankruptcy.

The rationale behind this entertainment/education effort remained obscure. In her report to Parliament, Dlamini-Zuma insisted, "Theatre, as an art form, is no doubt a very powerful instrument for spreading health messages." She accepted the charge "that there were problems with administrative procedures and financial controls" but concluded that "the play was a good idea."[29] Noting that HIV prevalence among pregnant women in KwaZulu-Natal was already 18.2 percent, and in Mpumalanga 16.2 percent, the health minister declared her wish to "recommit my Department to the struggle against HIV/AIDS, which is a deadly scourge in our society." She suggested that the criticism of the play by the public was because the play was about condoms. She countered that "it is not my intention to promote sex and promiscuity among teenagers" by advocating condoms, but insisted: "It should also be recorded that the message must also be very clear and simple. The major lesson from the play is indeed: "If you cannot abstain use a condom.' Considering that 392 out of 1,000 children are born of children and the use of condoms does prevent unwanted pregnancies, sexually transmitted diseases (STDs) and HIV/AIDS, I submit to you that even if that was the only message that the youth could learn, then that is possibly enough."[30]

Clearly, if the words of the minister of health can be taken to represent the views of the government of South Africa at the time, there was a large gap between the understanding of the enormity of the threat and the quality of the response. The slogan the government used, "if you cannot abstain, use a condom," had been borrowed from the Ugandan ABC program. Community theater, plays, and music had also been an exceptionally important tool in Uganda's AIDS programs, but *Sarafina II* was a far cry from what Uganda had done. An expensive, commercially successful play that had been a musical hit in New York was an unlikely vehicle to carry the AIDS message to all South Africans, most of whom did not speak English or live in areas where the expensive lights and sound equipment could even be plugged in. The health minister diluted the concern with AIDS in her justification of the expenditure by mentioning the high rate of teen pregnancy and the prevalence of other sexually transmitted diseases. In short, the South African government at that time had no clear policy direction and was not certain how to implement the limited policy that it had.

By contrast, the use of music, dance, and theater to transmit messages about AIDS was highly effective in Uganda because Uganda's efforts were entirely home-grown, low-tech, and easily accessible. Plays were written by school children and teachers, not professionals. Music was local, often based in local idioms and languages. Plays were scripted and performed by members of local communities in their communities. This was not the case in South Africa.

The scandal over *Sarafina II* and its technological and financial excesses were soon eclipsed, however, by events around fast tracking the so-called miracle cure for AIDS known as Virodene.

The Virodene Scandal

In 1997, Dlamini-Zuma formally accepted claims by a company called Cryopreservation Technologies in Stellenbosch, South Africa, that it had a cure for AIDS. The company called it Virodene. She and Mbeki, then deputy president, began to promote Virodene as a miracle cure for AIDS partly on the basis that this was a South African invention and represented an African solution to an African problem. They agreed to try to accelerate its acceptance by the Medicines Control Council (MCC), the statutory body charged with certifying the safety and efficacy of all new drugs, and awarded its developer 3.7 million rand for further research.[31] When the MCC refused to approve clinical trials on the reasonable grounds that there was no evidence of Virodene's effectiveness, but considerable evidence of its toxicity, they accused the MCC of unjustified interference in their scheme to promote the drug. This cure turned out to be a highly toxic industrial solvent, dimethylformamide. In tones that indicated Mbeki's sense of betrayal by the MCC, he wrote about the matter in the March 1998 ANC newsletter.

> More than twelve months ago, emanating from a request the Minister of Health [Nkosazana Dlamini-Zuma] presented through me [Thabo Mbeki], the Cabinet listened to a presentation by the Virodene researchers. Cabinet also had the privilege to hear the moving testimonies of AIDS sufferers who had been treated with Virodene, with seemingly very encouraging results. The Cabinet took the decision that it would support the Virodene research, up to the completion of the MCC processes. So far, this has not necessitated any financial or other material support. The Cabinet has not changed its mind on this issue. Those in Government, who deal with this matter directly, including the Minister of Health and myself, will continue to [promote Virodene] until Government policy changes. The importance of this is further emphasised by the fact that our entire system of government, from the national to the local level, has begun implementing a programme of action of sustained national mobilisation to intensify the offensive against the spread of HIV/AIDS.

Mbeki then cited some scientists who were willing to support the company's claims, and concluded his message,

> Alas, "the local review board," the MCC, still refuses to accept the application, despite its knowledge of the unanimous opinion of these "learned

and highly qualified professionals," and whose credentials it is perfectly aware of.

To confirm its determined stance against Virodene, and contrary to previous practice, the MCC has, with powers to decide who shall live or die, also denied dying AIDS sufferers the possibility of "mercy treatment" to which they are morally entitled.

I and many others will not rest until the efficacy or otherwise of Virodene is established scientifically. If nothing else, all those infected by HIV/AIDS need to know as a matter of urgency.[32] [All quoted phrases appear as in the original]

The details of any experiments or drug trials that may have taken place in the research on Virodene were never released. Dlamini-Zuma and Mbeki, as minister of health and deputy president, reacted to what they perceived as the arrogance of the MCC. They had presented Virodene as an indigenous discovery that promised, if not a cure for AIDS, then a mercy treatment to which those who were dying were morally entitled. Their willingness to believe that such miracles were possible, entirely outside of normal scientific practice, indicates the depth of their denial that AIDS was in fact the most serious epidemic facing South Africa. Although it was true that tuberculosis and malaria killed more people than AIDS at the time Virodene was being discussed, by 2004 AIDS had indeed become the leading cause of death in South Africa.[33] Their sense of *moral* outrage, too, strongly suggests that they continued to see HIV as a moral problem rather than a normal illness. Some years later, Mbeki spelled out the grounds for his moral outrage and most of the rationale for his apparent rejection of the science of HIV and AIDS (views he probably still holds) in an ANC document.[34]

In 1999, when Mbeki was elected president and Nelson Mandela stepped down, Dlamini-Zuma was "redeployed" (in the terminology of the ANC ruling party, which prides itself on its high degree of command and control from the center) as minister of foreign affairs.[35] In her place, Mbeki appointed Manto Tshabalala-Msimang, who has carried on the tradition of denialism.

While these dramas played themselves out at the top of the political hierarchy, considerable and extraordinary development of health care, including AIDS prevention and the provision of ARVs and highly active antiretroviral treatment regimes, had already begun in private hospitals and was carried out secretly in some public hospitals on a limited basis. This served as a kind of counterbalance to the misdirected leadership from the Department of Health and Office of the President. The process of grassroots development and civil society action in opposition to government, well established in apartheid South Africa, now began to grow in response to government attitudes to HIV and AIDS.

HEALTH LEGISLATION AND POLICY

In the period since 1994, the South African Parliament has passed twenty-nine separate pieces of legislation relating to health care providers and public health. These have covered important aspects not only of biomedical practice, nursing, and pharmaceutical provision and dispensing, but also alternative medical practices such as traditional healers, chiropractic, and homeopathy. These have transformed South African health care in profound ways by making many medications cheaper and improving service delivery to the poor and in rural areas. None of this legislation, however, has directly addressed HIV and AIDS.

The ANC government inherited a health care system that was highly fragmented and that emphasized curative care, high-tech urban hospitals, and the private sector.[36] Great strides have indeed been made to broaden the reach of public health initiatives and to make provision for primary health care clinics and better-serviced hospitals outside of the urban areas and for the poor.

In 2000, Minister of Health Tshabalala-Msimang approved a five-year plan that was meant to guide the government's response through 2005. The process began, when she came to office in 1999, with a meeting that was meant to draw on as many sectors of the population and stakeholders as possible. This included "faith-based organisations, people living with HIV infection and AIDS, human rights organisations, academic institutions, the civil military alliance, the Salvation Army, the media, organised labour, organised sports, organised business, insurance companies, women's organisations, youth organisations, international donor organisations, health professionals and health consulting organisations, political parties, and relevant government departments."[37] In addition, the resulting plan also noted that the minister consulted traditional healers in bilateral meetings. The new minister of health gave the impression that there had been a broad poll of public opinion and stakeholder interests. Conspicuous by their absence, however, were the AIDS Consortium and the TAC—both offshoots of the AIDS Law Project—and other civil society organizations that had begun to oppose the government. While sports organizations and the Salvation Army were given a hearing, the most active civil society organizations concerned with AIDS and most of South Africa's leading AIDS scientists were left out of the loop.

The HIV situation by then was already reaching extreme proportions in some places. In KwaZulu-Natal Province in 1997, a prevalence of 63 percent was reported in one pediatric ward in a tertiary hospital,[38] while an adult medical ward in the same province tested 54 percent HIV-positive[39] and a gynecology ward in a district hospital yielded a figure of 42 percent.[40] In Gauteng Province, in the pediatric ward in a tertiary-level hospital one study found 29 percent already infected in 1996,[41] while 18 percent of those in another pediatric ward were HIV-positive in 1998.[42] While overall HIV prevalence was found to be 22.4 percent and 32.5 percent in antenatal clinics in KwaZulu-Natal, according to the planning document,[43] many hospital wards already had a large burden of HIV-infected patients. The HIV/AIDS/STD Strategic Plan for South Africa, 2000–2005, committed the government to following the global guidelines for HIV and AIDS care, prevention, testing, and monitoring that had been provided by the United Nations General Assembly Special Session on HIV/AIDS, the World Health Organization, and the United Nations Programme on HIV/AIDS. HIV monitoring at antenatal clinic sentinel sites was augmented with strict data collection protocols that insured accurate data collection. Voluntary counseling and testing centers were set up at most major hospitals.

Review of the achievements since NACOSA, however, was disappointing. Lack of trained personnel, inadequate funding, failure to develop previously envisioned bureaucratic structures, lack of provincial level policies and people to drive them, and absence of management protocols for prevention, care, and testing, among many other failures, were highlighted by the five-year plan. To remedy this, the government appointed the deputy president and former husband of the minister of health, Jacob Zuma, to drive new initiatives within government and to strengthen an intersectoral and interdepartmental response with specific targets. There were also some shortcomings in the plan. As Leclerc-Madlala points out, the plan "appears to mean little more than improved co-ordination and collaboration between various government ministries."[44] It took almost no notice of civil society, or of organizations outside of the government and the ANC party structures.

The plan noted, however, "The immediate determinants of the epidemic include behavioural factors such as unprotected sexual intercourse and multiple sexual partners," while the "underlying causes include socio-economic factors such as poverty, migrant labour, commercial sex workers, the low status of women, illiteracy, the lack of formal education, stigma and discrimination." On paper, then, South Africa's plan for dealing with HIV and AIDS showed promise.

Just as the plan was being adopted, President Mbeki began to voice severe doubts about the direction the government was apparently taking.

CHAPTER 9

Imagining AIDS

South Africa's Viral Politics

MBEKI'S DENIALISM — ITS ROOTS AND BRANCHES

The roots of what has come to be called President Thabo Mbeki's "denialism" are undeniably deep in South African soil. Its branches are discernable in many aspects of health beliefs and medical practice in South Africa. It is far too simple to call it a denial. It points to a world of meanings—a worldview—that links almost every aspect of health and illness to the social rather than the medical. It is not a denial of knowledge or a denial of science and medicine. It is a refusal to bring into the mind's eye, the imagination, a vision of the community of sufferers and the cause of their suffering.

President Mbeki has been in the forefront of efforts to reduce violent conflict in Africa, and to reform governments across the continent. He led the continent in formation of the African Union (AU), a new continentwide organization that has replaced the old, corrupt, and somnolent Organisation of African Unity. The AU instituted a program of peer review of African governments by other Africans in order to lead the continent toward good government and economic development. In the eyes of many South Africans, Mbeki is more concerned with the rest of Africa than he is with his own country. In most areas of government, Mbeki's leadership has been excellent, and he has earned high approval ratings across the South African political and racial spectrum. Early in his presidency he announced the coming of the African

Renaissance. Although it was not entirely clear what this might mean, it has been taken as a call for African pride, African sovereignty, and a rebirth of African self-reliance. Mbeki has helped to negotiate peaceful settlements of several violent conflicts in Africa, set up the New Partnership for Africa's Development, was instrumental in development of the AU constitution and its institutions, and has campaigned strongly at world forums for reduction of debt and increased aid for African development.

As admirable as these efforts have been, they have had negative impacts, as well. The premise of solidarity between African governments, for example, has led him to ignore the steady decline into chaos, poverty, and starvation of Zimbabwe, South Africa's neighbor. With respect to AIDS, it has led him to recruit other African countries into his contrarian positions on HIV, use of antiretroviral (ARV) drugs, condoms, and educational interventions. The successes and the failures are part of a package intricately bound up with a commitment to Africanism—which implies finding a distinctive African way to solve problems of society and governance—and a politicization of most issues that might have simpler, more technical solutions.

Between 31 May and 5 June 2006, delegates from around the world met in New York for the United Nations General Assembly Special Session on HIV/AIDS (UNGASS). The meeting was meant to review progress toward goals set in 2001 for dealing with AIDS. There, a consortium of countries led by Gabon (as the current president of the AU) and South Africa sought to undermine previous agreements made in Abuja, Nigeria, in 2001 (the Abuja Declaration). This initiative by the UN offered progressive evidence-based methods and commitments for fighting AIDS. Gabon represented the concerns of African states with Islamic majorities. With the support of the South African government delegation, it sought to exclude reference to homosexuality, sex workers, and women and young girls, all of whom are especially vulnerable to HIV infection. The South African delegation has also sought to exclude mention of specific targets for provision of ARV therapy, suggesting that it did not want the government to be held accountable for the chronically slow provision of ARVs across South Africa.

Before the meeting, however, the South African Department of Health had already moved to exclude the AIDS Law Project (ALP) and the Treatment Action Campaign (TAC) from accreditation at UNGASS 2006. A number of civil organizations had also prepared a memorandum to Kofi Anan, the secretary general of the United Nations, to point out the inadequacies of the South African Department of Health's own report to UNGASS. Apart from its exclusion of key stakeholders, the report failed to include or misrepresented statistics on HIV mortality, HIV prevalence, tuberculosis and HIV incidence, and the total number of patients receiving ARV treatment. In keeping with the government's desire not to be held to promises, the report also omitted ARV treatment targets.[1] A representative from Open Society South Africa, Sisonke Msimang, commented, "Our [African] states have behaved in the most shocking fashion. . . . Our missions have been complacent and disorganised at best, and in the case of Gabon and South Africa, obstructionist."[2] The organization of African states that Mbeki had worked hard to create was now supporting him in his campaign to undermine AIDS prevention.

Just two weeks earlier, on 19 May, Nozipho Bhengu, the daughter of a South African member of Parliament, had died of AIDS and as a result of following the advice of the minister of health, Manto Tshabalala-Msimang. Nozipho's mother, Ruth Bhengu, had made headlines in 2001 by announcing in Parliament that her daughter was suffering from AIDS-related illnesses but was doing well because she was following the nutritional advice of the minister of health, eating a diet rich in garlic, ginger, olive oil, lemon juice, beetroot, and vitamins provided by Matthias Rath,[3] yet another charlatan offering an AIDS cure, like Virodene (see chapter 8), with the imprimatur of the South African government. The peculiar diet had been devised by Tine van der Maas, a former nurse and self-taught nutritionist, who managed to convince the health minister that it was an effective cure for AIDS. In 2005, an apparently healthy Nozipho had declared the diet effective after having been on it for three years. "It works. I am the scientific proof," she claimed.[4] Early in 2006, Nozipho had said that she was writing a book, *From Victim to Victor,* about the success of her diet. She died of AIDS before the book was completed.[5]

The vitamin salesman Matthias Rath has contributed to the deaths of many other AIDS victims. TAC has documented a number of these.[6] Seriously ill people have been recruited by Rath and his team at the Rath Foundation in Cape Town to participate in drug trials that are conducted illegally and without scientific protocols. These are apparently protected by the minister of health, who refuses to prosecute and continues to promote their products.

In spite of all this, in a letter to the *Mail & Guardian* newspaper published on 9 June 2006, Minister of Health Tshabalala-Msimang declared triumphantly, "We were right all along," referring to the views she and the president had expressed. She declared that her report to UNGASS had been an outstanding success. "Returning to New York last week for the review of the Declaration of Commitment on HIV/ AIDS was gratifying," she began. She said that the meeting showed "how far the world has come to accept what President Thabo Mbeki sought to highlight as early as 2000." She ignored the issue of treatment entirely in saying that "Secretary General Kofi Anan . . . recognised that poverty, underdevelopment and gender inequality are among the principal contributing factors to the spread of HIV and AIDS." This, she said, had been the basis of the South African government response all along. She also emphasized that "promoting a healthy lifestyle, . . . traditional medicine and other therapies" were the priorities of her department.[7]

At the International HIV/AIDS Conference in Toronto in August 2006, the minister further embarrassed South Africa by setting up an amateur-looking booth with bowls of beetroot, garlic, and lemons. The United Nations' special envoy for HIV/AIDS in Africa, Stephen Lewis, condemned Tshabalala-Msimang and President Mbeki, saying that their "theories [were] more worthy of a lunatic fringe than of a concerned and compassionate state." He added that, in his opinion, "they can never achieve redemption" and that they know "what they are doing is wrong."[8] Even Tshabalala-Msimang's deputy in the Department of Health, Nozizwe Madlala-Routledge, said that the booth was an "embarrassment."[9]

By the end of September 2006, there were movements to put South Africa on a better course. The powerful Congress of South African Trade Unions, a partner of the African National Congress (ANC) and the minuscule South African Communist Party in a tripartite alliance, voted at its meeting on 19 September to adopt a resolution that said, "the time for conflicting and confusing messages about HIV/AIDS is over."[10] The deputy president of South Africa, Phumzile Mlambo-Ngcuka, attempted to address the meeting to explain the new government position, but she was shouted down, as other members of government had been before. They blamed her husband, Charles Ngcuka, for the prosecution and removal of the former deputy president, Jacob Zuma.

By the middle of October, the minister of health was taken to hospital with what was described as an "acute respiratory illness." No further information was made available about her illness until March 2007, but in her absence, Deputy President Mlambo-Ngcuka moved to take over the government's AIDS programs. At a meeting of the South African National AIDS Council in later October, Mlambo-Ngcuka announced that a new five-year National Strategic Plan on HIV and AIDS would be announced on 1 December, World AIDS Day. The old plan had expired in 2005, without action from Minister Tshabalala-Msimang. At the end of October, the deputy minister of health, Nozizwe Madlala-Routledge, appeared to have taken charge of the department's AIDS program. She said that she and the deputy president had been in consultation with TAC for the past three months, and had obtained agreement from the Cabinet that foods such as garlic and beetroot, although good for health, are not alternatives to antiretrovirals. They announced new targets for action, to be achieved by 2011, including treating 650,000 people with ARVs (175,000 were being treated at that time), distributing 500 million condoms annually (340 million were being distributed annually), promoting mutual faithfulness, and reducing by a modest 10 percent the number of children under age 14 who engage in sex.[11] Nevertheless, a few days later, the Office of the President responded that Tshabalala-Msimang was still in charge of the AIDS programs, but by 10 December the Office of the President recanted, saying that Madlala-Routledge would maintain control even after the minister returned to work briefly from her extended hospital stay.[12] Her husband, Mendi Msimang, the treasurer-general of the ruling ANC, had intervened to prevent her being fired.[13] Apparently, the "time for conflicting and confusing messages" was still not over, and a TAC spokesperson said that the organization was "not popping Champagne corks yet."

Tshabalala-Msimang did not return to her ministry until June 2007. She was clearly still ill and was gravely thin, the nature of her illness still undisclosed. Although back at work, she refused to attend the Third South African AIDS Conference in Durban, convened 4–8 June, because she felt that the organizers had snubbed her by not giving her a major speaking role.[14] Her deputy, Madlala-Routledge, also withdrew, apparently in sympathy.

It is difficult to understand these tragedies and travesties, but the roots of Mbeki's denialism, and that of the two ministers of health in the New South Africa, can be traced to two things. First, there is a determination to find an "African solution to African problems." This is an oft-repeated slogan, to which President Mbeki and his government were deeply committed. On the positive side, this commitment has led to the founding of the new AU and to unprecedented economic and political development in South Africa. But, this commitment also helps to explain the *Sarafina II* and Virodene scandals (see chapter 8) and the government's denialism. This idea has close parallels with the thinking of South African traditional healers who say that if the ancestors (*madloti*) knew about AIDS, then surely they must know how to cure it from the resources of the African bush. In defense of her HIV salad display at the Toronto International HIV/AIDS Convention, Tshabalala-Msimang argued that "more than 80 percent of people on the [African] continent use traditional medicine," merging her own advocacy of an idiosyncratic diet with so-called traditional medicine.[15] It is also similar to the go-it-alone attitude during apartheid of the previous ruling party, the white Afrikaans-dominated National Party.

The era of government-approved efforts to create an African solution is by no means over. In July 2007, the University of Cape Town suspended Girish Kotwal, a chief of medical virology at the Institute of Infectious Diseases and principal investigator in the university's medical biotechnology program; he subsequently resigned. He and his laboratory staff had conducted unauthorized clinical tests of their herbal remedy called Secomet V—a plant extract—on HIV-positive people.[16] Kotwal had organized a conference on natural products and molecular therapy in South Africa in January 2005, which Tshabalala-Msimang attended. She claimed that research on natural remedies such as this "provide[s] an opportunity to reclaim our [African] scientific and socio-cultural heritage, which was stigmatised and discredited as primitive rituals and witchcraft during many years of colonialism and apartheid." She claimed that a false division between African traditional medicine and biomedicine had been created "by the need to make money from patented drugs through discrediting the use of natural products."[17]

In addition to the desire for African solutions, there is a belief that AIDS is some sort of trick foisted on Africa by major Western pharmaceutical companies. Many believe that, at best, this is rooted in racist myths, or, at worst, in actual racist agendas pursued by shadowy forces of multinational corporations. Many are suspicious of the methods used to combat AIDS, such as promotion of condoms (which some fear are dangerous) or promotion of abstinence (which some see as denigrating sex, and black sexuality in particular). This is similar to the discourse of the traditional healers who say that if AIDS is, in fact, incurable, then the African spirits and ancestors that guide African healing must not know about it, and therefore it must come from outside Africa. Far from being a wild and unmotivated invention of the political elite, then, Mbeki's denialism is consistent with at least some popular beliefs of the ordinary South African.

There has also been intervention, however, from a number of Western scientists, led by Peter Duesberg, of the Department of Molecular and Cell Biology at the University of California, Berkeley, and David Rasnick, who until February 2003 had been associated with the same department. Their papers and research in the late 1990s and early 2000s evidently convinced President Mbeki that HIV did not cause AIDS and that AIDS was a lifestyle disease caused by recreational drug use and by misguided use of AZT and other ARV medications. Duesberg and Rasnick denied that there was any connection between HIV and AIDS and that, in the words that President Mbeki used to paraphrase their findings, "a single virus cannot cause a syndrome [AIDS]." (In her 9 June 2006 letter to the *Mail & Guardian,* Tshabalala-Msimang reaffirmed this view, saying, "we could not blame the challenge of HIV/AIDS only on the virus.")[18] Given his Africanist ideology, Mbeki's reliance on Duesberg and Rasnick and the faith placed in Rath's vitamin cocktails and Tine van der Maas's diets may seem surprising, since none are South African. Duesberg is a German-born American and Rasnick is American, while Rath is German, and van der Maas is Dutch. Nevertheless, their message is consistent with Mbeki's beliefs and commitments. With much of the rest of South Africa, Mbeki appears to accept the view that disease and death are caused by social forces, including other people, lifestyle, witches, bad attitudes, and food. These beliefs are largely unchallenged by the high degree of medical pluralism that exists in South Africa: there is always another therapy. No system of healing or medical treatment appears to have hegemonic status in South Africa. Biomedical (allopathic) medicine competes with homeopathic, chiropractic, osteopathic, New Age, traditional African, Christian faith healing, Chinese, Islamic, and Hindu healing practices, and use of patent medicine, food supplements, and herbs (African, Asian, European), among many others. In this context, biomedical explanations, preventive strategies, and approaches are taken by the South African public as one option among many.

Duesberg and Rasnick's denialism was based on their observations about the course of the HIV epidemic, especially in the United States and Europe in the last two decades of the twentieth century (see chapter 2). They listed ten "facts" about the epidemic, including that it was not infectious since health workers in contact with AIDS patients had not been infected; that there was no one *defining* illness but rather a "syndrome," whereas other viruses caused a discrete disease such as chicken pox or poliomyelitis; and that the epidemic progressed nonexponentially, just like a lifestyle disease (such as lung cancer due to smoking, or obesity, or diabetes).[19] They believed that they could show that "recreational drug use was a common denominator for over 95% of all American and European AIDS patients" and, therefore, that "HIV proves to be an ideal surrogate marker for recreational and anti-HIV drug [ARV] use."[20] Their denialism was based on their misinterpretation of the HIV prevalence trends in the United States and Europe, but was wholly accepted by President Mbeki (see chapter 1). He included Duesberg and Rasnick on his Presidential International Panel of Scientists on HIV/AIDS in Africa to advise him on AIDS policy. Despite the presence of other scientists who conclusively disproved the denialist position, Mbeki has clung to his beliefs.

In a number of speeches between 1999 and 2001, Mbeki presented the denialist position to South Africa. He stopped just short of implementing the position in policy. In fact, the Department of Health, led by factions who disagreed strongly with the president and the minister of health, struggled to develop a rational AIDS policy in spite of their leadership. Mbeki was persuaded to keep his ideas to himself. Almost. In April 2002, Mbeki announced that the government would proceed with treatment based "on the premise that HIV causes AIDS."[21] Stopping just short of acknowledging that HIV causes AIDS *as fact*, the government agreed to proceed *as if* HIV caused AIDS.

In early 2002, an anonymous, forty-thousand-word document arguing the denialist position, titled "Castro Hlongwane, caravans, cats, geese, foot & mouth and statistics: HIV/AIDS and the struggle for the humanisation of the African," began to circulate within the ranks of the ANC.[22] The document was traced to Mbeki's computer by means of the document's Microsoft Word properties. A coauthor was also identified: Peter Mokaba, who died, probably of AIDS, the following year. The document has not been repudiated by the ANC or withdrawn from circulation.[23]

The effect of the document was dire. Edwin Cameron, now a justice of the Supreme Court of Appeal and founder of the ALP, wrote, "The distribution of the ANC document—and suggestions that its provenance commanded high approval—cast a sombre shadow over the AIDS debate in South Africa. Within influential government circles, for agonising months, eventually years, public debate about AIDS, its treatment and its causes seemed to come to a virtual dead stop. Support for the facts about HIV transmission and AIDS treatment seemed a heresy to which no government minister would adhere."[24]

The document begins with a number of quotations, including one from the author's preface to the novel *The Constant Gardener* by John Le Carré: "As my journey through the pharmaceutical jungle progressed (in which a number of people were murdered, others killed with experimental drugs, and governments and universities corrupted), I came to realise that, by comparison with the reality, my story was as tame as a holiday postcard."[25] The document takes this as its theme, and accuses the pharmaceutical industry of having "manufactured" the AIDS epidemic in order to sell highly expensive and ultimately toxic drugs to unsuspecting Africans.

The document is a jeremiad couched in the legalistic style of a formal petition for redress. The authors declare that the "monograph discusses the vexed question of HIV/AIDS . . . based on the assumption that to understand this matter, it is necessary to study it." Fifty-three "theses" are then proposed, in the manner of a constitutional preamble or of Martin Luther's ninety-five theses posted on the door of the Wittenberg Cathedral at the start of the Protestant Reformation in Europe. Each one begins with one or another of the phrases "It [the document] accepts . . . ," or "It rejects . . . ," or "It recognises . . . ." The leading thesis declares that the document "does not accept the assertion that only scientists and medical doctors are capable of understanding this medical condition" and that "there are many unanswered scientific questions about the HIV/AIDS thesis and many hypotheses about this matter that are falsely presented as facts."

Among the fifty-three theses are the following, which effectively summarize the thrust and intention of the document.

> It recognises the reality that there are many people and institutions across the world that have a vested interest in the propagation of the HIV/AIDS thesis, because they have too much to lose if any important element of this thesis is proved to be false.

> It accepts that these include the pharmaceutical companies, which are marketing anti-retroviral drugs that can only be sold, and therefore generate profits, on the basis of the universal acceptance of the assertion that "HIV causes AIDS."

> It also accepts that the HIV/AIDS thesis as it has affected and affects Africans and black people in general, is also informed

by deeply entrenched and centuries-old white racist beliefs
and concepts about Africans and black people. At the same
time as this thesis is based on these racist beliefs and concepts,
it makes a powerful contribution to the further entrenchment
and popularisation of racism.

It rejects as baseless and self-serving the assertion that millions
of our people are HIV positive.

It rejects as fundamentally incorrect and anti-democratic the
attempt to transfer the responsibility to look after oneself to
the state, which seeks to turn the state into an omnipotent
apparatus that must even police the sexual activities of every
individual South African.

It argues for loyalty to the truth and a refusal on the part of
the government and the people to succumb to pressures that
are directed at serving particular commercial and political interests at the expense of the health of our people.

It rejects the assertion that, as Africans, we are prone to rape and
abuse of women and that we uphold a value system that belongs
to the world of wild animals, and that this accounts for the alleged
"high incidence" of "HIV infection" in our country.

It enjoins all our people to think for themselves, refusing to be
intimidated or terrorised by those who have powerful voices
and the backing of the fabulous wealth we do not have, because
we are poor.

The document declares in the most forceful language possible Mbeki's
commitment to an "own way" of his own devising, one that is based
in an overwhelming fear of conspiracy by the pharmaceutical industries to sell drugs at any cost, and a deep loathing of what he sees as
a racist agenda behind it. There can be no doubt that in some cases,
international pharmaceutical companies have tested, marketed, and
even "dumped" drugs on poor populations in the third world, and that
there is more than a suspicion of blame. The movie version of John Le
Carré's novel is based on this premise. Both the movie and the novel
have sold exceptionally well, demonstrating that Mbeki is not the only
one to fear and loathe this fact. But there is no evidence that this has
actually happened in the case of AIDS and ARVs in Africa. In fact,
the South African government had already negotiated highly favor-
able price reductions for all AIDS medications. Boehringer Ingelheim

had offered the drug Nevirapine at no charge to government clinics for use in mother-to-child transmission (MTCT) prophylaxis, but the government had rejected its offer in the belief that it was toxic.[26] It is used (very successfully) for MTCT prophylaxis in all other countries, however.

The document also displays the personal pain of those who have watched their colleagues and friends die of AIDS. It tells in heroic terms the story of Parks Mankahlana, one of Mbeki's closest friends and advisors at the time, who, like Peter Mokaba, probably died of AIDS (though this was denied).[27] Mankahlana is portrayed as a loyal defender of the faith who sacrificed his life for truth.

> *Parks Mankahlana* rose from his deathbed to oppose this campaign against the President and the truth. He spoke in words that polite society, the friends of the Africans, considered unacceptable because they were not pretty.
>
> And then he died, vanquished by the anti-retroviral drugs he was wrongly persuaded to consume. He suffered from anaemia and received dedicated attention from his doctor. Nevertheless he died prematurely, because some, *other than his doctor* [emphasis in original], advised him to take anti-retroviral drugs.

The document concludes in the manner of the Communist Manifesto, rejecting the idea that Africans were, in the wording of the document, "sex crazy . . . and diseased," prone to "abuse women and the girl-child with gay abandon!" because Africans were a people among whom "rape is endemic because of our culture!"

> No longer will the Africans accept as the unalterable truth that they are a dependent people that emanates from and inhabits a continent shrouded in a terrible darkness of destructive superstition, driven and sustained by ignorance, hunger and underdevelopment, and that is victim to a self-inflicted "disease" called HIV/AIDS.
>
> *For centuries we have carried the burden of the crimes and falsities of "scientific" Eurocentrism, its dogmas imposed upon our being as the brands of a definitive, "universal" truth.* [emphasis in original]

Although there may indeed be people who believe such things, they were scarcely evident anywhere in South Africa. For evidence of racism, Mbeki quotes W. E. B. Dubois, the American writer and civil rights activist of the late nineteenth and early twentieth centuries, and Angela Davis, an American radical activist of the 1960s. The Castro Hlongwane of the title was a black child who was excluded from a caravan camp (a holiday destination) on the South African coast, where he had gone with his white school friends for an end of year party in December 2001. According to the *Sunday Times* newspaper, "Schoolmate Ryan Templar, 18, said he was told by [park owner] Theresa Smit that Hlongwane had AIDS and would rape other campers."[28] Although the document acknowledges that the proprietor of the holiday camp was "unsophisticated," it attributes these beliefs to "mature practitioners of the deceits of the sophisticated," by which it apparently means the president's critics.

These moral and ideological beliefs had little bearing on the public health crisis that AIDS presented. There is no evidence that South Africans, or black people in general, are "sex crazy . . . and diseased," as Mbeki asserted, and this document certainly does not present any convincing evidence. The source of Mbeki's fury expressed in the "Castro Hlongwane" jeremiad must lie in the models of struggle against and resistance to apartheid. But that battle had already been won. Mbeki's own presidency was proof of that.

The legacy of conflict between government and civil society is deeply etched in South Africa's politics, but Mbeki's document also strongly reflects his own educational background as a University of Sussex student and as political leader of the ANC's struggle against apartheid. His inspiration lies as much in English Romantic and revolutionist rhetoric as in South Africa. A quotation from the poet and Irish republican W. B. Yeats is the source of the "geese" in the title, while the American author and satirist Mark Twain is the source of the "cats." The Marxist humanist Herbert Marcuse is liberally quoted in the document, and the American anthropologist Paul Farmer's book *AIDS and accusation*, published in 1992, is given credit for showing that AIDS is a disease of poverty, a "misery seeking missile." The document states that "the South African Government has nevertheless put in place 'an anti-AIDS programme as good as any other anywhere in the world,' "[29] a view that Mbeki and his minister of health have restated many times since then. Their denialism or dissent, however groundless, cannot be attributed to anything but their best intentions for the country.

The denialist response to AIDS that Mbeki and those around him espouse repeats the pattern of political struggle rather than active engagement with good governance. Its effect has been to allow the needless deaths of many people; in fact, far more have died of AIDS than died during the violent period of armed resistance against apartheid, and far more than ever die of poverty in South Africa.[30] This claim was made by Costa Gazi, a medical doctor who worked in a government hospital and served as health secretary for the Pan African Congress. In April 1999, Dr. Gazi had said that the health minister, Nkosazana Dlamini-Zuma, was guilty of manslaughter as a result of her refusal to use AZT to prevent mother-to-child transmission of HIV. Dr. Gazi was fired by the enraged minister of health. After lengthy court proceedings, it was not until 24 March 2006 that a full bench of the Transvaal Provincial Division of the High Court handed down judgment in an appeal by Dr. Gazi against the minister of public services and administration and others.[31] The judgment concurred with Dr. Gazi's statements, noting that the minister of health's decision "amounted to a conscious, deliberate and informed policy to sacrifice the [lives] of babies that would contract HIV/AIDS because their mothers were not treated with AZT, in order to save the expense. . . . It is hardly surprising that some members of the medical profession and of the public at large would describe this policy as a murderous one."[32] TAC had also made formal charges of culpable homicide against the ministers of health (Tshabalala-Msimang), and trade and industry (Alec Erwin) in March 2003, but these were eventually dismissed by the court.

Mamphela Ramphele, a former colleague of the Black Consciousness leader Steve Biko (and the mother of his two children), a former head of the University of Cape Town, and a World Bank vice-president, has also called Mbeki's denialism "irresponsibility that borders on criminality."[33] The title of Catherine Campbell's 2003 book, *"Letting them die"*, echoes the words of the South African satirist and actor, Pieter-Dirk Uys: "In the old South Africa we killed people. Now we're just letting them die."[34] Campbell exposes the reasons for the failure of many AIDS programs in South Africa. She places great emphasis on the failure of government to build "bridging capital," consisting of "state-society synergy." Such synergies were vastly important in Uganda's reduction of HIV prevalence. She points to "national government disunity and vacillation over the existence and causes of AIDS" as major factors in the failure of an AIDS control project aimed at sex workers around a mine complex.

With more and more people suffering from AIDS or living with HIV, Mbeki and the minister of health sought to preserve the illusion of a well-mannered debate. They blamed the epidemic on "scientific Eurocentrism" and toxic ARVs, while their critics decried their stance as "murderous" and blamed government intransigence. Where government failed, nongovernmental organizations (NGOs) and organizations of civil society stepped in.

TREATMENT ACTION CAMPAIGN:
CIVIL SOCIETY'S RESPONSE

Despite the government's five-year plan of action for 2000 to 2005, most important steps against AIDS would not have been taken without strong pressure from outside of government and the ruling party. Foremost among these pressure groups has been TAC, which first appeared on the scene on Human Rights Day, 10 December 1998, with a manifesto to government to end "unnecessary suffering and AIDS-related deaths of thousands of people in Africa," which was caused, the manifesto said, by "poverty and the unaffordability of HIV/AIDS treatment."[35] TAC was, like the AIDS Consortium, a spinoff of ALP and initiated by the National Association of People Living with AIDS/ HIV. TAC was led by Zackie Achmat, who was himself living with HIV. The organization was launched on the steps of St. George Cathedral in Cape Town, the launching site of some of the most important social movements and civil disobedience campaigns against apartheid. As in the struggle against apartheid, the country's independent judiciary soon became one of the most important avenues for seeking redress.

In its initial statement, addressed to the then minister of health, Nkosazana Dlamini-Zuma, and the minister of finance, Trevor Manuel, the TAC manifesto demanded treatment, but not prevention. It held common cause with what then Deputy President Mbeki would later emphasize as his chief concerns: poverty and the power of the pharmaceutical industries. Despite this, the movement became deeply embroiled in constant protests, petitions to government, court action, and marches to protest government action or inaction regarding HIV/ AIDS, and to seek redress.

In May 2000, the five pharmaceutical companies that produced the major AIDS drugs (Glaxo Wellcome, Bristol Meyers Squibb, Roche, Merck, and Boehringer Ingelheim), together with the World Bank and UNAIDS, began negotiations to radically reduce the price of these drugs to South Africa and other needy countries. Access to the antiretroviral drugs—AZT, 3TC, DDI, and D4T—was TAC's primary goal, but provision of Diflucan (fluconazole), produced by Pfizer, was also essential for treating thrush and other fungal and yeast-type secondary infections. Early the next year, TAC staged mass demonstrations against the price of AIDS drugs. Led by Mark Heywood of ALP, a TAC team began negotiations with Pfizer to reduce the price. In October, when negotiations proved unsatisfactory, Zackie Achmat, the director of TAC, flew to Thailand, where locally produced generic fluconazole was sold for two rand per capsule, one-fortieth of the cost of Diflucan in South Africa. On his return, he brought three thousand capsules back with him in an act of civil disobedience—generic fluconazole was not registered in South Africa and therefore was illegal.[36] Courts declined to prosecute Achmat, however, and Pfizer agreed to donate fluconazole to four hundred of South Africa's three thousand public health facilities. A compromise was reached that did not flout patents protecting Pfizer's rights to Diflucan/fluconazole but did make it available to many of those who needed it. Supplies fell far short of total demand, however.

In August 2000, TAC took the minister of health to court to force the government to provide Nevirapine for prevention of mother-to-child HIV transmission, and won the case. The government initially consented, and then appealed the decision and referred the matter back to the Cabinet. After more than a year's delay, on 14 December 2001 TAC won the appeal against the minister of health and nine provincial members of executive council (MECs) for health, forcing the government to begin implementation of Nevirapine programs in all public hospitals that were equipped to do so. Then the government back-pedaled again (see figure 16). The case was eventually heard by the Constitutional Court, the highest in the land. The Constitutional Court issued an interim order and, in July 2002, issued a final order against the minister of health requiring the government to protect newborns from perinatal HIV infection by the best means possible, including (but not exclusively) the use of Nevirapine. The government was finally defeated in court, and effective drugs began to be used in government hospitals.[37] Despite continuing resistance from the Department of Health, by the middle of 2006 Nevirapine was finally available in all government hospitals to prevent mother-to-child HIV transmission, but only with a single dose at birth, and another at a six-week follow-up appointment, which few poor women attended. As one of only seven countries worldwide in which child mortality was rising, and in which ninety thousand children were infected with HIV each year, it was clear that the intervention was either already too late or insufficient. Medical researchers recommended using AZT with Nevirapine over a longer treatment period, but government healthcare workers were too fearful of "angering the health department" to implement the new program.[38]

By 2005, TAC and other organizations were more concerned with treatment than with prevention. Suzanne Leclerc-Madlala, an anthropologist whose research on AIDS and public response has often been essential to support for public action, expressed the view that the technical language of prevention—terms such as *risk profile, awareness,* and *sexual negotiation* for condom use and safer sex—"seemed to be from an age of innocence." With AIDS now infecting or affecting nearly everyone, the terrain had shifted from an emphasis on prevention to treatment as the only hope. Prevention seemed to be failing; treatment for those living with HIV and AIDS was now paramount.[39] Against this, the government continued to resist campaigns for treatment and continued to promote prevention with the bulk of the resources at its disposal. In this, the government was no doubt correct, but it seemed to flout the demands of the public, especially as represented by TAC, ALP, the AIDS Consortium, and other major NGOs.

As a result of pressure from the press, TAC, other NGOs, and professional organizations, on 8 August 2003 the South African Cabinet committed itself to the provision of ARV treatment in public hospitals. Three months later, the government published the *Operational plan for comprehensive care and treatment for people living with HIV and AIDS,* which was meant to guide the process. The plan stated that at least one ARV treatment point would be available and stocked in each of the fifty-three administrative districts in the nine provinces. The rollout, however, was unconscionably slow. The first public ARV service point was established in Gauteng Province in March 2004, and it was not until the end of 2005 that all fifty-three districts were served by at least one hospital. Still, it was not enough. Approximately 85,000 people were receiving treatment by the end of 2005, out of the 5.2 million who were infected. At least 520,000 of those infected required immediate ARV therapy at that time, but the model proposed in the operational plan suggested that 120,000 should be reached.[40] The results of the rollout were well below the target specified in the operational plan.[41] This failure was without doubt the primary reason that statistics were not reported to UNGASS in May 2006, and why all mention of specific targets was strenuously resisted by the South African delegation led by the minister of health.

TAC, often in association with other organizations, has continued to bring action against members of the government and others who

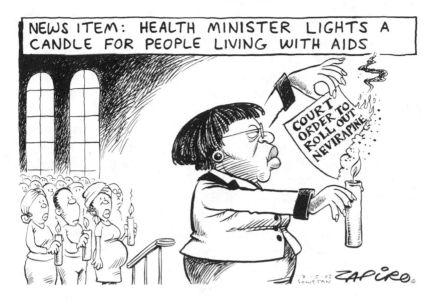

FIGURE 16. The minister of health, Manto Tshabalala-Msimang, defies court order requiring state provision of Nevirapine in cases of potential mother-to-child HIV transmission at birth. (© Zapiro and *Sowetan*)

refuse, or appear unable, to contribute to the rollout of treatment. For instance, in association with the South African Medical Association (the largest and principal organization of South African medical practitioners), TAC filed court papers against the minister of health, the Medicines Control Council (MCC), the Western Cape MEC for Health, the megavitamin promoter Matthias Rath, and the AIDS denialists Dr. David Rasnick and Dr. Sam Mhlongo, a professor of family medicine at the Medical University of South Africa. They also assisted prisoners in the Westville Correctional Centre in Kwa-Zulu Natal Province to file papers with the court requesting immediate access to ARV for prisoners. The case was filed in early May, and by the end of June the court issued orders compelling the provincial government to provide ARV therapy to prisoners. The Jali Commission, set up to investigate allegations of mismanagement in the South African Correctional Services Department, found that up to 90 percent of prisoners in South Africa were HIV-positive, due in large part to gang rapes and overcrowding in prisons.[42] These and other court actions have been exceptionally important in moving treatment ahead.

While resisting treatment with ARVs and promoting alternative therapies, including traditional healing, special diets, vitamins, and others, the government has invested heavily in prevention. The effectiveness of these efforts has remained difficult to measure, but the continuing rise in HIV prevalence and stable levels of incidence suggest that they may well be ineffective. Prevention messages have almost entirely been delivered by high-end media, such as large billboards erected and maintained by Primemedia and other major players in the entertainment and media industry. Many members of the new black middle and upper classes are heavily invested in these companies. The costly prevention strategy fits nicely with ANC policy aimed at rapidly developing a black managerial and professional class. Though billboards developed by LoveLife are often obscurely worded and overly clever, and often appear in languages inappropriate for their locations, South Africans are all highly mobile and this method does reach a large percentage of the public. The use of television is also justified by high levels of access across South Africa. In 2001, 44 percent of black African households had television sets, and this percentage has certainly increased greatly in subsequent years.[43] While LoveLife addresses the outdoor advertising, print, and other awareness programs targeted at schools and rural areas, Soul City produces and presents extremely popular TV programs. Due to questions about the effectiveness of LoveLife's approach, the Global Fund to Fight AIDS, Tuberculosis, and Malaria cut its funding to LoveLife at the end of 2005. Nevertheless, both programs continue to dominate the prevention scene in South Africa.

Although late in developing, there has been a powerful and more positive response to AIDS mounted by many organizations, churches, NGOs, and service organizations around South Africa. Their growth in numbers has been almost exponential (unlike the more linear progress of HIV prevalence), but not quite as rapid as the Ugandan response. For example, figure 17 shows the rapid increase in organizations dealing with children who are either infected with or affected by HIV and AIDS.

As the *Lancet* editorial suggests (see chapter 8 epigraph), something like a Truth and Reconciliation Commission is required not only to make AIDS appear as a clear and present danger to the fabric of South African life and livelihood, but also to compel action. The South African judicial system has played a central role in the response to AIDS. Court action has been constantly required to force government to take responsibility. The courts have acted as the primary interface between civil society awareness and government action. The

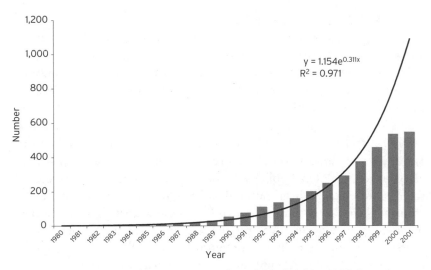

FIGURE 17. Exponential increase in number of South African NGOs and private organizations dealing with children and HIV/AIDS. (Data from the Children's Institute, University of Cape Town)

struggle against AIDS in South Africa, in other words, has taken on the dynamics of the struggle against apartheid, in which broad-based social movements, NGOs, and external donors have had to struggle against an intransigent government. Despite the "gulf of incomprehension that divides the African National Congress policy makers from their critics,"[44] the struggle against AIDS in South Africa has also been a struggle that engaged the modern institutions of a highly bureaucratic but democratic state. The sources of conflict lay in competing versions of modernity,[45] especially in differing understandings of how social factors generated the conditions and the causes of disease. The denialists seem truly to believe that poverty caused AIDS, a result of poor nutrition, a heavier burden of other diseases among the poor, and their victimization by powerful and wealthy multinational pharmaceutical corporations. They believe that their action is justified by an alternative science and by an astute political analysis of the effects of globalization, especially the greater threat posed by unscrupulous capitalists.

AIDS in South Africa has been understood, too, in terms of competing concepts of human rights. President Mbeki has couched his approach to AIDS in a commitment to an ideology of Africanism that prioritizes the right to an autonomous African identity that can create its own solutions for its own problems.[46] His Africanism, however, is predicated on a modernist discourse of development and self-determination. This places Africa at odds with the developed West while it seeks to achieve similar levels of social and economic development that will lead to full sovereignty, that is, to full power of self-determination as an autonomous actor in world politics. This also frequently places the government at odds with TAC and other NGOs and social movements that are rooted in the discourse of human rights, specifically the rights to life, health, and livelihood, which are guaranteed by the South African constitution. The president and his minister of health are involved in a global politics, then, while their opponents from civil society are engaged in a national politics of and for human rights. Ironically, this dichotomy is not unlike the one that divided government and people during the struggle against apartheid. These two differing visions of the political community and of South Africa's place in it have had profound implications for the way the struggle against AIDS has been fought.

The original Truth and Reconciliation Commission was set up by Bishop Desmond Tutu and others in order to present the truth of what happened during the struggle against the previous government for universal democracy and human rights. It aimed to normalize relations between government and the South African people, on the one hand, and to seek reconciliation between groups of people that had formerly been in deep and violent conflict. It also attempted to ensure justice, recommending punishment when this was appropriate and practical, and forgiveness wherever possible. But the Truth and Reconciliation Commission concerned itself with the past. AIDS is very much of the present.

IMAGINATION AND AIDS

Among other lessons, the South African experience of AIDS in the decade and a half of its ascendancy teaches us that, alone among epidemics, AIDS requires a tremendous feat of imagination. Imagination is required because the infection is not immediately manifest in its host. It takes imagination to visualize the impact of the epidemic before anything much has happened, and to shape an effective response. While the consequences of each infection are readily apparent to those who suffer and eventually die, and for those around them who are either infected or affected as a result, it is not obvious that a political response is the only effective response that can be made. To understand that

AIDS—both a medical and a social condition—requires a political solution takes a leap of imagination. The imagination must be shaped by its political and cultural context. Yet AIDS is not itself of political origin.

AIDS requires a political response because it affects the foundations of social order at the level of the family whose members and their labor are lost, and of individuals who feel the sting of prejudice or stigma. Because it is a slow epidemic, developing over many years, with an effect on the population as a whole, it becomes a feature of daily life. Its impact on lifestyle and life expectancy is like the impact of poverty, war, civil disorder, administrative collapse, or other political catastrophes. The connection that Duesberg and Rasnick saw between lifestyle and AIDS exists, but the denialists had the direction of the causal arrow reversed. The overall ability of a society to care for its members affects the ability of those who are afflicted to survive or to maintain an acceptable quality of life for as long as possible. Although South Africa's failure to provide adequate care for people living with AIDS is not in itself the consequence of poverty or war, the effects on society are the same. Mbeki's stated belief that AIDS is a disease of poverty, although not true in itself, has the same effect on HIV-positive people as pervasive poverty would. AIDS *causes* poverty, and as much as denialism leads to further death and higher HIV prevalence, it causes greater poverty. This is a failure of imagination with powerful political consequences.

Any political order stands or falls on its ability to shape and change certain behaviors of its members who are the citizens or subjects of that order. We also expect a democratic state to provide security and to guarantee the human rights of its citizens. Another irony emerges. While Uganda is ruled by a sort of benevolent dictator who came to power through force of arms, it has provided significant civil benefits through an effective response to AIDS. It did this largely through popularly approved social mobilization around the threat of AIDS, which was presented as a political problem to be solved politically. South Africa, though triumphantly democratic after 1994, has often failed to provide the means for securing its citizens' right to health, security and welfare by failing to mobilize society effectively. The effort to make democracy work in the New South Africa diverted attention from AIDS: during Nelson Mandela's stewardship, AIDS simply fell off the political radar for all practical purposes. More than this, however, the patterns of South African politics that emerged over the last quarter of the twentieth century seem to have dictated a politics founded on adversarial relations—as if history was coming back to haunt those who did not understand it—rather than solidarity and common purpose.

Both Uganda and South Africa evolved political responses, but in entirely different ways. These differences reflect different histories, social organizations, and cultures. Uganda moved in a way that allowed the struggle against AIDS to be incorporated into a general social movement of reconstruction and nation building in the aftermath of war and civil collapse. Levels of social integration were possible in Uganda because of its relatively smaller size and limited diversity, while South Africa's response has been characterized by a culture of conflict between civil society and the state that has not been transcended, despite the end of apartheid as the manifest target of civil resistance. The tradition—or better, the pattern or structure of conflict—has been a characteristic feature of South African politics from at least the beginning of the twentieth century.

This epidemic, unlike others, confuses categories of the personal and the public. HIV infects individuals, but is transmitted through social structures (that is, sexual networks). It infects us at our most intimate moments, but changing the overall course of the epidemic is only possible through massive public effort. Its first and most obvious consequences are personal, as an affliction of the body, but its broader implications exist at the level of national economies that lose labor, productivity, commitment, and trust.

This opposition between the personal and public has to be resolved through a social imaginary that can unite the large scale of political order with the small-scale personal experience of sex, illness, and death. Conceptually, this book has sought to do this by showing how individuals are linked in larger networks. But practically, this must be done through political mobilization and political vision. Ultimately it depends on the quality of political community and moral purpose.

South Africa has attempted this through an approach based in human rights (and cultural rights), on the one hand, and one based in large-scale public messages, on the other. This has been far less effective, evidently, than Uganda's approach, which has directed its messages at the most local level: the school classroom, the office and workplace, the church or mosque congregation. While not ignoring human rights issues entirely, Uganda set its anti-AIDS agenda in terms of achieving a collective objective of national survival and reconstruction by building its AIDS programs into national reconstruction. During South Africa's reconstruction of national identity and social transformation, efforts to stem the tide of AIDS were perceived as an impediment and burden.

South Africa's responses to AIDS have been highly politicized. But because AIDS has been cast as a political cost, the political process became adversarial rather than cooperative. Its cost lay not only in the financial outlay that would be required to provide adequate means for testing, care, treatment, and social change, but in the leadership's perception of the burden of the past, of apartheid, and its racialized discourse of sexual shame. First, the Office of the Public Protector's action in the *Sarafina II* scandal, then the action of the Medical Control Council in quashing plans for the development of Virodene as a miracle cure, and finally, the action of TAC in opposing the minister of health's foot dragging in provision of ARV therapies were all perceived by the national leadership as threats to the political ascendancy of the ANC, and as virtually treasonous questioning of the legitimacy of the minister of health and the then deputy president, Mbeki. (For better or worse, Mandela remained aloof throughout, taking a critical stance only after the end of his presidency. He was the only one who could do so without being accused of obstructionism.) This perception created an adversarial relationship between national leadership and civil society. This in itself was all too familiar to all South Africans.

When Mbeki then seized on the dissident notion that HIV did not cause AIDS and that ARVs were too toxic to administer on a national scale, he seemed to take a position against normal science and common sense. His tirade in "Castro Hlongwane" demonstrated that he had a deep fear that South Africans, especially black South Africans, would be seen as savages with unbridled sexuality. Although there are those who may believe this, they are scarcely in a position to make their views known, still less to have a political effect. This fear seems to loom large in the political imagination of Mbeki and his group, and has thus had an ironic political effect: shame. Whether or not a robust belief in the value of sex and the participation of many South Africans in dense networks of sexual relations is anything to be ashamed of, shame has apparently led the national leadership to deny the very existence of AIDS. It is especially ironic because the Mbeki government represents the rationalist and moderate side of the ANC on most other issues, especially with respect to economic policy. Mbeki's position has deflected South Africa from effective political action, but it is ultimately rooted in rational assessment of the costs, risks, and evidence, however misguided this now seems. The primary value appears to be a commitment to a romantic revolutionism that justifies an intransigent Africanism. Like the apartheid government that he fought for so long, Mbeki has chosen a nationalist go-it-alone policy that neglects evidence in favor of ideology. He represents this policy as a renaissance of African responsibility and action that grows out of an authentic African experience and knowledge.

Another faction in the ruling party, led by the former deputy president Jacob Zuma, acts as a counterpoint to Mbeki's position. Despite allegations of rape and corruption, Jacob Zuma continues to occupy a populist position that calls for a return to African tradition and culture. In opposition to Mbeki's perceived "Englishness," Zuma presents himself as a "100% Zulu boy."[47] Despite his appeal to tradition, and his adherence to a strong ethnic and working-class identity, Zuma led the government's AIDS campaign before leaving the deputy presidency. He continues to support treatment and an aggressive AIDS policy as leader of the ANC, recognizing the deep resonance this will have with many of South Africa's poor who support him. In the next chapter we will see how these contradictory positions are also rooted in South African tradition.

In attempting to explain South Africa's partial failure of social policy, political imagination, and collective action against AIDS, I have tried to portray the contradictory meanings that lie beneath the surface of nearly incomprehensible complexity, folly, and often futile conflict. This is not adequate to the task of achieving a more positive understanding of AIDS in South Africa, however. To do this, we must explore further the cultural meanings of sex in South African life and the nature of the sexual networks that provide the channels through which HIV moves. With this done, we shall finally be in a position to make some suggestions about how a new approach can be structured around a deeper, culturally informed, and politically embedded understanding.

CHAPTER 10

Flows of Sexual Substance

The Sexual Network in South Africa

THE MEANING OF SEX IN SOUTHERN AFRICA

Expressions of sexuality and acts of sex have been treated as behavior—that is, as individual acts primarily motivated by internal psychological states of mind or body—in most of the social scientific and psychological literature, while cultural studies and literary approaches have treated it in categorical (as gender) or cultural (representations) terms, or as discourse (after Foucault). A cultural anthropological model, by contrast, must seek to understand the symbolic and semiotic dimensions of sex and sexuality in southern Africa. Here I examine the traditional culture of sex and sexuality, relying in large part on data from traditional healers (*sangomas*) in order to discover the deeper meanings of sexuality that link it to marriage and marriage payments (*lobola, bogadi*), gift exchange (payment, exchange of services such as cooking or use of accommodation, or affection), reproduction, and recreational uses of sex.

Sex can be better understood as being *productive* of identities rather than a reflex of gender (masculinity, femininity), and its social function in traditional southern African societies can be better understood in terms of flows of sexual substance (sexual fluids) between males and females, with concomitant flows of material goods. We can see that sexual substance flows along the same traces of the sexual network that HIV does; it is part of the same linked system of social relations.

Where anthropologists have studied flows of gifts, property, wealth, and value through the legitimate network of sexual relations that we call kinship systems, in this case we observe a broader field of relations that go beyond kinship but have many of the same characteristics.

Incidents

Several incidents over the last five years focus our attention on aspects of sex and notions of blood, body and sex in South African culture—what we might call the national consciousness of sex and AIDS.[1] These incidents concern the rape of children, the fear that a group of female *sangomas* expressed about the danger to men of sexual fluids, and accusations of rape against Jacob Zuma, the former deputy president, former chairman of the South African National AIDS Council, and former husband of the first African National Congress minister of health. These incidents expose issues involving sex and the flow of sexual fluids, or sexual substance, concepts that are crucial components of the structure of kinship and family, the continuity of generations, and, above all, the configuration and durability of South African sexual networks.

Baby Tshepang   In the remote city of Uppington, in the far north of the sparsely populated near-desert province of Northern Cape, four men went on trial in 2001 for the rape of a nine-month-old baby. On 27 October 2001, in Louisvale, a small township near Uppington, the mother had left the child alone while she was drinking, and came back to find her crying and bleeding. The baby survived after reconstructive surgery, and the men were eventually found not guilty. The baby became known as Baby Tshepang. Later in 2001 in the Johannesburg neighborhood of Joubert Park, another baby was raped when her mother left her in a squalid room in the tenement near downtown Johannesburg in which they lived. No arrests were made. These two cases stirred, not for the first time, a huge outcry in the press and in Parliament about how and why these horrible crimes could have happened.

These stories quickly became part of the South African social consciousness. The incident near Uppington inspired a play, *Tshepang: The third testament,* by Lara Foot Newton.[2] The play, though based on the true story, is fictionalized in a way that generalizes its content because in that year (2001), approximately twenty-one thousand rapes of children were reported.[3] The play is a restrained yet harrowing, brutal yet sensitive response to these facts. It exposes the poverty of emotional resources as much as the economic poverty of the main protagonists, and it attempts to explain the rape as a consequence of the previous severe childhood abuse of the rapist, who turns out to be the impoverished mother's boyfriend. A repeated line, as if from the chorus of a Greek tragedy—"Nothing ever happens here"—exposes the social, economic, moral, and emotional dimensions of poverty. The play is powerfully effective in conveying a sense of the weight of past abuse and violence that must be carried by those who have suffered it. In the play this is dramatized for the mother by making her carry a baby's cradle strapped to her back, a symbol of both her embodiment of the violence, her shared guilt, and grief.

Although addressed to, and experienced by only the very small theatergoing audience in South Africa, the play does suggest the cultural significance that events of this kind have come to have in South Africa in the first decade of the twenty-first century. It makes an effort to come to terms with sexual brutality of this kind, an effort that is also seen in other aspects of South African life, from the popular press, such as *The Sun* (a sensationalist tabloid popular in Soweto), to community radio stations that are heard by the majority of people in South Africa. The incident, once brought to the public attention, soon elicited many other stories of the rape of children in South Africa. Baby Tshepang was placed in foster care. In the play, as in the press, the cause of the evil is held to be social rather than individual, collective rather than personal. Blame is not assigned to a specific person but rather to "the people."

The outcome of the second high-profile case in Johannesburg has been extensively discussed by Claudia Ford, who adopted the baby and wrote a book about the process.[4] This child is now healthy and happy after reconstructive surgery and loving care. These cases are exceptional, however: the vast majority of children who are raped are not cared for in any way out of the ordinary. Very few prosecutions result in conviction.

From these cases, a consensus formed around the notion that many men—especially poor, uneducated black men—believe that AIDS could be cured by having sex with a virgin. It was believed that they had selected babies of around one or two years old to have sex with because they were guaranteed to be virgins. This "explanation" has never been confirmed as a motive by the actual perpetrators of these crimes, and may therefore be an urban legend. Whatever the status of this belief,

and whether or not it actually motivates rape of this kind, it has cap-
tured the South African imagination. The claim that some people hold
the belief has, at least, the *status* of fact. It has been targeted by AIDS
interventions and education programs. The newspapers and TV channels carry educational messages emphasizing that "sex with a virgin
will not cure you of AIDS." Community education literature on HIV/
AIDS similarly carries warnings that the belief that sex with a virgin
will cure AIDS is false. Whether or not people actually hold this belief,
or this belief actually motivates some criminals, the public apparently
considers the existence of such a belief to be plausible.

The intense focus on this apparent absurdity, in any case, directs
our attention to the connections made between sex and healing and
between sex and age or life stage, and to the values attached to the presence or absence of sex in the process of healing and illness. Specifically,
it points to the notions that sex has a power to heal and that some
power or substance in female virgins can effect changes in the male.
The healing takes place through flows between people, not within any
single person. Healing, like illness, has social causes.

"We are killing our men"   In another time and place, I sat with a group
of *sangomas* who were attending a training workshop on HIV/AIDS in
Acornhoek, a small town in the lowveld region of Limpopo Province.
The facilitator told them that they should advise all of their clients to
use condoms, and as is usual in such workshops, he demonstrated how
a condom should be put onto the penis. He used a broomstick to demonstrate, although this caused much derisive laughter about how unrealistic a broomstick was as a model. Since a great deal of the healers'
work concerns sexual or romantic problems, they were scarcely naïve
about penises. In particular, the healers declared, the condom could
interfere with sex, and cause poor health or even disease and madness.
Discussion centered on the dangers of condoms. Condoms, it was
declared, could cause a dangerous backup of semen in the male and
therefore lead to dangerous illness. Furthermore, condoms could come
off and disappear inside the woman. It was held, however, that condoms could be useful in preventing male contact with menstrual blood,
a substance that was truly dangerous, and could also prevent contact
with women who had recently attended funerals and thus carried a dangerous impurity that could kill men. "We are killing our men," one
woman declared, by not being sufficiently careful about preventing such
dangerous contact. The discussion of HIV had been sidetracked into

discussion of other kinds of dangerous substances that could be absorbed by men through sexual contact with women.[5] None of the women spoke of specific incidents, but rather of categories (men and women) and of flows between them. There were no specific shocking instances or couples named; talk was of general flows through networks of lovers. They might have been epidemiologists talking about randomized contagions. In fact, they were concerned with their own networks of relations.

Many, if not most, African traditional healers prefer not to recommend condoms, not only because they believe that condoms present significant dangers, but also because they believe that their own medicines are more effective in preventing HIV transmission or sexually transmitted infections (STIs). Many people in South Africa believe that the lubrication on condoms, or so-called condom oil, is absorbed by both men and women during sex with condoms and that this leads to impurity of the blood that can be treated only with traditional medicines.[6] I have heard, too, that some people fear "worms" in packaged condoms that can be seen if a small amount of water is placed in the condom and it is held up to the sunlight.[7] Others say that condoms can get inside women or that they can blow up in the uterus and cause damage or death. Some fear that the semen that ought to flow out is forced back into the man's blood by the condom, and thus causes a new form of illness. All of these beliefs limit use of condoms, and thus may have consequences for public health, but they also point to some important cultural truths. These cases and beliefs suggest strongly that substances—menstrual blood, pollution from death and funerals, or substances from the condoms themselves—can be absorbed into the bodies of both sexual partners. Some informants suggest that sex with a condom is not really sex at all.[8]

Jacob Zuma's shower   At the beginning of 2006, the rape trial of the former deputy president, Jacob Zuma, brought sex and beliefs about sex to the forefront of South African public consciousness. Sex and AIDS these days is never far from the public consciousness in South Africa, but the Zuma trial brought anxieties about politics, power, gender, and sex into close connection with one another and raised interest to a fever pitch. The judge delivered his decision on Monday, 8 May 2006. Millions of South Africans tuned in to hear the entire reading of the judgment, which was publicly broadcast on several of South Africa's leading radio channels. After six weeks of hearings in the Johannesburg

High Court, the judge found Zuma not guilty of rape. There was never any question that penetrative sex had occurred and that Zuma had not used a condom. The judge ruled, however, that the sex appeared to have been consensual.

Although the judgment evoked some surprise, especially among the AIDS activists and women's groups that had held demonstrations in the street outside the court building in downtown Johannesburg through-out most of the court's proceedings, most people agreed that the judg-ment itself was correct: although there were many ambiguities involved in the testimony about the event, there was simply not enough evidence to convict Zuma of rape, and much circumstantial evidence to suggest that the woman had not explicitly resisted sexual intercourse or had implicitly consented. What emerged from the case was evidence of a different kind—evidence of beliefs about sex, desire, and the body that might have been difficult to elicit in any other way. Before his removal from the government as the result of an indictment on corruption charges, Zuma had been a member of the presidential AIDS commis-sion and had declared himself to be a force for moral regeneration. In the aftermath of the Baby Tshepang rape stories, he had told reporters that he blamed apartheid for "sowing the seeds for the breakdown of the institution of the family," and explained that the molestation of children and infants today is a symptom of this degeneration.[9] Such generalities are simply not helpful in advancing our understanding of the rape "epidemic" in South Africa; significantly, Zuma did not attempt to use this logic in defending himself.

The thirty-one-year-old woman who accused Zuma claimed that she thought of him as a father figure. In his defense, Zuma made several revealing claims. First, he said that the woman had sexually enticed him by wearing what he called a *kanga* (also called *lihia* in Zulu), which is a brightly colored piece of cloth measuring approximately 1.8 meters by 1.2 meters. These are used and worn by women throughout eastern and southern Africa, and usually signify respect. In rural areas, they are worn over the clothing as a symbol of modesty, and in Zulu, Swazi, and Xhosa custom particularly, no woman should greet a chief of village headman without wearing one. Thus, the idea that wearing this type of cloth suggested sexual availability provoked outrage.

Second, when Zuma was questioned about whether he was aware that his accuser was HIV-positive and was known as an AIDS activ-ist, he declared that he had known, but he had taken a shower after sex so that he would not be infected with HIV. Even after the trial he defended this statement, saying that he had showered "for hygiene" and "because I knew the type of person I was sleeping with."[10] He also said that he thought the risk of infection was sufficiently low to be worth taking the chance.

Finally, Zuma told the court that according to Zulu culture, he was obligated to have sex with a woman whom he believed to be aroused. Not to do so, he stated, would have been disrespectful of the woman and would have made her angry with him. He testified under oath that when he perceived her to be ready, "I said to myself, I know as we grew up in the Zulu culture you don't leave a woman in that situation, because if you do, then she will even have you arrested and say that you are a rapist."[11]

Although the judge's verdict was widely accepted by the South African public, Zuma's comments about HIV and sex during the trial and afterward caused reactions ranging from debate to outrage. The popular cartoon series *Madam and Eve*,[12] which runs in many of South Africa's newspapers, lampooned Zuma's remarks about his shower and the confusion and misdirection they caused. In his comment on the trial and the verdict, Stephen Lewis, the United Nations special envoy for AIDS in Africa, spoke out against Zuma's "ignorance." Speaking in Nairobi, Kenya, at the meeting of the African Union, Lewis said, "I feel embarrassed for the African leadership and, if you will forgive me, that has been the situation in South Africa where the voice of political leadership has been both confused and confusing. . . . I don't think anything can compensate for the damage that [Zuma] has done."[13]

Zuma's case shows the degree to which "tradition"—in this case, Zulu culture—has entered mainstream national discourse on sex. Here tradition is held to legitimize sexual behavior that would perhaps ordinarily be considered out of the ordinary, if not perverse. It also points to the way in which the discourse about sex has entered the national mainstream. On the main page of www.IOL.com, one of the leading South African Internet sites and service providers, "The Zuma rape trial" was *the* main index heading, followed by "Development," "Education," "Environment," "Finance/Labour," and other topics. Indeed, even Lewis stepped into the debate. He compared Zuma's comments with President Thabo Mbeki's idiosyncratic view that poverty, not HIV, causes AIDS, and with Minister of Health Manto Tshabalala-Msimang's controversial promotion of a diet of olive oil, garlic, and beetroot to cure HIV. Zuma's comments, Lewis remarked, demonstrated that the South African leadership is "confused and confusing."[14] Their beliefs are sincerely held, however, and, I argue, based on deep cultural understandings of sex and AIDS (which they share with the larger South African public).

Unlike Uganda, then, where the biomedical view of AIDS has been fully accepted and Ugandans do not deny the existence of AIDS and its causes, South Africa remains deeply ambivalent about the existence, nature, causes, and treatment of AIDS, and poorly led in its response to the epidemic.

TOWARD A MODEL OF SEXUAL MEANINGS

These notions of sex and sexuality point toward a cultural understanding of sex and sexuality—widely current in southern Africa—in which some sexually transmitted substance flows between both sexual partners. It is embedded in a *cultural*—or, as this is coded in South Africa, "traditional"—discourse of persons, values, bodies, and exchanges rather than in the biomedical discourse of bodies as biological organisms, or the psychiatric and psychological discourse of cognition, desire, and repression.

In anthropology we already have a rich tradition of theory about the person, values, and exchange, but this body of theory has not been widely applied to the understanding of sexuality in Africa.[15] This theoretical tradition may help to expand our conceptualization of sexuality *as* culture in a way that goes beyond the more simplistic notions of cultural influence.[16] A theory of cultural influence holds that culture, as an external domain separate from sexuality, may *influence* the specific content of sexuality, but the theory maintains the essentialist premise that sexuality is ultimately universal and biological. A theoretical position that holds that sexuality is part and parcel of culture, and that sexuality itself has its own cultural tenets and structures, goes beyond such a cultural influence model toward a model of sexuality embedded in culture and culture embedded in sexuality.

Based on extensive conversations with traditional healers and other South Africans of many backgrounds, and using evidence from the press and radio, I describe a model that will help to explain what may be local and culturally different meanings associated with sexuality and the practices of sex in southern Africa. As a model, it is necessarily abstract—a conceptual or heuristic system developed on the basis of observations, interview data, and casual conversation with diverse people, and from the sources of popular culture. Like other models—the Protestant ethic and the spirit of capitalism, the Iroquois system of kinship, the law of supply and demand, the theory of contagious magic, or monotheism—it is rarely, if ever, found in a pure form, fully instantiated in practice. Instead, it seeks to isolate a set of related phenomena and to construct an explanation based on rules of internal consistency and critical coherence rather than empirically demonstrable truth. The power of such models is their heuristic value in discovering underlying (that is, not empirically visible) orders of meaning that can be said to shape life in complex ways. This is also the weakness of the model in social science: it is often difficult, if not impossible, to fully evaluate its validity. This is true of most of the grand narratives as well as of lower-level theoretical constructs that seek to deal with issues such as witchcraft, interpersonal violence, or literary genres, since these take their form through practice and their own genealogies rather than through specific command or explicit specification (as law or bureaucratic order does, for instance). Nevertheless, the model that is developed here is intended to explore specific areas of cultural difference associated with a geographical and cultural community, that of southern Africa. As such, it does not specify race. The actual distribution of meanings associated with this model's system remains an open question.

South African Conceptualization of Sexuality and the Body

Contemporary southern African representations of the body and practices of sexuality point toward a concept of flows of bodily substance and gifts that go both ways in the (hetero-)sexual[17] encounter, that is, both men and women absorb each other's sexual fluids during sexual contact. This implies a concept of the person that is permeable to both physical and spiritual substances of other persons, rather than—or perhaps in addition to—a Western concept of the individual.[18] Specifically, South Africans seem to understand sex as involving a permeation of the body by any substance involved in sexual contact, and therefore as a potential threat to both males and females. It suggests a different concept of the biological boundaries of the person that is rooted in cultural concepts of the body, especially the sexual body. This has far-reaching effects in decisions about use of condoms, but more than this, it points to a set of distinctive beliefs about sex that must be understood in terms of representations of the body, of sex and sexuality, and of the notion of the nature of the person in southern African society.

According to the cultural precepts of South African traditional culture, sex itself is part of human nature, something everyone engages in. Traditional healers expressed this in various ways in interviews:

> People do have sex because it is nature and it was created. It is part of life. Women and men . . . it really does not matter who you are.[19]

> Sex is for pleasure. It is for the nation and people.[20]

Typically, South Africans believe that the body fluids that result from sexual arousal and orgasm derive from the blood. Blood is hot and is heated by sexual desire and arousal, causing a portion of it to be secreted. In a study of adolescent sexual attitudes and behavior in Acornhoek, Limpopo Province, Collins and Stadler concluded that male "sexual desire was considered to stem from the need to drain . . . increased volume of blood from the body [while] semen and vaginal secretions were believed to be 'blood that is hot.'" They found that the group of adolescents with whom they worked believed that "during sexual intercourse the 'blood' of a woman and a man were . . . exchanged or mixed together."[21] In the same context, female desire is similarly understood as deriving from the blood: "Her blood will tell her how to act," said one young woman in Acornhoek. "She will think she is old enough for sex once she begins to menstruate."[22] Jeannerat reports that older Venda women say that once she stops menstruating a woman no longer has sexual desire since "her blood is no longer coming." Sex under these circumstances becomes dangerous: "If she would engage in sexual intercourse, the semen of her husband could no longer be washed out of her uterus by the menstrual flow and its accumulation would cause her stomach to swell up as if she were pregnant. After nine months the stomach would burst and the woman would die."[23]

Thus semen and vaginal fluids are no different from menstrual fluids, or blood itself, in the folk models of their derivation. The SeSotho word *madi* may mean both blood and semen,[24] as does *igazi*, the Zulu word for blood/semen. Since blood is also what is passed down to subsequent generations through conception and birth, and since this is what connects the ancestors with the living, it is a source of power that is comprehended cosmologically.

According to traditional healers and, therefore, to many ordinary South Africans, the flow of blood across the generations, from grandparents to children and to subsequent generations, is understood to be literally physical. It is not blood as spiritual symbol or as some transcendent substance that represents the continuity of the blood line, but actual blood that flows from one generation to another. Since vaginal fluids and semen are identical to blood, the conception of a child from the blood of the mother and of the father allows the blood to flow directly across the generations. The ancestors are physically connected to the living through this link constituted by the real flow of sexual substance. This conception is illustrated in figure 18. Sex is implicated in flows that move in two directions: through the generations and through time (shown in figure 18 as the vertical axis), and across space and society through the medium of networks of sexual partners (shown on the horizontal axis in the diagram). In cultural terms, of course, time is not necessarily seen as vertical since people are linked to the graves of the ancestors and to living sites that have previously been occupied. Flow of blood across generations and flow of sexual substances between persons represent different dimensions of relationship in the same social universe. These constitute a landscape of both the living and the dead, of the ancestors (*amadloti*), and of people (*abantu*), which is, like the physical earth, a physical connection between different kinds and orders of being.

In everyday life, the dimension of generational time is embodied in the imagined landscape of the space of life and death. The landscapes that most people imagine are networks of places where ancestors and elder family members live, or have lived and are buried, and include the places where kin and children currently live, have sex and babies, and eventually die. Pathways (roads, highways, footpaths) and frequent travel to visit the living or graves of the dead make this network real. Similarly, the domain of social relations, including sexual relations, is not separable from time, since sexual and other social relations change through time. The model presented here is meant to indicate the nexus between two separate dimensions in which the sexual act necessarily takes place (that is, at a particular moment in time and with certain cultural intentions and social implications). Each sex act is the nodal point in a network of relationships that exists in a landscape of meaning.

In this worldview, the ancestors are still with us and influence us not only because their blood is our blood, but also because their earth is the earth we also walk on and in which we also will eventually be buried. Sex lies at the center of this. Blood or semen that flows—both over time from generation to generation, and across partners from male to female and female to male—is not conceptualized as a metaphor. It is real, physical blood that is transferred through sexual exchanges.

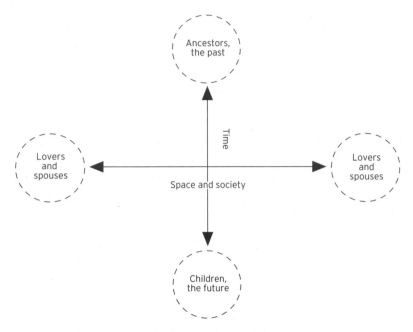

FIGURE 18. Flows of sexual substance in social time and space.

When sex results in the conception of a child, the child's blood is therefore also the ancestors' blood, which the child will ultimately pass on
to subsequent generations.

In the temporal dimension, blood/semen flows down from previous
generations to future generations through the medium of those currently
alive. This is understood to be a real flow of real substances that actually and materially constitute our bodies. The blood of the ancestors is
our blood, and it will be passed on to future generations as the same
blood. Implicitly, it seems that blood and semen are transmitted from
one person to another through sexual reproduction (and other forms of
sexuality), through time and across generations and therefore are also
permanent—enduring as long as life endures. They are transmissible but
nontransitory substances. As such, they constitute a flow of value across
generations and can be thought of as a kind of currency that is exchanged
across generations. They are the wealth of the nation (*mali ya sechaba*)
that enables people not only to survive, but also to understand their survival as part of an ongoing exchange across time that links generations
in a permanent and enduring way. The sexual networks of South African

society, then, are not limited to the living since they also include, implicitly, the blood/semen of the ancestors as well. When relationships break
down between lovers or within the family, first the ancestors should
be asked to intervene. This is done by calling them at the grave side, if
possible, or by offering them the blood of sacrificial chickens, goats, or,
in extreme cases, a cow or bullock. This is called *kupahla*, to call the
ancestors with a gift. Thus, a gift of blood and value flows back to them
in a counterexchange within the network. This is the first resort advised
by southern African traditional healers, since ancestors particularly keep
watch over social relationships, including sexual ones.

In the social (horizontal) dimension, people who are living today—lovers
and spouses—exchange their substance through sexual acts that link
persons in networks of relations that involve exchanges of other kinds
of currency in addition to the sexual currency of semen and vaginal
fluid. In other words, sex is not held to be merely or even primarily for
reproduction, but is itself a legitimate part of daily transactions among
persons in which things of value are exchanged. The sexual exchange
is necessarily implicated in a broader flow of values, some of which are
physical or economic values (such as use of a car or cell phone, a place
to sleep, a new dress or clothes) and some of which are intangible values
(such as a good conversation, a shared joke, a good time, or a sense of
closeness and intimacy). Sexuality participates, in other words, in a
network of reciprocal exchange of gifts that link people as lovers, just
as the gift of blood and life from the ancestors links them to the living
and to their potential descendants in a reciprocal exchange network
across time. Since blood/semen is both transmissible and nontransitory,
it can play a role like that of other durable goods in such an exchange,
and it creates the same sense of reciprocal rights and obligations that
exchange of other durable goods creates. A link created through sexual
action is an enduring social relation that connects people who have sex
(or who have had sex) with one another in an enduring networks of
relations. This is represented in figure 18 as the horizontal dimension.

Thus, the South African sexual network is sustained by constant
flows of sexual substance, but also of many other kinds of value, things
and services. This takes place within a cosmology that understands the
ancestors as being among us, albeit unseen. These acts of exchange
allow people to imagine their communities of kin, comrades, and fellow citizens, but the sexual network itself is never imagined, never represented. It remains a hidden, occult structure, which is nevertheless

responsible for the transmission of HIV. The unseen structure of the sexual network is the *unimagined* community.

In these terms, Jacob Zuma's declaration that he would be violating the woman's "human right to sex" if he refused what he took to be her advances, is not as absurd as it might at first seem. The right to sex, although not generally articulated as one of the principle human rights upheld by the United Nations or the South African constitution, can be understood as a right to engage in the fundamental exchanges of a valued substance that sex entails. Taken in this way, Zuma was invoking South African ideologies of sex, kinship, and *Ubuntu* (humanity). Other testimony in the trial showed that Zuma had already helped his accuser with cash and efforts to find her a place in an overseas educational establishment. It would not be unusual to expect an exchange of sex for such services in many similar South African situations. Although his invocation of Zulu culture scarcely excuses the unprotected sex with whatever coercion he may have used, the continued acceptance of Zuma as a leader in South Africa suggests that he had indeed struck some cultural chords that resonated with many ordinary South Africans.

Several authors have pointed to the significance that fertility has in many African cultures. This has been most comprehensively summarized by the Caldwells and their collaborators in a series of articles that highlighted the significance of sexual networks in the AIDS epidemic.[25] While reproduction and fertility are important in South Africa, and children are certainly welcome, compared to the ritual emphasis placed on fertility in many other parts of Africa, South Africans seem to see sex in broader terms. The role that sex plays in South Africa is far more than just a reproductive one. Since South African societies, especially as they exist today, often place little importance on lineage or clan—except, perhaps, in chiefly and royal families such as that of the Zulu king, among others—fertility as such has less to do with maintenance of kinship and property regimes, and more to do with contemporaneous exchanges in networks of relations.

This helps to lay the foundation for the extent and interconnection of sexual networks that has been discussed in previous chapters. This linkage puts sexuality, and the partners involved in sexuality, at a crucial cosmological nexus that involves the flow of blood through generations and the flow of sexual substance across social networks of persons that are linked through sexual contact and all of its implications,

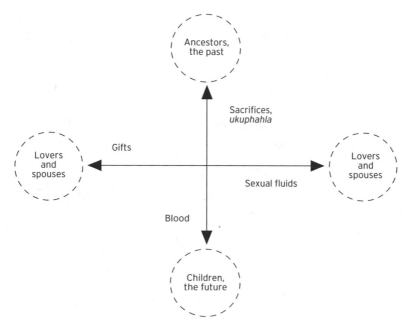

FIGURE 19. Sexuality as exchange of blood and gifts.

including trust, mistrust, jealousy, mutual powers and vulnerabilities, and love (or hate). It also places sex at the juncture between the power of the ancestral spirits and the power of the bush, or nature, that lies in the broader landscape. This is represented in figure 19.

Sexual flows among the network of lovers or spouses also involve concomitant flows of other kinds of valuables, such as cattle, money, clothes, and other objects of value. This is especially true in bride-wealth payments, called *lobola* in the Nguni languages[26] and *bogadi* in the Sotho-Tswana languages. These payments involve an exchange of wealth (generally expressed in terms of cattle as units of value, but paid in currency or other items of value) that formally passes from the bride-groom's family to the bride's family. Other gifts from the bride's family also pass to the bridegroom, and since the *lobola/bogadi* is rarely paid in full, the exchange is often nearly balanced between the two families. The promised but unpaid *lobola* stands as a contingent debt. The flow of gifts from the living to the ancestors is similar: never fully complete, always contingent, and ideally balanced. Similarly, the flow across generations should be acknowledged—and often is—with appropriate and regular sacrifices of animals for the ancestors in exchange for blessings,

protection, and luck that only the ancestors (or other spirits) can ultimately bestow. The gifts given to the ancestors through sacrifice involve
both the actual blood of the animal as well as the animal's value. They
are thought of as being equivalent to the exchanges of goods that take
place at marriages. *Lobola* exchanges, in other words, are the same
as the exchanges involved in *kupahla* (gift exchange with ancestors).
Both create and maintain relationships through flows of substance and
value. The ancestors are therefore party to every exchange of a sexual
or kinship kind.

The two flows may interact disastrously as, for instance, at times
of death when contact with a corpse pollutes one's body and makes
sex with others dangerous. At this point of rupture at the end of life,
sex must also be interrupted. This can also be understood in terms of
exchange of substances that occurs in all social interactions, including
those involved with death. People infect one another on a daily basis,
not just through sexual contact, but also through their other personal
substances—breath, spirit, and presence or shadow (*seriti* in Sotho, or
isithunzi in isiZulu). As long as these substances are shared in daily
life, life goes on. But death interrupts these flows and thus leads to
contamination since the reciprocity of exchanges of substance through
normal interaction is interrupted, too. If the contamination of death is
not removed by means of ritual intervention, then it can be transmitted
to others, especially through sexual contact. This causes illness and
might even lead to death.

The *sangoma*'s fear of condoms, then, can also be seen in this
light. Both condoms and death interrupt the flow of sexual substance.
Although death does so permanently, interrupting the flow of substance
in daily life, the condom does so temporarily. Both death and condoms, then, constitute rupture of the social fabric and, ideally, should
be avoided. When the female *sangomas* said that women were "killing
their men," they meant that rupture of flow of this kind leads to illness,
morbidity, and ultimately to death.

An act of sex is, therefore, both a personal joining together of bodily
substance and a simultaneous conjuncture of cosmological principles.
These two flows implicate and entail each other and create life in several ways. Any sexual act is potentially a procreative act, but also helps
to mutually create the partners themselves through mixing of their
bodily substances, through creating new social identities (as lovers),
and through affirmation of each partner's own sexuality and sense
of masculine/feminine identity. As a potentially pro-creative act, sex

creates the children through whom one's own blood will continue to flow. As a re-creational act, that is, one that reaffirms and possibly elaborates on one's own social identity, recreational (as opposed to procreative) sex is also a creative act. The two acts of creation exist as a single bodily performance—sexual intercourse—that lies at the juncture of two dimensions in the work of making persons.

Sex, therefore, is imbued with curative or healing powers but, precisely because of this power, presents special dangers and requires certain avoidances (taboos). It is never simply an act of pleasure divorced from the universe of kin, friends and lovers or from the universe of spirits, god(s) and witches. Both appeals to ancestors and medicines from the bush (nature) have significant powers to influence the outcome of sexual acts: to protect against sexually transmitted infections, to cleanse pollution that derives from sexual acts, to cleanse unclean conditions that interfere with sexual relations (such as attending a funeral), to capture a lover's affections, to prevent intercourse with someone else's lover, and many other kinds of love magic. The herbal medicines (*muti*) of the bush are used to treat sexual dysfunction (such as impotence), STIs, and infertility, and as love magic because the power of herbs is linked both to the ancestors and to the landscape in which the herbs are found. Their powers derive, that is, from both the flow of spirit through generations and the flow of spiritual influences across and through the landscape.[27] Sexually transmitted diseases are communicated through the blood, too, according to traditional healers and traditional health beliefs. South African traditional healers say, for instance, that "STDs are caused by the uncleanness of the blood such as when people sleep together and one party is not pure you can transmit the disease to the next person."[28] Or, "STD can be transmitted sexually but basically it is the impurity of the blood."[29] The power of herbs in treating sexual problems is thus also linked to the two dimensional flow of blood and spirit that characterize the African cosmological conception of man's place in nature.

Sexuality is thus not natural in the Western biological sense, but specific to human nature as a social being. It is experienced as an organic need, such as hunger. Like hunger, it can be controlled, satisfied, or thwarted by products of the land. In African languages, pervasive metaphors for sex involving food, foodstuffs, and eating testify to this. Yet, it is fundamentally interorganic, taking its form through multiple organic persons, and transcends the mere organic by involving spirits of ancestors and the creation of children for whom one's (sexual, reproductive) self will eventually stand as ancestor. It is creative of humans and created by them, but not by them alone. Sexuality provokes intense arousal and desire, but also dread, fear, and loathing. The act of sex creates bonds between persons, but also dissolves them through jealousy. It is, like most other human or spiritual powers in the southern African cosmologies, inherently socially unstable and morally ambiguous. It is both bad *and* good, desired *and* feared, therapeutic *and* pathogenic.

Sex also creates personal identities. A female virgin becomes a woman through sex, but more than this, a wife. When a female person's identity changes from girl to woman she acquires not only an identity but also a role. She enters into a web of diffuse and multiplex relations with the man with whom she has had sex. Except for thoroughly modernized or Westernized women, this implies a complex set of duties and obligations. There is little sense in more traditional African communities of an isolated sexual act merely for the sake of pleasure. The exchange of bodily substance implies other exchanges and the relationship thus constituted is open-ended and multistranded. Minimally, a woman who has sex with a man—unless it is a purely commercial transaction, that is, prostitution—is expected to cook for him, clean for him, and above all respect (*ukuhlonipa*) him. Such relationships may segue into what is regarded as traditional marriage or customary marriage if they endure long enough. They do not necessarily imply sexual exclusivity. Thus, a woman may have such a set of complex duties and expectations with several men. This is part of being a woman, that is, playing the role that the identity conferred by sex entails. While male persons acquire their identity as men in some black South African communities through circumcision, they acquire their masculinity—and through this, their respect—through sex. They also acquire a set of diffuse, usually unstated, obligations to support their woman by giving them gifts such as clothes, food, and other benefits. Stereotypically, these are the three Cs: cash, cars, and cell phones. Ultimately, should they formalize their relationship traditionally, they pay larger sums of bridewealth to the woman's family. In all cases, sex creates social identities and embeds persons in dense social networks of duties, expectations, and obligations that are all held to be creative of the true (African) person (Nguni/Zulu: *umuntu*; Sotho/Tswana: *motho*).

These concepts are fundamentally the same as those that inform the work of traditional healers, whose indigenous knowledge system[30] is shared by all types of traditional healers, that is, the *isangoma*, who heals through possession of spirits that enable him or her to dream and

	Enduring	Transient
Substance	**Blood** (*madzi/igazi*)	**Body** (*mzimba/mmele*)
Nonsubstance	**Spirit** (*moya*)	**Shadow** (*seriti/isithunzi*)
	Fluid	Immanent

FIGURE 20. The diviner's (*sangoma*'s) model of the body.

to perceive illnesses in clients, and the *inyanga* (SiSwati/isiZulu) or *din-gaka* (SePedi), who is not possessed by spirits but uses knowledge of the indigenous pharmacopeia in healing with herbs. Both types of healers preserve African traditional philosophies and medical knowledge and elaborate on them.[31] The South African indigenous healing system with which I am most familiar is the widespread *ndzau* cult of the lowveld and the urban Johannesburg/Pretoria/Soweto area in the highveld.[32]

In synoptic form, the work of the traditional healer in the South African lowveld generally involves manipulation of four coordinated substances of the body. These are the spirit (SePedi: *mmoya*, Zulu/Swazi: *umoya*), the body (SePedi: *mmele*, SiSwati: *umtimba*, isiZulu: *umzimba*), the blood (SePedi: *madi*, SiSwati: *ingati*, isiZulu: *igazi*), and the aura (SePedi: *seriti*, SiSwati: *sitfunti*, isiZulu: *isithunzi*, also translated as shadow, moral weight, influence, or prestige).[33] These substances interact in ways that are similar to the sexual system of flows that I have already outlined. This is represented in figure 20 as the *sangoma*'s model of the body.

The body (*umzimba*) itself consists of flesh (*inyama*) and is the transient locus of the other substances that can be thought of as flowing through the body and, at the same time, constituting it. Blood and spirit are both enduring substances that survive the death of the transient body in which they reside. Spirit, *umoya* (also meaning air, wind, or breath)—a nonmaterial substance or essence—comes from the ancestors (*amadlozi*) and passes on to the succeeding generations through birth, growth of children, and the next generation's own subsequent procreation. Blood passes in the same way, but unlike spirit it flows only through direct lines of (biological) procreation. Spirit, especially the ancestors, also follows the lines of blood, but it can be selectively activated through ritual and/or prayer or deactivated by ignoring it until it possibly makes its presence felt by demanding attention. Spirits, however, can cross lines and flow across the landscape. They can be detained at specific geographical points where people have met unexpected death, such as in automobile accidents or in battle. They can thus flow across bloodlines and affect others who may not be directly related to them. Thus, several different spirits of different ethnic/linguistic groups may possess *sangomas,* those who are possessed by spirits and heal through possession trances. Like the body, which dies, the shadow is a nonmaterial presence or aura that the body projects. It is identified with the smell of the person, by the bodily dirt that is present in the person's clothes and living space, and by the sense of presence, character, or charisma that the person has.

Each of these substances is used in different ways in healing. The body and blood may be treated with herbs that are drunk or rubbed into small cuts. The shadow and spirit are treated through washing with herbal baths, steaming and sweat baths, and by smoke or foam made from plants that produce froth when infused and stirred. Each must be balanced in the person to ensure health, with excesses of blood or spirit being purged (through enemas, vomiting, or sweating), and with deficits being made up through ritual treatments involving calling of the spirits (*pahla*), sacrifice, or herbal and ritual strengthening treatments. All of these entail an adjustment of flows of substance (material or nonmaterial/unobservable) through and in the body. Health results from a balance of substances both within the body and between others involved with the person's social and sexual network of kin, friends, lovers, and associates.

Like the healing system, the sexual system is similarly conceptualized as balancing flows of substance. Health requires adequate sexual activity that allows the person to absorb the sexual substance of others and, for men especially, to drain excess substance (sperm as hot blood) into others. Both women and men acquire the shadow of their partners in this way, and thus augment their own bodies with the valuable substance of others. According to an often-quoted proverb, "a person is a person through other people." This applies in particular to the sexual exchanges that create flows of substance among one's lovers, since they also create the person. Sexuality and healing, then, are parallel systems of flows that create healthy persons just as they create babies who become persons through continued interaction. Without either sex or traditional healing, traditionalists maintain, the person will sicken and die. Nevertheless, sexual flows must be contained and channeled. If the person is ill and being treated by a traditional healer, engaging in sex is generally forbidden. Sexual exchanges and the linkages of one's own shadow and blood with others can interrupt the healing process that attempts to balance and manipulate these flows in order to achieve health. The parallel nature of these systems of flows can be seen from the proscription on sex while being treated or healed. In effect, one can either be healed or have sex, but not both. The practice of both would produce unpredictable results since they are part and parcel of the same bodily systems.

Through every act of sex, then, a person not only expresses desire and receives pleasure, but is also received into the social networks of interdependency and trust that permit the expression of one's own character. The southern African conception of the person as always a creation of and through other people means that networks of social relations are the matrix out of which people achieve their sense of worth and identity. Sex is also part of this, and sexual networks link not just people but also generations and, through them, nature, the environment, and the cosmos. For traditional healers, this is symbolized by the ocean (*lwandle*), the limitless water to which all rivers flow and from which all rivers obtain their source. The flows of sexual substance ultimately link to greater flows, with other people as their channels.

With the coming of the New South Africa, the vast majority of South Africans experienced a rapid emergence of freedom. This freedom was often interpreted as freedom to consume the fruits of democracy and modernity as symbols of participation in the new state. With standards of living rising rapidly for black people, new avenues of political and economic participation opened. Among these was sexual freedom. In the New South Africa, Deborah Posel has pointed out, "Consumption—as an affirmation of life and marker of progress—in turn folds into imaginaries of sexual consumption and sexual freedom."[34]

Sex itself became an object of free and public consumption, especially after 1992 when laws against pornography, prostitution, and brothels were scrapped or no longer enforced, and freedom of movement and residence was restored. In other respects sex has always been the principal and most highly valued consumable in South Africa. The rapid extension of social grants from government to mothers of young children, the unemployed, the retired, the disabled, the landless, the homeless, and many other categories has pumped cash into an economy in which sex is one of the objects of consumption. Although sexual freedom was once primarily restricted to men,[35] the new sense of

political and social freedom has also permitted women to express their
freedom through sexual consumption. Legislation aimed at empower-
ing women means that more and more women are employed in salaried
positions, and many use their disposable income to attract men and
engage in sexual recreation. This also is not entirely new, though it has
become more prevalent. In a sympathetic and detailed study of the sex
life of Bantu women in 1950s Johannesburg, Laura Longmore points
to the predominance of "highly sexed" men in the "Eastern Native
Township" where she conducted her research, and she remarks that
this "must have a positive effect upon the relatively few women who
become equally stimulated" by their interest.[36] This leads to women
having one or more "back door husbands" as "women realise they can
support themselves and begin to show a spirit of independence."

Sex, then, is far more than mere expression of desire and its cul-
mination in pleasure. It is also not primarily focused on fertility or
fecundity, although this is a welcome and important aspect. Each
sex act is a value that is transacted in complex networks of exchange
through any instance of lovemaking, but also through bride-wealth or
sex that is exchanged for goods in a noncommercial way as gifts, and
in prostitution or other forms of transactional sex. Sex creates and
sustains networks of friendship, influence, mutual support, trust, and
love. It also creates networks of jealousy, suspicion, gossip, envy, and
evil. These overlap and interpenetrate.

The consequences of this are not all bad, but the southern African
sexual networks do provide wide-open pastures for sexually transmitted pathogens of all kinds. The high rates of rape and sexual violence
are probably also supported, if not directly caused, by these concepts
and practices. The rape of Baby Tshepang is an instance of this.

SEXUAL CULTURE AND AIDS

Although sex takes place between bodies that are everywhere fundamentally the same, it does so within a context of meanings that change
over time and across different communities of meaning. We have called
this the culture of sexuality, but the senses of this use of the term *culture* are different. The culture of sexuality is largely nonverbal, and
though it is shared, it is shared through networks of contact and communication between couples themselves. The discourse of sexuality in
South Africa is a discourse of acts rather than of words. It takes place
between two people who do not generally discuss their acts with others

or with each other. These acts link lovers in large, silent concatenations of sexual networks and constitute the community of shared sexual links and substance. This in itself is essential to the imagination of community, the so-called *ubuntu,* or African humanism, but it is never visible as such.

The overt meanings of sexual transactions are also public, and therefore shared as other aspects of culture are, but they are not publicly shared in the same way that other cultural meanings are. These meanings are specifically performed in the nonverbal discourse of bodies in which pleasure is taken and shared, and in which persons are produced. The production of persons in this cultural discourse of sexual bodies occurs in three ways. Procreative sex creates actual physical human beings and the social networks of family ties and kinship. Recreational sex recreates the person through social affirmation, and embeds its participants in widespreading cross-linked chains and circuits of exchange. This exchange is conducted through multiple media: objects that represent wealth, status, and prestige; practical services such as loans or transportation; gifts of money, food, or clothes; and intangible values such as trust, love, affection, and esteem. Finally, there is the role-creative aspect of sex, in which we become who we are as (gendered) men and women through sexuality. Sex is the act through which males become men and females become women. This necessarily takes place within the cultural categories that constitute gender at its deepest and most fundamental level. These three aspects of sexual values—the procreative, the recreative, and the role-creative—generate compelling motives to act. These motives lead people to link up to the wider social-sexual network. As we have seen, this network of exchanges is not just of the moment, or even of this world alone: it has cosmological and religious implications and is part of the deep structure of southern African culture over the long term.

Although social and political roles make use of the distinction that the discourse of sexuality creates (masculinity and femininity, or male and female), the culture of sexuality itself must be seen as a relatively autonomous domain of human experience. It constitutes a set of patterns of behavior that form root metaphors for most other aspects of political and social life but itself exists partly isolated from the broader sets of cultural categories and social practices that constitute the rest of daily life. This makes it especially difficult to study as another aspect of human social behavior, or as a domain of culture, but it remains as a fundamental raw experience of life itself that must be constantly interpreted through cultural frameworks of meaning, and actualized through sexual expression and activity as a part of everyday social life.

Sex, then, has its own cultural dimensions that shape its practice and the values associated with it. While many aspects of actual sexual practice are universally human, preferences and frequencies of acts are not. More important, the meaning of sexuality differs. Sexual meanings are central to concepts of self and of the person, and to the values we associate with others. The values we attach to pleasure also differ. Accordingly, where social structures, concepts of the person, and values differ, we may find differences in sexual culture that coordinate with these differences. Since some aspects of sexuality are certainly universal, however, we must expect that sexual cultures will differ, not absolutely, but as a matter of degree and emphasis.

This model of the traditional notions of sex and healing helps us to understand crucial aspects of the three cases with which this chapter began. They are linked by the underlying notions of flows of sexual substance, on the one hand, and the dual nature of sexual contact as both dangerous ("we are killing our men") and healing (Baby Tshepang), on the other. It is the flow of sexual substance that is held to heal AIDS in the case of having sex with a virgin, since the virgin's substance is pure. The discourse of healing cannot be separated from the discourse of flows because each constitutes the condition that makes the other possible. The women who feared they were killing their men, by contrast, feared that their own pollution through contact with death, stillbirths, and abortions could kill by virtue of their dirty blood. Zuma believed that the woman he is alleged to have raped—a young woman who was simultaneously his houseguest, a woman who called him father, a long-standing friend of the family, a member of his party, a friend of his daughter, a client, and a friend—required sex to keep her sane and healthy, according to his culture. Jacob Zuma's shower, although scarcely effective against AIDS, seems to have been a ritualistic act of cleansing and strengthening, and it is consistent with the notion of dirt, pollution, and contamination that are implicit in flows of sexual substance. The sex in this case was both healing and polluting, both decreed by culture and illegal, both a crime and its own punishment.

These concepts are powerful and contribute significantly to South African ideas of sex, its dangers, and its healing effects. Since sex is both harmful and healing in the traditional sense, the danger of HIV simply adds another burden of danger to the act but does not change the calculus of risk. Its danger does not cancel the healing effect it is also believed to have. Sex is essential to health, and if this means that it also presents certain new dangers, many appear to believe that the danger is just one more risk they have to take. Jacob Zuma did not reject unprotected sex with his houseguest merely because he knew she was HIV-positive. He took the risk . . . *and* a shower afterward. The centrality of sex in relationships of all kinds means that it links people in complex networks of sexual relations. As we have seen, these ideas also shape the social terrain through which HIV can spread so efficiently. Understanding these concepts is not going to stop the spread of HIV, of course, but it can help us to formulate more effective and culturally sensitive means of dealing with the epidemic.

CHAPTER 11

Preventing AIDS

A New Paradigm for a New Strategy

THE ANXIETY OF KNOWLEDGE

Science builds on what is known, but assessing the epistemological status of our knowledge is still one of the most difficult tasks. What we think we know can stand in the way of knowing more. This is especially true, perhaps, in this time of AIDS, and with respect to sex. Knowledge about sex is hedged with many constraints—moral, linguistic, practical, social, and cultural. And because HIV is sexually transmitted, knowledge of AIDS is limited by similar constraints, giving rise to new limits on language, knowledge, and action: stigma, secrecy, disclosure, "coming out," disclosing one's status, the ethics of disclosure, the ethics of sexual research, and so on. These aspects of the AIDS epidemic are problems not just of knowledge, but of knowledge about the kinds and limits of knowledge. There is, in other words, an epistemological crisis. Words such as *disclosure* and *stigma* have, in effect, been newly coined for this epidemic: their meanings today are so closely associated with AIDS and HIV that their previous usages and contexts (legal and religious, respectively) have been all but forgotten.

Claude Levi-Strauss pointed out that a "native theory" of something is often very difficult to rethink because everyone already knows. This is especially true of sex, and is increasingly true of HIV prevention strategies and theories of how the virus came to be, and how it might one day go away. "Conscious models, which are usually known as 'norms,'" said Levi-Strauss, "are by definition very poor [models of social realities] since they are not intended to explain the phenomena but to perpetuate them."[1] Everyone, it seems, already knows about sex, and to develop new models of it has proven extremely difficult, despite the apparent failure of many of the intervention methods based on previous models. Similarly, strategies for HIV interventions have become almost fossilized around the ABC approach. The notion of abstinence, in particular, has been taken up into religious systems of self-justification and ideology that resist even the most robust scientific evidence that it does not work.

The issues surrounding the global epidemic of HIV and AIDS, then, are increasingly about knowledge, what counts as knowledge, and how knowledge might be applied. Prevention strategies aim to increase the knowledge that people have about the virus and its consequences, despite the evidence that knowledge — especially knowledge about sex — does not necessarily influence sexual behavior. We reason, often without evidence, that the more people know, the more they will seek to change their attitudes toward sexuality and the more they will adhere to safer sex practices. Antiretroviral (ARV) treatment strategies rely on patients being sufficiently knowledgeable to motivate themselves to stick rigidly to the daily timetable of the daily treatment regimens.[2] Without this, the treatment runs the risk of producing more resistant strains of the virus in the body and in the population at large. Strategies aimed at getting people to test themselves voluntarily for the presence of the virus in their bodies are based the notion that knowledge of one's status will allow a person to adapt to the infection in ways that maximize his or her own health and that of others. Some intervention strategies have relied on what has come to be called "disclosure" — evidently based on the idea that knowledge of one's HIV status is at first necessarily secret — disclosure of a new and different state of being as a result of being infected by HIV. Consistent and honest disclosure would certainly help those concerned with public health to know the scale of the problem and help those who are infected or affected to deal knowledgeably with their own status.

The medical and biological sciences struggle valiantly against a growing tide of infection in order to increase their knowledge about a virus that is too small to see with ordinary microscopes, and whose very success (as a virus) relies on its protean and changeable nature that uniquely equips it to ride the sexual network. We believe that ultimately more complete knowledge of the chemistry and biology of the virus will enable us to destroy it, or at least to limit its damage. Political leaders in democracies build their strategies on what the public knows and believes about political issues that affect them. Citizens' knowledge about HIV and AIDS is a critical part of any social or political strategy aimed at coping with its menace. Finally, production and management of knowledge about the epidemic itself has become a significant part of global health care and information systems, and plays a role today in most of the social science, medical, health care, and public health disciplines. Vast databases are maintained by the United Nations, by governments, and by research institutes. Much of this is made available on the Internet, and research continues to fill specialized AIDS journals as well as many other journals in many disciplines.

It seems that the more knowledge we have about HIV/AIDS, the more anxious we become. One of my students in Johannesburg, Zodwa Radebe, who has worked in AIDS research and prevention, once remarked to me, "The more I learn about HIV and the more people I work with who are HIV-positive, the less I seem to know; the more my understanding is shaken."

Knowledge of AIDS is like knowledge of sex, then: it is anxious knowledge.

President Thabo Mbeki's attitude toward AIDS is scarcely influenced by science—indeed, it has been antiscientific—but many South Africans are sympathetic with it. His political instinct tells him that people cannot easily be led in directions they do not want to go. The majority of the South African population does not want to face the terrible facts any more than the president does. The anxiety about knowledge of AIDS comes in part from the political and cultural divisions about what kind of knowledge about AIDS should count, and how it should be used. Medical pluralism in South Africa has allowed a considerable range of therapeutic responses to AIDS. Traditional healers, and even Minister of Health Manto Tshabalala-Msimang's special diet and emphasis on good nutrition, have helped some, it appears, while others have died. But ARVs do not cure AIDS, either, and they do not work for everyone. The ongoing debate about the legitimacy of science, though a disaster for disease prevention, has deep roots in southern African culture. These are symptoms of a pervasive anxiety of knowledge.

By the time HIV was discovered, Uganda already had a native category for it and an established discourse. We have seen that HIV was already endemic in southwestern Uganda for some time before science identified a causative agent. This appears to have given Ugandans a head start in knowledge and allowed them to understand it as a "normal illness." It meant that they were able to "adopt" the affliction as their own and deal with it honestly, with clear political leadership, within familiar cultural frameworks, and using science and medicine. The contrast between this and the politicized and adversarial response in South Africa is sharp and clear.

Paradoxically, however, knowledge of AIDS has not, for the most part, halted its advance, especially in South Africa. The central role that knowledge has assumed in the development of epidemic—in charting its advance and impact, in finding and implementing ways to combat it, and, above all, in the knowledge of one's own HIV status and the decision to disclose or to deny—has become as problematic as the disease itself. Today, HIV is as much a disease of knowledge as it is of the body.

In the case of other medical conditions, knowledge has increased our capacity to treat and to deal with them to the extent that most diseases and conditions are treatable. This is true of HIV infections and of AIDS, too, but medical knowledge alone has not been enough to turn the tide. Communication technology has also blossomed over the same period. Almost no one is beyond its reach. Multiple channels of public communication bathe nearly everyone in oceans of information every day. Perhaps in no other case has knowledge been mobilized so forcefully and at such cost as in the struggle against AIDS . . . and with so little effect.

It is now clear to science that more knowledge about HIV and AIDS does not lead to change in attitudes or sexual behavior. It is increasingly apparent that knowledge about sex is part of complex, culturally elaborated codes of behavior concerning gender, personal identity, community morality, status, prestige, family and household organization, and much else besides, including politics and economics. While it is not enough simply to know more about HIV and AIDS, it is also clearly detrimental to personal and public health to know nothing at all, to know only a little, or to know the wrong things.

In considering the HIV/AIDS epidemic, we need to be strict about the domains of knowledge and the types of logic and argument that pertain to them. On the one hand, we must be clear that the inexorable progress of the virus is a purely biological phenomenon, not a moral one. People are infected without regard to their moral status;

viruses are not moral agents. In the case of flu, no one is blamed when the fever and chills start, and no one is blamed for the coughs and runny noses. Fortunately, we do not die from the ordinary kinds of flu, and this evidently lightens its moral loading. But even in the great flu epidemic of 1918, moral evaluation was not a part of the diagnosis. This, unfortunately, is not the case with HIV infections. The virus is sexually transmitted, for most part, and sex is always beset by moral strictures. But the moral part of it has nothing to do with the actual biological processes involved in the epidemiology and biology of the virus.

On the other hand, we need to be strict in understanding that the sociology of sexuality is not biological. Although desire for sexual contact, touch, and love are certainly biologically rooted and essential for our sense of well-being and physical health, the ways in which they are achieved are highly variable. The existence of desire, we have learned, does not determine the shape of the institutions, stratagems, or behaviors that satisfy those desires, any more than the apparently biological capacity for language in humans determines what language any one of them will speak. The variety of ways in which the sexual impulse is expressed—or suppressed—is vast and apparently unlimited. Thus, we cannot reason from biology to the sociology of sexuality. Nevertheless, when people make statements about uncontrolled sex, promiscuity, or immorality being the cause of the HIV epidemic, they are often reasoning—if *reasoning* is the right word—from the notion that sex is biological and, for some, uncontrollable.

To moralize about the biology of sex and epidemiology, or to biologize the sociology of it, are equally disastrous options. But we often do not know where the boundaries between sociology and biology might be "in fact," or where they—morally, or politically, or philosophically speaking—should be.

The ABC approach has been called a "social vaccine," thus medicalizing a complex sociology. It is a suggestive metaphor, a misapplication of medical approaches to what is in fact a complex sociological phenomenon. It attempts to apply a reductive and deductive methodology inappropriately to a domain that can best be approached ethnographically and historically as a complex set of meanings and interactions. The reduction of this to a medical methodology that attempts to isolate single causes of symptoms in a functionally closed system of the body does not allow us to adequately conceptualize the complex open systems of social and cultural life.

BEYOND ABC

Until now, the ABC approach—or one or another of its components—has formed the basis for prevention strategies. These methods attack the HIV transmission network only indirectly.

It is increasingly clear that our effort to halt or even slow the progress of AIDS is failing. This is especially true in southern Africa, the region that has the largest number of people living with HIV in the world. This is not because people do not know what causes AIDS, that HIV is transmitted through sexual contact, or that it is incurable and eventually fatal. Surveys show us that nearly 100 percent of people living in southern Africa know this. The vast majority of southern Africans also know at least some ways to prevent it. Campaigns often seem feeble and misguided in South Africa, but surveys show us that almost no one is ignorant of AIDS, its causes, and its consequences. Why, then, has this knowledge failed to have an effect?

In some categories and age groups in South Africa, nearly one in two people is likely to be infected. Overall, the rate is much lower, but chances are at least one in ten that a new partner will be HIV-positive. If the chances of contracting a fatal disease are so high, why do so many continue to have unprotected sex?

It may be true, of course, that education campaigns are having an effect, and that HIV prevalence would be worse if not for the fact that everyone is so knowledgeable. But this is scarcely adequate. In South Africa alone, HIV is still infecting an estimated two thousand people per day. Each day, too, one thousand people die of AIDS, despite a much-delayed, but now functioning, rollout of ARVs in government clinics across South Africa. In fact, many people have changed their sexual behavior, but even the changes that have occurred are not sufficient. Why?

To answer these questions requires a shift in perspective. Strangely, we must turn away from the obvious facts that sex provides personal pleasure, that people desire fulfillment through passion, and that most people wish to have children. Desire and pleasure do not cause AIDS, and they do not transmit it. The moralizing discourse that frequently accompanies AIDS education campaigns often makes it seem as if they do. Religious groups that advocate abstinence, for instance, often stress the importance of controlling desire, or delaying pleasure. This resonates strongly with the high value that religion—especially Judaism, Christianity, and Islam—places on resisting temptation, self-denial, and sacrifice. The virgin is the symbol of all of this, and the paragon of purity. Associated as it is in public opinion with sexual excess and unbridled passion, AIDS appears to be custom-made for recruitment to these religious sentiments. The Abrahamic religions, rooted in the Book of Genesis and the idea of the fall from grace, praise the denial of desire as the root of virtue. None of this is relevant to AIDS and its prevention. Excessive and inappropriate moralizing may even hinder effective prevention.

The logic for abstinence is primarily religious, not epidemiological. Sexual desire and passion lead to sexual contact, but transmission of the virus only occurs if sex is part of a much larger network, and only under certain conditions. The high and rising birth rate in Uganda alongside falling or stable HIV prevalence, versus the low and falling total fertility rate alongside rising HIV prevalence in South Africa, demonstrates this. Appeals for abstinence are heeded primarily by those who are already inclined toward it for other reasons, usually religious. The Nelson Mandela 2005 AIDS survey in South Africa, for instance, reported that only 10 percent of youths who had never had sex said that they were abstaining because of fear of HIV or other STIs; most were just not ready or lacked a partner.[3] While abstinence from sex protects absolutely against sexual infection, the abstinent also do not transmit sexual infections. The truly abstinent few, then, are largely irrelevant to the problem of HIV transmission. For the rest, abstinence is only temporary, and their limited removal from the sexual network—or delayed entry—has a negligible impact on the transmission of HIV. Money and effort spent on promotion of abstinence, even if and where it is effective, is therefore wasted.

The role of sex in procreation—making babies—is also largely irrelevant in the quest to control AIDS. The fact that fertility fell in South Africa while HIV advanced unchecked shows this truth conclusively. The two "side effects" of unprotected sex—pregnancy and HIV (or other STI) infection—are apparently unrelated.

The knowledge people have about sex and its consequences does not necessarily translate into self-protective action. Is this merely fatalism? To a degree, the answer is yes. Many people do express the opinion that now that AIDS is so common, there is little they can do to prevent it.

But this points to an even stronger desire to engage in sex than we can account for through our ordinary theories of human behavior. People are willing to risk their lives for it. Is it merely a biological drive that we can do little to control? The history of humanity gives us many examples of religious groups and cultures that have successfully imposed cultural or religious restrictions on sex. In some cases, such as the most puritanical sects of early Shakers in America, this has been so effective that the lack of sex has caused them to die out entirely. Other sexually puritanical religious sects must constantly recruit new members to compensate for their inability to reproduce themselves. So, the answer to the question about whether sex is an uncontrollable biological drive is no. It can be controlled by exceptionally strong cultural—especially religious—beliefs, and by powerful policing of these beliefs. But such control is only desired, and possible, in small, strongly motivated groups of people. Apart from this, sex is far too important to the vast majority of people to be controlled in this way.

It may seem to some that the current epidemic must be caused by an over-indulgence in unprotected sex. This seems unlikely. Judging from surveys of sexual behavior, albeit limited and incomplete, South Africans do not appear to have any more sex than, say, Norwegians or Americans.[4] Since pregnancy is the other main consequence of unprotected sex, if South Africans were having unprotected sex more than others, then the birth rate would also be high. In fact, this is not the case. Thus it appears that the amount of unprotected sex South Africans engage in cannot be the reason for rising HIV. Why then is HIV so prevalent?

ASKING THE RIGHT QUESTIONS

When science fails to answer questions such as these, it is often because the wrong questions have been asked. Since the beginning of the HIV epidemic more than twenty years ago, research on AIDS and approaches to combating it have focused on the behavior and psychology of the individual. This is hardly surprising because sex occurs between individuals, not social structures. The obviousness of this fact has blinded nearly everyone to the larger picture.

Since sex has been seen as behavior, preventive measures have been based on getting individuals to make isolated decisions. This has failed. We can begin to see this larger picture when we understand that sex is in fact a relation between two or more people. In other words, it is a social relation. This allows us to see sex acts as building blocks of social structures, and to develop prevention strategies that aim at the social level at which HIV is transmitted across populations.

The ABC approach to prevention relies on the individual's moral

decisions. It was first formulated by a Catholic priest in Tanzania in the
1980s, and was popularized by Uganda. The United Nations agencies
and the U.S. Agency for International Development further promoted
it as the Ugandan solution to HIV reduction. The first two terms in
this approach, *abstinence* and *being faithful*, rely primarily on religious
precepts. In its original formulation, the C (condoms) was promoted
only for those who could not abstain or be faithful: they were the last
resort for moral failures. This "original" interpretation is again gaining
ground in Uganda, where evangelical Christianity, driven by wealthy
American fundamentalists, is sweeping the nation. Whatever its effect,
this moralist approach neglects the fundamental social values of sex,
and it is not informed by an understanding of the importance of sexual
networks. Where interventions by so-called faith-based organizations
have been successful, it probably has more to do with the fact that they
address cultural issues within the context of relevant social groupings
and structures than with anything having to do with abstinence or even
moral positions.

Sex is the basis for all primary social bonds in human society. The
relationships formed by sex are probably more important than the
momentary pleasure any individual derives from it, and it is this that
drives our need for sex. In fact, primates, including humans, spend
more time having sex than any other animals. Decades of anthropological research on mankind's nearest genetic relatives, the bonobo
chimpanzees, show that they spend a great deal of their time engaged
in sex and sexual play. Humans, like their primate relatives, "naturally" engage in sex because we are the most social of animals and sex
is a fundamental part of our social nature. Sex, then, is a relation, not
just behavior.

This insight helps us to understand why calls for abstinence are not
effective. Although abstinence from sex does guarantee immunity from
infection, it is a price few are willing to pay. This is not a moral failure.
It is, anthropologically speaking, what makes us human, perhaps all
too human. A shift toward seeing the fundamental social value of sex,
however, can also shift our perspective in the effort to stem the tide of
HIV.

This new understanding is to be found not in individual behavior,
but rather in how people are linked into larger structures as the result
of social relations that sex creates and sustains. Anyone who has sex
with more than one other steady lifetime partner (one who also *only*
has sex with his or her steady partner) is necessarily involved in a

sexual network that links that person's sexual relationships with his or her partners to all the other sexual contacts those partners have had or will have with other partners. Depending on how many partners people have, this network can quickly grow to encompass virtually an entire nation of sexually active people.

HIV is an infection of sexual networks as much as it is an infection carried by people. Looked at in this way, the motives for sex, or characteristics of gender and sexual orientation, do not matter. Rather, the shape, timing, and extent of the sexual networks are of paramount importance. Similarly, whether sex takes place in marriage or outside of it is less important than the sexual links that are formed. This perspective moves our attention away from the moral decisions individuals make to the more abstract level of the network.

Judgments about the morality of sex are important to preserve human dignity and the value of sex itself, but often hinder the effectiveness of programs aimed at limiting HIV. Suspicions about condoms, religious strictures on talking honestly about sex, and the high moral value placed by some on abstinence have all been counterproductive. A focus on networks may obviate some of these concerns.

Sexual networks are formed and given shape by the number of sexual partners people have, the frequency with which they have sex, and the timing of their sexual encounters. This determines how efficient the network will be in transmitting the virus. For instance, a person who has sex in the month after being infected him/herself will be vastly more likely to pass on the infection than will those who have been infected longer, up to a point. If a newly infected person has sex with more than one person during this time, the chance of passing HIV on to the wider sexual network is huge. Sexual networks in which each person is linked to multiple others, or in which people switch between several "steady" partners over a short time, are much more likely to transmit HIV. When people have sexual contacts in many different places, perhaps quite distant from one another, the network becomes a highly efficient transmitter of the virus to all parts of the network.

These networks function like highway networks, electrical transmission networks, or even the Internet: every point in the network is reachable from any other point. Moreover, such networks remain highly efficient transmitters of people, goods, power, or HIV, even when many links may be broken. The Internet was designed specifically to be resistant to attack. Some sexual networks may be like the Internet.

The South African sexual networks are clearly highly efficient transmitters of HIV. This can be accounted for by the fact that the population is highly mobile and closely interlinked in dense, overlapping sexual networks.

By contrast, networks that are highly localized, or clustered, with few connections to the outside, or in which people do not change partners frequently, will be very slow to transmit the virus. It now appears that HIV was already endemic in small human populations in central Africa for many decades before the virus was first identified in the early 1980s. It remained limited to small populations, however, and did not escape from these isolated clusters of sexual partners.

This was the case in Uganda. Uganda has been hailed as the only African country in which HIV prevalence has fallen. Attempts to discover why this happened have been inconclusive. In fact, the decline in HIV prevalence in Uganda was so sudden that ordinary epidemiological models cannot account for it. This sudden drop in HIV prevalence, as we have seen, reflected a comprehensive and sudden collapse of the nationwide sexual network that was caused by many factors: death from AIDS, some of the ABC factors, and, above all, the intensive involvement of all aspects of society, government, business, labor, schools, churches, mosques, traditional healers, chiefs, and others. The sexual network suddenly stopped transmitting HIV efficiently and HIV prevalence fell faster than could be accounted for either by individual decisions to practice safer sex or by death alone. Ultimately, it was the collapse of the sexual network that led to Uganda's apparent success.

For many reasons, HIV went global in the 1980s, however, and spread around the world. Can HIV now be put back into the bottle of small local populations? The answer does not lie in individual decisions about whether to have risky sex, but rather in how the broader sexual networks—now nationwide and global—might be reconfigured to make them more resistant to transmission of HIV.

A NEW PARADIGM

With these perspectives in mind, we can return to the question with which we began: Why do AIDS education campaigns apparently have so little effect? To the extent that they fail to change the configuration of sexual networks, AIDS education campaigns alone are unlikely to change the progress of the epidemic. This is true for all networks. For instance, if a few substations in an electrical transmission grid fail, the entire network does not crash, though it might be less efficient in transmitting electricity to all parts of the grid. If the long-distance power lines fail, however, the entire electrical transmission network can collapse. As long as the transmission lines remain up and functional, the failure of a few, or even many, substations can be compensated by rerouting the flow of electricity around them. The same effect can be seen in road networks. For an ordinary network of local roads, if storms damage a section of roadway, cars and trucks can go around the problem on other roads and reach their destinations. The disrupted roadway may slow them down, but they will still get where they are going. If, however, the channel tunnel that now connects England and France were blocked, it would no longer be possible to drive between the two countries. The two national road networks would be isolated from each other.

The same effect can be seen in sexual networks. Two countries have had exceptional success in controlling infection: Uganda and Thailand. Thailand's HIV problem was primarily restricted to prostitutes and their clients, and AIDS education campaigns were effective in getting them to use condoms in their transactions. This interrupted the network that might have allowed HIV to flow freely into the larger population. Increasing the resistance of the network to HIV caused the network to stop transmitting HIV so easily, and HIV prevalence fell rapidly.

Uganda's situation is more complex because the epidemic encompassed the entire sexually active population. Large-scale and integrated programs across all sectors of society and government were effective in changing sexual behavior. But Uganda is also highly differentiated by class, ethnicity, status, residence, and religious affiliation, among other things. The population is largely rural and not very mobile. There were also many deaths from AIDS. All of these factors had the effect of eliminating links between clusters of previously sexually linked people, and the whole network collapsed. HIV was no longer transmitted efficiently throughout the network, and HIV prevalence fell dramatically. The clustered or "lumpy" shape of Ugandan sexual networks multiplied the effects of death and individual decisions to use condoms or reduce the number of sexual partners.

In South Africa, there are few social differences that prove to be barriers to sexual contact. The population is highly mobile, relatively wealthy compared to Uganda and the rest of Africa, and highly urbanized. Its sexual networks are extremely efficient. Even though education campaigns have been effective—and surveys show that they have been at least as effective in South Africa as they were in Uganda—they have had little effect on the network. This is because the South African network is highly interconnected, like a local network of roads or a regional power grid. Even though many links in the sexual network have been eliminated, there are still enough links to ensure efficient transmission of the virus throughout the network.

It is clear that merely the accumulated effect of individual decisions, or levels of knowledge, cannot be effective unless they change the shape of the network. Sexual networks, not individuals, are the transmission lines through which HIV flows across a country. Education and awareness campaigns that miss these facts are likely to fail. So far, especially in southern Africa, they have failed.

A NEW STRATEGY

The perspective developed in this book shows us a new direction for AIDS prevention, one that focuses on the sexual networks that are largely hidden from view. This new direction should not replace the efforts that are already being made, but rather build on these by shaping sexual networks to make them less efficient at transmitting HIV. Preventive strategies must still rely on the knowledge, choices, and practices of individuals, but the new approach is oriented toward rational engagement at the social level rather than isolated decision making at what are, inevitably, inconvenient moments of sexual arousal.

This approach does not ask people to abstain from sex. We now know that this has had little impact. Instead, it seeks to limit exposure to the broader sexual networks of a region, a nation, and the world. The new approach also seeks to avoid moral imperatives and moralizing. Instead, it seeks to expose the hidden sexual networks that transmit HIV and to change them into less efficient transmitters.

There are a number of new preventative measures that can be put into practice. First, we must encourage people to limit themselves to one partner at a time. Overlapping sexual involvements create highways for HIV, especially if shifts between partners occur more rapidly than a month or two. This is similar to the "be faithful" message of the ABC mantra, but it avoids the moralistic overtones of the call for abstinence, the first letter of the triad.

Second, we must make people aware that the timing of their shifts to new partners is especially dangerous. If people would wait for at least a month between new partners, the sexual network will be much more resistant to the flow of HIV. This is because newly infected people are more likely to infect others in the first month or so after infection has occurred. Once in the blood, the concentration of virus rises rapidly until the immune system begins to respond. After about a month, the quantity of viral copies falls to a point where the chance of infecting others is relatively small. Studies of so-called discordant couples (in which one partner is HIV-positive and the other HIV-negative) who continue to have regular unprotected sex show that the chance of infection for the uninfected partner is usually small, depending on their sexual practices (anal sex increases the risk of infection). Eventually, the viral load rises to high levels again as the HIV-positive person develops AIDS. HIV may eventually be passed on in these couples, of course, but if no new partners are involved, especially during the period of high viral load, then transmission to the larger population can be avoided.

Third, the efficiency of HIV transmission across large-scale sexual networks is greatly increased if people have sex far from their own locale. Keeping sex close to home makes long-distance jumps across the larger network more difficult for HIV. Eventually, as in Uganda, the efficiency of HIV transmission in the sexual network collapses.

A new approach to prevention that takes these facts to heart can be simply expressed.

- *One at a time.* Having multiple sexual partners within a short period of time provides multiple links in the sexual network through which the virus can spread rapidly. The one-at-a-time message avoids the moralizing that is inherent in the call for abstinence, and does not deny the value and importance of sex itself. It reduces the density of the sexual network, and thus increases its resistance to the flow of infection.

- *Give it a break.* Waiting at least a month before starting sex with a new partner helps to ensure that a newly infected person is less likely to pass on the virus during the period of high viral load at the beginning of an infection. Timing is critical.

- *Keep it close to home.* This message operates on the diameter of the sexual network. It can be interpreted literally as keeping sex in the home (that is, in the marriage or with one steady partner). Again, it avoids the moralizing message. More than this, however, long-distance links are most likely to connect pools of infection to parts of the network that are not yet infected by bringing everyone closer to everyone else in the network. Pools of infection occur among those who travel. Research has identified long-distance truck drivers and migrant workers as relatively high-prevalence groups. Sexual contact far from home is equally likely, however, for those who travel on business or to seek work, or during travel for funerals, rock concerts, visits to family, or even religious pilgrimages. Although keeping sex local may rule out the fabled one-night stand at a conference in a distant city, it would have a powerful effect on making the sexual network more resistant to transmission of HIV.

The approach can also be packaged as *One, One, One:*[5]

· One at a time,

· One month between, and

· One locale or community.

Built on a conceptual platform different from that of the familiar ABC set of preventive measures, this new approach can greatly increase the effectiveness of prevention. Rather than relying on the cumulative effect of many individual decisions to practice safer sex, this strategy acts on the configuration of the network itself. It does not rely on moral judgments and commitments, but on more practical considerations. As the network becomes more resistant to the flow of infection, it will have a multiplier effect on each individual decision that decreases each person's risk.

Because sex is inherently a social act, rather than merely a behavior, this approach can refocus prevention efforts on a social ethics, in addition to an individualistic morality. Crucially, this approach does not replace other approaches, but works synergistically with them. Its *multiplier effect* increases the impact of any individual decision. Together with the ABC message, this approach to prevention could help to turn the tide of HIV/AIDS epidemics in Africa and beyond.

Notes

PREFACE

1. Ingold 1992.
2. Anderson 1983.

CHAPTER 1

1. I assume comparability despite the fact that comparative studies involving South Africa and other African countries are extremely scarce. I cannot argue the case more fully here due to limits of space, but merely assert it on the basis of years of experience.

2. "HIV/AIDS barometer," *Mail & Guardian,* 18–24 May 2007, 45. According to this news item, estimates indicated that 2,133,490 people had died of HIV/AIDS by noon on 16 May 2007. The source was cited as Plusnews (www.plusnews.org), but the article did not discuss the methodology used to arrive at this estimate.

3. Dorrington et al. (2006) show that 47 percent of all deaths in 2006 probably were due to HIV/AIDS although they were classified under several different categories in the Statistics South Africa report on causes of death for the years 1997–2003 (Statistics South Africa 2005). This statistic rises to 71 percent of deaths in the 15–49 age group.

4. By mid-2006, approximately 350,000 people annually, or around 960 per day, died of AIDS, according to an estimate of the Actuarial Society of South Africa (2006); the South African Institute of Race Relations (2007) gives a figure of 393,777 deaths in 2006, or 1,078 deaths per day.

5. Actuarial Society of South Africa (2006) reports that life expectancy had dropped from 63 in 1990 to 51 in 2006, while the Integrated Regional Information Network (2008) reports life expectancy for men as 47 years and

for women as 49 years. The South African Institute of Race Relations (2007) gives a life expectancy at birth of 50.4 years. UNICEF reports a life expectancy of 46 years (www.unicef.org/infobycountry/southafrica_statistics.html).

6. Under-five mortality in 2007 was 71 annually per thousand live births (South African Institute of Race Relations 2007) compared with 59.4 in 1998 (South African Institute of Race Relations 2002). According to UNICEF, under-five mortality was 60 in 1990 versus 68 in 2005; most of the increase occurred in the first years of the twenty-first century. By contrast, Uganda's under-five child mortality rate fell from 160 in 1990 to 136 in 2005 (www.unicef.org/infobycountry/southafrica_statistics.html, accessed 24 May 2007).

7. South African Institute of Race Relations 2006: 2.

8. Beresford 2006; Green et al. 2006; Ssewanyana and Younger 2005.

9. See Wasswa 2005; Kaplan 2006; Baryarama et al. 2007. United Nations Program on HIV/AIDS (2006: 6, 17, 19–20) points to "discrepant trends in rural areas" of Uganda, where HIV prevalence is apparently rising slightly. "Prevalence rose from a low of 5.6% in men and 6.9% in women in 2000, to 6.5% in men and 8.8% in women in 2004, according to data gathered in a study done in 25 villages" (United Nations Program on HIV/AIDS 2006: 17). This report was based on Shafer et al. (2006) and Ministry of Health, Uganda, and ORC Macro (2006). The latter report, however, gives a prevalence of 7.5 percent for women and 5.0 percent for the age group 15–49 in 2005 (Ministry of Health, Uganda, and ORC Macro 2006: 101). It is not yet clear how significant these data are. These levels are still at or below the prevalence levels reached in 2002 after a period of declining prevalence since 1992. Baryarama et al. (2007) report, however, that prevalence rose to 15 percent in 2003 from 13 percent in 1999 for clients of voluntary counseling and testing facilities, and that incidence rose from 0.9 percent (95 percent confidence interval [CI]: 0.8 to 1.1) in 1993 to 2.3 percent (95 percent CI: 2.2 to 2.5) in 2003.

10. See Motsei (2007) for a comprehensive discussion, especially from the viewpoint of a black South African feminist writer. News stories include: (1) Gordin 2006; (2) "Zuma rape case 'investigated' " ["According to Beeld the complainant is a 31-year-old HIV-positive AIDS activist"], News24 .com, 19 November 2005, posted online at www.news24.com/News24/South_Africa/Zuma/0,,2-7-1840_1837093,00.html (accessed 30 January 2006); and (3) Evans and Rampersadh 2005. Zuma was found not guilty of the rape charge in June 2006, and his trial for corruption has been indefinitely postponed. His alleged accomplice in the corruption case, Schabir Sheik, was found guilty in late 2005, and the court recorded that there was a "generally corrupt" relation between them.

11. Green et al. 2006.

12. Museveni 1997: 1.

13. Museveni 1997: 7.

14. South African Institute of Race Relations 2004: 297. Since these provinces did not yet exist in 1994, however, these figures are reconstructed based on generalizations from prenatal clinic (pregnant women) data. In view of the subsequent progress of the disease and later population-based seroprevalence surveys, these figures are approximately correct.

15. African National Congress 1994.

16. Despite the lack of action, Minister of Health Tshabalala-Msimang stated that this document "has guided the health sector for 10 years and is still relevant today. Almost everything we have done is in there, and we intend to continue with the unfinished business" (Tshabalala-Msimang 2004).

17. African National Congress 2002b.

18. African National Congress 2002b.

19. Centre for Development and Enterprise 2005: 12.

20. Centre for Development and Enterprise 2005: 17.

21. Marks 2002: 16; Posel 2003a, 2003b.

22. Lemey et al. 2003; Zhu et al. 1998.

23 Caldwell and Caldwell 1996: 563.

24. Mann 1989; Mann, Netter, and Tarantola 1992.

25. Marx 1982.

26. Gottlieb et al. 1981; Masur et al. 1981. Although Gottlieb et al. 1981 was one of the first published notices of the syndrome, Gottlieb and his coauthors were not yet aware of the causal agent involved. They suspected that the immune suppression among homosexual men in San Francisco was due to high levels of infection by cytomegalovirus.

27. Centers for Disease Control 1982; Centers for Disease Control and Prevention 2001; Guérin et al. 1984; Liautaud et al. 1992; Pape and Johnson 1988.

28. Marx 1982.

29. Centers for Disease Control 1984.

30. Serwada et al. 1985.

31. Barnett and Whiteside 2002.

32. Sahlins 1981, 1983; Comaroff and Comaroff 1992.

33. Turner 1969.

34. Sahlins 1985.

35. Weber 1979.

36. Gluckman 1963, 1965; Thornton 1994: 151–152.

37. Thornton 1994.

38. Geertz 1983.

39. Farmer 1995.

40. Farmer, Lindenbaum, and Good 1993.

41. Asamoah-Odei, Calleja, and Boerma 2004.

42. Nattrass 2004.

43. Parkhurst and Lush 2004.

44. Vance 1999 [1991].

CHAPTER 2

1. Commission for Africa 2005, chap. 6, para. 6

2. Serwadda et al. 1985. The origins of HIV, however, have been traced to areas farther to the west, in northern Democratic Republic of Congo (Zhu et al. 1998).

3. Stoneburner and Low-Beer 2004: 715; Asamoah-Odei, Calleja, and Boerma 2004.

4. Measure DHS+ 2002.

5. UNICEF, online at www.unicef.org/infobycountry/uganda_statistics
.html.

6. The South African TFR in 1970 was 5.6, and in 1990 it was 3.6
(UNICEF, online at www.unicef.org/infobycountry/southafrica_statistics
.html).

7. South African Institute of Race Relations 2003: 30.

8. Morris et al. 1995; Morris 1997; Rothenberg et al. 1998; Rothenberg
et al. 2000; Aral 1999; Liljeros, Edling, and Amaral 2003; Wohlfeiler and
Potterat 2003; Low-Beer and Stoneburner 2003.

9. Brown 2005.

10. I use the terms *transmission* and *transmitters* here rather than *infectiv-
ity* or *infective agents* in order to emphasize the differences between transmission of pathogens through a connected network of susceptible persons and the
random infection of populations by pathogens that travel through air, water,
or food resources, as most other pathogens do.

11. The standard epidemiological model is presented clearly and simply in
Gouws and Abdool Karim 2005.

12. Stoneburner and Low-Beer 2004.

13. Stoneburner and Low-Beer 2004: 717.

14. See also Low-Beer and Stoneburner 1997 (figure 1), which shows a
similar model with presumed incidence made to fall from 1985–1987, and then
with an incidence reduction of 3 percent per annum. Neither model approximates the reality. This model is also presented in Stoneburner et al. 1996: 691
(figure 5), with more elaboration, and again, more briefly, in Stoneburner et
al. 1998.

15. Gray et al. 2006: 348.

16. Hogle et al. 2002; Green et al. 2006; quotation is from the latter publication. This research involved twenty-four focus groups selected from different social strata and residential areas in three Ugandan cities—Mbarara,
Kampala, and Mbale—with fully transcribed records, and thirty intensive
interviews with major social actors including educators; medical, military, and
government personnel; Christian priests; Islamic imams; traditional healers;
journalists; and others.

17. Green et al. 2006: 337.

18. Baryarama et al. 2007.

19. Gray et al. 2006: 347.

20. Hart 2004.

21. Rasnick lost his affiliation with the University of California in 2002,
but as late as 2006 he was still claiming to be affiliated with that university.
He has been repeatedly warned by the University of California to cease using
its name in his publications and pronouncements. See the Treatment Action
Campaign Web site, www.tac.org.za/newsletter/2006/ns09_05_2006.html.
Rasnick currently works in Pretoria with Matthias Rath, selling high-dose
vitamins that are alleged to cure AIDS or to be useful in treating it (Farber
2006).

22. Duesberg and Rasnick 1998.

23. Duesberg and Ellison 1996; Farber (2006) provides a more recent but no less flawed restatement of this position. See Gallo et al. (2006) for detailed refutation, and the AIDS Truth Web site, www.aidstruth.org/harper-farber .php.

24. Duesberg and Ellison 1996: 5, 1.

25. According to Duesberg and Rasnick (1998), diseases caused by viral agents have the following characteristics.

(i) They rise exponentially and then decline within weeks or months as originally described by William Farr in the early 19th century (Bregman & Langmuir, 1990). The rise reflects the exponential spread of contagion and the fall reflects the resulting natural vaccination or immunity of survivors. (ii) The epidemics spread randomly ("heterosexually" in the words of AIDS researchers) in the population. (iii) The resulting infectious diseases are highly specific reflecting the limited genetic information of the causative microbe. As a consequence the viral diseases are typically more specific than those caused by the more complex bacteria or fungi. It is for this reason that the viruses and microbes are typically named for the specific disease they cause. For example, influenza virus is called after the flu, polio virus after the poliomyelitis, and hepatitis virus after the liver disease it causes. (iv) The microbial and particularly the viral epidemics are self-limiting and thus typically seasonal, because they induce anti-microbial and viral immunity and select also for genetically resistant hosts.

All of this is certainly true.

26. According to Duesberg and Rasnick (1998), diseases caused by environmental or toxic chemical factors have the following in common: "(i) They follow no specific time course, but one that is determined by the dose and duration of exposure to the toxin. (ii) They spread according to consumption or exposure to toxic agents, but not exponentially. (iii) They spread either nonrandomly with occupational or lifestyle factors, or randomly with environmental or nutritional factors. (iv) They range from relatively specific to unspecific depending on the nature of the toxin. (v) They are limited by discontinuation of intoxication, but not self-limiting because they do not generate immunity." Duesberg and Ellison (1996) correctly claimed that medical researchers had a duty to consider the alternative hypothesis that "some noninfectious cause such as poor diet or some toxic substance present in the environment or a toxin consumed in an unusually large quantity" had also to be considered for the science to be valid.

27. Duesberg 2000. Duesberg and Ellison (1996: 6) wrote: "The single flaw that determined the destiny of AIDS research since 1984 was that AIDS was infectious. . . . The only solution is to rethink the basic assumption that AIDS is infectious and caused by HIV." President Mbeki appears to have accepted this position completely.

28. Mbeki was not alone in this, as Farber (2006) shows, and many, including Duesberg and Rasnick, among others, still assert this position.

29. Van der Vliet 2004: 59. The letter can be found online at www.wash ingtonpost.com for 19 April 2000.

30. Duesberg 2000; see also Duesberg and Rasnick 1998. Duesberg (2000) refers specifically to two other supporting papers (Anderson 1996; Seligmann et al. 1984), one published four years earlier and the other sixteen years earlier, and both having been superseded by newer, more accurate research. Brook-

meyer (1996) had already discussed the causes of such statistical false reasoning in 1996, effectively refuting the denialists.

31. Duesberg 2000.

32. Duesberg and Rasnick (1998: 86) wrote, "the long-term consumption of recreational drugs (such as cocaine, heroin, nitrite inhalants, and amphetamines) and prescriptions of DNA chain-terminating and other anti-HIV drugs, cause all AIDS diseases in America and Europe."

33. See The Virus Myth Web site, at www.virusmyth.net/aids/index.htm. According to its index page, it contains more than 1,200 Web pages and 850 articles. It was last updated 7 July 2003 (accessed 31 May 2007).

34. Bregman and Langmuir 1990. Also see Brookmeyer 1996: 784.

35. In fact, poverty and HIV prevalence are slightly negatively correlated for large populations; see Stanton 2006. In other words, it can be shown that the greater the wealth, the higher the HIV prevalence, or the less poverty, the greater the HIV prevalence. The relatively high wealth of South Africa and Botswana, both with extremely high HIV prevalence, tends to skew this correlation for Africa toward a stronger positive correlation between wealth and HIV than may exist elsewhere.

36. The only detailed tracing of a significantly large sexual network that I am aware of to date is Kohler and Helleringer 2006. This is for an island, Likoma, in Lake Malawi.

37. Caldwell, Caldwell, and Orubuloye 1992: 385.

38. Jonathan Stadler's work in the Bushbuckridge area of Limpopo Province, South Africa, is promising. See Kaufman, de Wet, and Stadler 2001; Collins and Stadler 2001; Stadler 2003.

39. Faloutsos, Faloutsos and Faloutsos 1999; Barabási 2002; Buchanan 2002; Watts 2003; Strogatz 2003; Leskovec, Kleinberg, and Faloutsos 2005.

40. Buchanan 2002; Strogatz 2003.

41. Asiimwe-Okiror, Musinguzi, and Madraa 1996; Hogle et al. 2002; Ministry of Health, Uganda 2002.

42. Caldwell and Caldwell 1996: 563.

43. See chapter 1, note 9.

44. As of May 2007, there were not sufficient data to suggest anything but fluctuating stability within a range of 5–7 percent.

45. Human Sciences Research Council 2002; Dorrington, Bradshaw, and Budlender 2002; Asamoah-Odei, Calleja, and Boerma 2004.

46. These are Jinja, Mbarara, Tororo, and Mbale.

47. Probable errors exist in all of the data points for many reasons. A trend line tends to even out the errors and show the data's overall tendency to change in a particular direction at a particular rate. Since the entire data set is taken into account, the errors involved in each point are less important than the overall picture.

48. South African Institute of Race Relations 2004: 297, table "Antenatal Clinic Surveys: HIV infection rates of women attending public antenatal clinics by province, 1991–2002," citing Department of Health, South Africa 2002.

49. Asamoah-Odei, Calleja, and Boerma 2004; Kirby 2004.

50. Leskovec, Kleinberg, and Faloutsos 2005; Hart 2004.
51. Eglash 1999.
52. Ministry of Health, Uganda 1992–2002.
53. Wasswa 2005.
54. Leskovec, Kleinberg, and Faloutsos 2005.
55. Leskovec, Kleinberg, and Faloutsos 2005.
56. Barabási 2002: 91, 80.
57. Barabási 2002: 20.
58. Gladwell 2000.
59. Strogatz 2003: 255.
60. Bishai et al. 2006.

CHAPTER 3

1. Gray et al. 2006: 348.
2. This is primarily because statistical methods (and the epidemiological methods that are based on them) assume that HIV prevalence is a function of one variable or some set of the identified variables (abstinence, condom use, etc.), and that these can be measured within reasonable limits on error. We assume that these variables are independent and can therefore be separated from one another by mathematical methods. We also have to assume that probabilities are distributed normally, that is, according to a Gaussian or Weibull distribution. None of these assumptions, however, is necessarily valid.
3. Measure DHS+ 1998.
4. Dorrington, Bradshaw, and Budlender 2002; Kirby 2004.
5. Konde-Lule, Musagara, and Musgrave 1993; Hogle et al. 2002; Stoneburner and Low-Beer 2004; South African Institute of Race Relations 2002; Wellings et al. 2006.
6. Wellings et al. 2006.
7. Wellings et al. 2006: 1723.
8. Stoneburner and Low-Beer 2004: 717, figure 3(A). See chapter 2 for a fuller discussion.
9. Wohlfeiler and Potterat 2003.
10. Caldwell, Caldwell, and Quiggin 1989, 1991; Caldwell, Caldwell, and Orubuloye 1992; Barnett and Whiteside 2002; Gray et al. 2006; Green et al. 2006.
11. Thornton 2003a; Parkhurst and Lush 2004; Kirby 2004.
12. Barnett and Whiteside 2002: 295–306.
13. Goody 1976; Caldwell, Caldwell, and Quiggin 1989.
14. Weber 1979; Goody 1976.
15. Cronje 2005.
16. Reid 2002; Roberts 1962.
17. South African Institute of Race Relations 2003: 376.
18. South African Institute of Race Relations 2005a. The owners of these "farms" are often corporations.
19. South African Institute of Race Relations 2003: 376.
20. South African Institute of Race Relations 2003: 376–378.

21. Buchanan 2002; Strogatz 2003; Barabási 2002.

22. Fallers 1964.

23. Maquet 1961.

24. Beattie 1971: 7.

25. Bishai et al. (2006) find "a robust association between residing in rural Ugandan communities where multiple languages are spoken and the odds of non-spousal sex for unmarried women and for married men." Specifically, they found that "for unmarried women rates of sexual activity were significantly higher, 26% in multilingual compared to 13% in monolingual clusters (Z = 3.01, p < 0.01). But rates of extramarital contact were significantly higher for married men with 29% in multilingual clusters compared to 16% in monolingual clusters (Z = 3.59, p < 0.01)." Men had from four to twenty extramarital partners in these multilinguistic communities, whereas sexually active unmarried women reported from three to five partners in the previous twelve months.

26. Measure DHS+ 2002: 75.

27. Mukyala-Mukiika 2000: 105.

28. The kingdom of Ankole is the sole exception. President Museveni felt that the traditional social structure of this kingdom, with its racial/ethnic hierarchy of BaHima and BaIru, was too similar to that of Rwanda and Burundi to be allowed to reconstitute itself. Conflict between people labeled Tutsi (linked to the BaHima in Ankole) and those labeled Hutu (linked to the BaIru in Ankole) has led to extreme bloodshed in Rwanda and Burundi in the past, and Museveni intended to avoid this in Uganda. Doornbos (2001: v) notes, "Particularly to Buganda, where the idea of kingship could count on broad popular support, social relations and perception of history in the Ankole region have rather appeared to militate against re-acceptance of monarchical institutions."

29. Mukyala-Mukiika 2000: 96; Doornbos 2001.

30. The Ganda kingdom has been dominated by Protestants since the late nineteenth century, when the Protestant faction won an internal struggle against the Catholic faction. Thus, the display of a Ganda kingdom flag at a Catholic school is significant in showing the broad appeal of the Ganda monarchy.

31. Richards 1966.

32. Wrigley 1996: 238; Reid 2002: 36.

33. Asamoah-Odei, Calleja, and Boerma 2004: 36.

34. Bessinger, Akwara, and Halperin 2003; Udjo 1998.

35. Brown 2005.

36. Lwanga and Othieno 2005.

37. Udjo 1998.

38. Measure DHS+ 2002; Kirby 2004.

39. Thornton 2005.

40. Beattie 1971: 7.

41. Budlender, Chobokoane, and Simelane 2004.

42. Thornton 2001.

43. Kaufman, de Wet, and Stadler 2001.

44. Thornton 2003b.

45. Karlström 2004.

46. Thornton 2002.

47. South African Institute of Race Relations 2005b: 375. *Working vehicle* is defined in the statistics as a road-worthy, licensed vehicle with four or more wheels. There are, in fact, many more that are not road-worthy or are unlicensed, in the rural areas especially, and this does not include motorbikes and motorcycles.

48. South African Institute of Race Relations 2005b: 385.

49. South African Institute of Race Relations 2005b: 377.

50. South African Institute of Race Relations 2005b: 519.

51. South African Institute of Race Relations 2005b: 518.

52. South African Institute of Race Relations 2003: 10; South African Institute of Race Relations 2004: 12–13.

53. Measure DHS+ 1998.

54. Budlender, Chobokoane, and Simelane 2004; Statistics South Africa 1998.

55. Karlström 2004: 598.

56. Karlström 2004: 598.

57. Wasswa 2005; United Nations, Uganda 2005.

58. Human Sciences Research Council 2002.

59. Low-Beer and Stoneburner 2003; Stoneburner and Low-Beer 2004: 714.

60. Caldwell, Caldwell, and Orubuloye 1992.

61. Low-Beer and Stoneburner 2003.

62. Asamoah-Odei, Calleja, and Boerma 2004: 35.

63. Asamoah-Odei, Calleja, and Boerma 2004.

64. Asamoah-Odei, Calleja, and Boerma 2004: 35.

CHAPTER 4

1. Kiwawulo (2006) reports an increase from 10 percent to 25 percent in one year in the Kawempe District. Mulondo (2006) reports that, with HIV infections rising slightly, Museveni warned against complacence. The Uganda AIDS Commission director, Dr. Kihumuro Apuuli, reported an increase in new infections from 70,000 in 2003 to about 130,000 in 2005, according to KaiserNetwork.org (www.kaisernetwork.org/daily_reports/rep_index .cfm?DR_ID=37396, report dated 22 May 2006, accessed 7 November 2006). Merson (2006), citing Wakabi (2006), notes, "HIV prevalence is no longer on the decline and, in fact, may be increasing in some parts of the country and particularly in adults aged in their 30s." See also Gray et al. 2006: 349.

2. Baingana 2005: 70.

3. Loconte 2003.

4. Loconte 2003.

5. Loconte 2003.

6. Hogle et al. 2002.

7. Whitworth et al. 2002.

8. Whitworth et al. 2002: 1048; Kamali et al. 2000.

9. Kamali et al. 2000.

10. Turyasingura 1989.

11. Van Dijk 2000; Meyer 2004; Rice 2004; Epstein 2005.

12. Ministry of Health, Uganda 2001.

13. Whitworth et al 2002; Kamali et al. 2000.

14. Asiimwe-Okiror et al. 1997; Lyons 1996; Kagimu and Marum 1996; among others.

15. Hogle et al. 2002; Bessinger, Akwara, and Halperin 2003.

16. Hogle et al. 2002: 3.

17. Interview with Emmanuel Sekatawa, Institute of Statistics and Applied Economics, Makerere University, 4 July 2003.

18. Hogle et al. 2002.

19. Kagimu and Marum 1996.

20. To the best of my knowledge, the raw data are held to be confidential.

21. Ministry of Health, Uganda 2002: 7.

22. Ministry of Health, Uganda 2002: 8–9.

23. Whitworth et al. 2002.

24. Whitworth et al. 2002: 1048.

25. Whitworth et al 2002.

26. Hogle et al. 2002.

27. Interview with Dr. Samuel I. Okware, commissioner of health services/ community health, Ministry of Health, Kampala, 24 July 2003.

28. Asiimwe, Kibombo, and Neema 2003; Kirby 2004; Thornton 2003a.

CHAPTER 5

1. Idi Amin Dada, who had been president of Uganda since overthrowing Milton Obote on 25 January 1971, was known as one of the bloodiest dictators that Africa has seen. Some four hundred thousand died under his rule, and the entire "Asian" population (as those descended from original immigrants from India were called) of some twenty thousand people was driven out in the early 1970s. Amin was forced to flee Uganda after an attack by Tanzania in 1979 succeeded in restoring Milton Obote to the presidency. Amin died in Saudi Arabia on 16 August 2003.

2. Dr. Samuel Ikwaras Okware, born 16 August 1948 in Tororo, Uganda, received a master's in public health and epidemiology at the University of Minnesota in 1979 as a World Health Organization fellow, after studying for a doctorate in public health and an MB ChB (equivalent to the MD degree in the United States) at Makerere University from 1968 to 1976. During the last years of the Obote and Tito Okello regimes he was assistant director of medical services/public health. In 1985, he became director of the National AIDS Control Programme in the Ministry of Health, and chairman of the National Committee for the Prevention of AIDS. In 1990, he was made deputy director of medical services in charge of public health, and from 1995, as commissioner of health services/communicable disease control and AIDS, he continued to oversee the AIDS programs together with all other communicable disease pro-

grams. Since 1998 he has been commissioner of health services for community health. See www.health.go.ug/okware.htm.

3. Interview with Dr. Samuel I. Okware, Ministry of Health, 25 July 2003. Although Dr. Okware said this to me in July 2003, he was repeating words quoted by *New Vision* on 4 September 1993. See Iliffe 1998: 223, where they are quoted again.

4. Interview with Dr. Samuel I. Okware, 25 July 2003.

5. Inside headline: "*Abakazi abakuba abasajja kibook*" (Women whip their men), *Bukedde*, 5 July 2003, 14.

6. Interview with Dr. Samuel I. Okware, 25 July 2003.

7. Interview with Dr. Nakanyike Musisi, professor at Makerere Institute of Social Research and member of the Uganda AIDS Commission, Makerere Institute of Social Research, 26 July 2003.

8. In 2006, Professor John Rwomushana was director of policy advocacy and knowledge management at the Uganda AIDS Commission.

9. In 2006, Dr. Kihumuro Apuuli was director general of the Uganda AIDS Commission.

10. Kagimu et al. 1998: 215. The percentage of Muslims was greatly increased during the Amin regime, when considerable economic incentives to convert were offered. The businesses and properties confiscated from Indians and Europeans after 1972 were preferentially handed out to political supporters and to Muslims by Amin.

11. Interview with Emmanuel Sekatawa, Institute of Statistics and Applied Economics, Makerere University, 4 July 2003.

12. FGD: born-again Christian women, 45–60 years old, Ibanda County, Kabingo cell, Mbarara District, 16 July 2003.

13. FGD: men, 36–73 years old, Naguru, Kampala, 8 July 2003.

14. FGD: men, 35–64 years old, Kakoba, Mbarara, 17 July 2003.

15. Interview with Mrs. G. Goretti, community counselor, Kikyenkye, Mbarara, 16 July 2003.

16. FGD: women, 46–60 years old, Igorora, Mbarara, 16 July 2003.

17. Iliffe 1998: 150.

18. Iliffe 1998: 151.

19. FGD: professional women, 31–65 years old, Bumulyanyuma, Mbale, 17 July 2003.

20. Interview with Dr. Cissy Kityo Mutuluuza, deputy director (clinical and research), Joint Clinical Research Centre, 5 July 2003.

21. FGD: poor women, 18–50 years old, Kifumbira, Kampala, 9 July 2003.

22. FGD: male youths, 18–30 years old, Bungokho, Mbale, 18 July 2003.

23. FGD: professional women, 31–65 years old, Bumulyanyuma, Mbale, 17 July 2003.

24. FGD: professional women, 31–65 years old, Bumulyanyuma, Mbale, 17 July 2003.

25. FGD: professional women, 31–65 years old, Bumulyanyuma, Mbale, 17 July 2003.

26. FGD: male youths, 18–30 years old, Bungokho, Mbale, 18 July 2003.

27. FGD: male youths, 18–30 years old, Bungokho, Mbale, 18 July 2003.

28. Interview with Jessie Kagera, AIDS advisor to the president, conducted by Daniel Halperin, U.S. Agency for International Development, July 2003.

29. Interview with Jessie Kagera conducted by Daniel Halperin, July 2003.

30. Uganda AIDS Commission 2002; Kagimu and Marum 1996; Barnett and Whiteside 2002: 28–29.

31. Bayley 1983.

32. Barabási 2002: 123; Shilts 2001.

33. Barabási 2002: 124.

34. Kagimu and Marum 1996.

35. FGD: men, 22–54 years old, Kifumbira, Kampala (Ankole and Kiga, western Uganda), 11 July 2003.

36. FGD: poor women, 18–50 years old, Kifumbira, Kampala, 9 July 2003.

37. Interview with Dr. Samuel I. Okware, 25 March 2003.

38. FGD: unemployed men (mostly from the north, Acholi, Lango), Naguru (slum), Kampala, 8 July 2003 (in English).

39. This phrase was seen on a billboard in Mbarara advertising the services of the Counselling and Testing Service.

40. *Ukimwi* is an acronym in KiSwahili, standing for *Ukosefu wa kinga mwilini* (a shortage of protection in the body).

41. Hooper 1990: 38.

42. FGD: unemployed men (mostly from the north, Acholi, Lango), Naguru (slum), Kampala, 8 July 2003 (in English).

43. FGD: unemployed men (mostly from the north, Acholi, Lango), Naguru (slum), Kampala, 8 July 2003 (in English).

44. FGD: unemployed men (mostly from the north, Acholi, Lango), Naguru (slum), Kampala, 8 July 2003 (in English).

45. FGD: unemployed men (mostly from the north, Acholi, Lango), Naguru (slum), Kampala, 8 July 2003, (in English).

46. 1982: Hooper 1990; 1983: Schopper et al. 1995: 171.

47. Iliffe 1998: 222, citing A. M. T. Lwegaba, "Preliminary report of 'an unusual wasting disease' complex nicknamed 'slim,' a slow epidemic in Rakai District, Uganda" (November 1984), photocopy of typescript, Ministry of Health Library, Kampala.

48. Iliffe 1998: 222, citing Olweny in Parry 1984.

49. Iliffe 1998: 223 n. 7, citing Sewankambo et al. 1987: 9.

50. Iliffe 1998: 223 nn. 11, 12, citing Serwadda et al. 1985, and Carswell et al. 1986.

CHAPTER 6

1. Kagwa 1905.

2. Kagwa 1900.

3. *Munno,* 13 April 1985, 1 (translation by the author).

4. Iliffe 1998: 223, 333. Iliffe credits the *Weekly Topic* as being the first to publish on slim, but *Munno* preceded this by five months, albeit in Luganda.

5. Serwadda et al. 1985.

6. Kreiss et al. 1986.

7. Serwadda et al. 1985.

8. Joseph Tamale Mirundi, "Siliimu avudde kuki Rakai?" *Munno*, 6 June 1985.

9. "Siliimu tava ku mwenge gwa kayinja," *Munno*, 19 June 1985.

10. "Ku bya siliimu nzikirisiganya ne Kafeero," *Munno*, 20 June 1985.

11. "'Siliimu' abatuuza bufofofo," *Munno*, 17 February 1986 (translation by the author).

12. "'Siliimu' abatuuza bufofofo," *Munno*, 17 February 1986 (translation by the author).

13. *Munno*, 25 April 1986 (translation by the author).

14. *Munno*, 26 April 1986.

15. *Munno*, 26 April 1986 (translation by the author).

16. *Munno*, 26 April 1986 (translation by the author).

17. "Ekyuma kya 'Siliimu' kigobye," *Munno*, 26 June 1986, 1. Nsambya Hospital an Anglican mission hospital, is one of the antenatal clinic sentinel sites.

18. "Eddagala lya siriimu linaatunaibwa mu maduka," *Munno*, 22 September 1986 (translation by the author).

19. "Bannauganda bassiddwako ekiragiro ku siliimu," *Munno*, 25 September 1986.

20. "Kampeyini ku kuwanisa siliimu yagguddwawo," *Munno*, 3 October 1986 (translation by the author).

21. "Omusaserdooti abagumizza kusiriimu," *Munno*, 14 March 1986, 3.

22. Interview with Emmanuel Sekatawa, Institute of Statistics and Applied Economics, Makerere University, 4 July 2003.

23. Hooper 1990: 40.

24. Focus group discussion (FGD): women, 33–58 years old, Mbarara, 17 July 2003.

25. FGD: men, more than 35 years old, Kifumbira, Kampala, 10 July 2003.

26. FGD: young men, Bungokho, Mbale, 18 July 2003.

27. United Programme on HIV/AIDS 2002: 6.

28. FGD: male youths, 18–30 years old, Bungokho, Mbale, 18 July 2003.

29. This may refer to the caliber of the guns or to the fact that the Tanzanian national independence day is called *saba saba,* after the seventh day of the seventh month (July) in KiSwahili, the national language of Tanzania. I was not able to determine the origin of the name for the heavy artillery.

30. FGD: men, 36–73 years old, Naguru, Kampala, 8 July 2003 (in English).

31. FGD: women, 36–60 years old, Mbale, Namukwekwe,16 July 2003.

32. Hooper 1990: 103.

33. Carswell et al. 1986.

34. Hooper 1990: 104.

35. Hooper 1990: 104.

36. FGD: women, 46–60 years old, Igorora, Mbarara, 16 July 2003.

37. *Munno*, 23 January 1989 (translation by the author).

38. United Nations Development Programme 2002. The global strategy was updated in 1992.

39. Kagimu and Marum 1996.

40. Uganda AIDS Commission 2002.

CHAPTER 7

1. Kagimu and Marum 1996. From 1989 to 1999, USAID provided $4.2 million to projects concerned with orphans.

2. Interview with Dr. Dorothy Balaba, THETA, Kampala, 3 July 2003.

3. Uganda AIDS Commission 2002.

4. Uganda AIDS Commission 2002.

5. Interview with Emmanuel Sekatawa, Institute of Statistics and Applied Economics, Makerere University, 4 July 2003.

6. Uganda AIDS Commission 2002.

7. Kagimu and Marum 1996.

8. Interview with Dr. Dorothy Balaba, 3 July 2003.

9. Kagimu and Marum 1996.

10. Kagimu and Marum 1996.

11. Kagimu and Marum 1996.

12. Kagimu and Marum 1996.

13. Uganda AIDS Commission 2002; Kagimu and Marum (1996) give the date of founding of the AICs as 1991.

14. Uganda AIDS Commission 1993: 7.

15. Ministry of Health, Uganda 2002: 6–7.

16. Konde-Lule, Musagara, and Musgrave 1993: 679, citing Wawere et al. 1991.

17. Uganda AIDS Commission 1993: 8.

18. Uganda AIDS Commission 1993.

19. Uganda AIDS Commission 1993: x–ix.

20. Kagimu and Marum 1996.

21. Uganda AIDS Commission 1993: vi–vii, para. 7 and 8.

22. Uganda AIDS Commission 2002; Uganda AIDS Commission 1993: vii, para. 13.

23. Uganda AIDS Commission 1993: vii.

24. Uganda AIDS Commission 1993: vii.

25. Uganda AIDS Commission 1993: para. 21.g.

26. Uganda AIDS Commission 1993: para. 21.f.

27. Museveni 1997: 217.

28. There is no attribution of source for this figure.

29. Uganda AIDS Commission 1993: 26–27.

30. Uvulectomy is the removal of the uvula, or soft tissue at the back and top of the throat, something like a tonsillectomy.

31. Uganda AIDS Commission 1993: 27.

32. Uganda AIDS Commission 1993: 36.

33. The removal of the foreskin of the penis (male circumcision) is practiced

in some areas in Uganda, but not all (especially not in Buganda). Removal of teeth and the uvula are related to traditional medical beliefs. Female circumcision is not practiced traditionally in Uganda, but may exist in Muslim-majority parts of the north due to contact with Islam in the Sudan.

34. Interview with Dr. Dorothy Balaba, 3 July 2003.

35. Interview with Dr. Dorothy Balaba, 3 July 2003.

36. Interview with Dr. John Rwomushana, Uganda AIDS Commission, Mmengo, 29 July 2003.

37. Interview with Dr. Dorothy Balaba, 3 July 2003.

38. Uganda AIDS Commission 1993: 33.

39. Kagimu and Marum 1996.

40. The Heritage Foundation briefing document, cited by the Bush administration in support of its negative policy on condoms, said, "Condoms do not play the primary role in reducing HIV/AIDS transmission" (Loconte 2003).

41. For a summary of condoms distributions and sources, see Kirby 2004.

42. Kagimu and Marum 1996.

43. Uganda AIDS Commission 2002.

44. Ministry of Health, Uganda 1996.

45. Uganda AIDS Commission 1993: 7.

46. Kagimu and Marum 1996.

47. Kagimu and Marum 1996.

48. Kagimu and Marum 1996.

49. Kagimu and Marum 1996.

50. Uganda AIDS Commission 2002.

51. Uganda AIDS Commission 2002.

52. Uganda AIDS Commission 2002.

53. 427,153 women, 425,644 men; 852,797 adults, 94,755 children.

54. 531,909 women; 413,591 men; 945,500 adults; 105,055 children less than 15 years of age.

55. Ministry of Health, Uganda 2002: 22; United Nations Development Programme 2002: 27.

CHAPTER 8

1. The History of AIDS, 1987–1992, AVERT, online at www.avert.org/his87_92.htm; Bureau of Hygiene and Tropical Diseases, *AIDS Newsletter*, issue 16 (1987); Cameron 2005: 79.

2. Cameron 2005: 79.

3. United Nations Programme on HIV/AIDS 2002.

4. The United Nations Program on HIV/AIDS (2006) estimated the number of people in South Africa living with HIV to be 5.5 million, with an error range of 4.9–6.1 million.

5. Actuarial Society of South Africa 2006. This model shows total accumulated deaths from AIDS by the middle of 2005 to be 1,477,556 for South Africa, based on earlier statistical trends. See www.assa.org.za/aids/content.asp?id = 1000000449.

6. BBC.co.uk, "Mandela's eldest son dies of AIDS," 6 January 2005, online at http://news.bbc.co.uk/1/hi/world/africa/4151159.stm.

7. "The South African response to the HIV epidemic has been characterised by a unique form of denialism in the highest echelons of political power" (Abdool Karim 2005: 31).

8. Address to CODESA by Nelson R. Mandela, president of the African National Congress, 20 December 1991. Posted online at www.anc.org.za/ancdocs/speeches/1991/sp911220.html.

9. Department of Health, South Africa 2000.

10. Van der Vliet 2001; van der Vliet 1994: 119; van der Vliet 1996.

11. The principle recent works on AIDS in South Africa include, among others, Abdool Karim and Abdool Karim 2005; Barnett and Whiteside 2002; Cameron 2005; Campbell 2003; Chirambo and Caesar 2003; Dorrington, Bradshaw, and Budlender 2002; Dorrington, Bradshaw, Johnson, and Budlender 2004; Heywood 2004; Iliffe 2006: 33–47; Kauffman and Lindaur 2004; Nattrass 2004; and van der Vliet 2001. In addition, a book of poetry and stories, Rasebotsa, Samuelson, and Thomas 2004, gives deep personal and literary insight into South Africans' experiences of living with HIV and dying of AIDS.

12. Van der Vliet 2001: 152.

13. Heald 2006.

14. Ijsselmuiden et al. 1993.

15. Baqwa 1996.

16. Ijsselmuiden et al. 1993.

17. Seidel 1996; Whiteside 1993.

18. Whiteside 1993.

19. Whiteside 1993.

20. Cameron 2005; AIDS Consortium Web site, www.aidsconsortium.org .za/.

21. The AIDS Charter, in Zulu, English, Afrikaans, Sotho, Tsonga, and Venda, is available on the AIDS Consortium Web site, www.aidsconsortium. org.za/index.php?option = com_content&task = view&id = 12&Itemid = 41.

22. African National Congress 1955.

23. De Cock, Mbori-Ngacha, and Marum 2002.

24. De Cock, Mbori-Ngacha, and Marum 2002; Nattrass 2004: 143, 146.

25. Nattrass 2004: 43; van der Vliet 2001: 160.

26. The ecu, or European currency unit, was the predecessor to the euro.

27. Baqwa 1996.

28. The public was never informed of who or what group had been involved in this subterfuge. Eventually, it appears, a consortium of "South Africans from the private sector" came up with the funds to support the minister and "pledge[d] to support and pay for the play and support future endeavours that deal with AIDS" (South African Communication Service 1996).

29. South African Communication Service 1996.

30. South African Communication Service 1996.

31. Deane 2005.

32. Mbeki 1998.

33. Doherty and Colvin 2004.

34. The document was circulated among ANC party members and through email. It has been posted on the Internet (www.virusmyth.net/aids/data/ancdoc.htm) together with other documents pertaining to AIDS denialism, including those of Rasnick and others (African National Congress 2002b). Microsoft Word's properties menu gives the name Thabo Mbeki in the author field of the document downloaded (September 2006) from the ANC Web site and reports that the document was created in April 2002. It is approximately forty thousand words in length. Under the title, the document is dated "March 2002." The South African government has made no effort to deny it or withdraw it.

35. Mbeki 1998.

36. Forman, Pillay, and Sait 2004.

37. South African Government 2000.

38. Pillay et al. 2001; 160 patients were tested. Cited in Doherty and Colvin 2004: 207, table 17.

39. Colvin et al. 2001; 507 patients were tested.

40. Wilkinson, Wilkinson, and Connolly 1999; 196 patients were tested.

41. Meyers et al. 2000; 507 patients were tested.

42. Johnson et al. 2000; 176 patients were tested.

43. South African Government 2000: 7.

44. Leclerc-Madlala 2005: 846.

CHAPTER 9

1. Letter to Kofi Annan, Secretary General, United Nations, from Joint Civil Society Monitoring Forum (JCSMF), re: United Nations General Assembly Special Session on HIV/AIDS (UNGASS)—South Africa's Progress Report, dated 6 April 2006. Document posted online at www.tac.org.za/Documents/JCSMF_letter_UN_govt%20report_re_UNGASS_7_april_2006.doc (accessed 25 June 2006). The JCSMF was founded in 2004 by several organizations including the Treatment Action Campaign, AIDS Law Project, Health Systems Trust, Centre for Health Policy, Institute for Democracy in South Africa, Open Democracy Advice Centre, University of Cape Town School of Public Health and Family Medicine, Public Service Accountability Monitor, and Médecins sans Frontières in South Africa.

2. "PanAfrica: Politics override the needs of vulnerable people at UNGASS UN integrated regional information networks." African News Service, 1 June 2006. Posted online at http://allafrica.com/stories/200606010192.html. Palitza Kristin, "South Africa: AIDS gathering highlights tensions between government, NGOs," Inter Press Service News Agency, 18 June 2006. Posted online at www.ipsnews.net/africa/nota.asp?idnews = 33502.

3. Rath describes his product as "micronutrients" that are "key factors to fight immune deficiencies." Pharmaceutical companies providing antiretroviral drugs are described as engaged in "pharmaceutical colonialism." See www4.dr-rath-foundation.org.

4. "AIDS patient backs Manto [Tshabalala-Msimang]," News24.com, 6 May 2005. Posted online at www.news24.com/News24/South_Africa/Aids_Focus/o,,2–7-659_1700611,00.html.

5. "Nozipho Bhengu" [obituary], *The Economist*, 8 June 2006. Posted online at www.economist.com/obituary/displaystory.cfm?story_id = 7033269. "TAC [Treatment Action Campaign] statement on the death of Nozipho Bhengu," TAC electronic newsletter, 24 May 2006. Posted online at www.tac .org.za/nl20060524a.html.

6. "Analysis of deaths on Matthias Rath illegal clinical trial," TAC electronic newsletter, 2 November 2005. Posted online at www.tac.org.za/ ns02_11_2005.html.

7. Letter to the Editor, "We were right all along," from Dr. Manto Tshabalala-Msimang, minister of health, to the *Mail & Guardian*, 9–15 June 2006, 23.

8. Westhead, Carter, and Momberg 2006.

9. Cullinan 2006.

10. Monare and Daniels 2006.

11. Cullinan 2006; Adams 2006; Monare and Daniels 2006; Westhead, Carter, and Momberg 2006.

12. "Manto still in charge of AIDS programme," South African Press Association, 6 November 2006, posted online at www.iol.co.za/index.php?set_id =1&click_id=125&art_id = qw1162827362448B243; "New plan for AIDS in South Africa," Africa News Dimensions, 5 November 2006, posted online at http://southafrica.andnetwork.com/index;jsessionid=6E76B05C195EA6 A211EE520578B2B488?service=direct/1/Home/older.fullStory&sp=l55345; "Manto's deputy will be her voice on AIDS," originally published by *The Star* (Johannesburg), 10 November 2006, 7, posted online at www.iol.co.za/index .php?from=rss_South%20Africa&set_id=1&click_id=&art_id=vn20061110 011955724C801675; "Manto's absence a boon for TAC," originally published by *Cape Argus*, 9 November 2006, 7, posted online at www.iol.co.za/index .php?set_id=1&click_id=125&art_id=vn20061109134229846C354511.

13. Zukile Majova, "How Manto dodged axing," *Mail & Guardian*, 18–24 May 2007, 2.

14. "Manto snubs AIDS conference," *The Star* (Johannesburg), 6 June 2007.

15. Westhead, Carter, and Momberg 2006.

16. See www.secomet.com/pages/science.php. Secomet V is an "acidic plant extract from the *trifollium* species" (Kotwal et al. 2005)

17. "UCT acts against academic associated with AIDS tonic," Mail & Guardian Online, 3 July 2006, www.mg.co.za/articlePage.aspx?articleid=27 6134&area=/breaking_news/breaking_news__national/; "UCT prof resigns over HIV 'concoction,'" *Cape Times* (Cape Town), 26 October 2006, 5.

18. Letter to the Editor, "We were right all along."

19. Duesberg and Rasnick 1998; Duesberg 2000.

20. Duesberg and Rasnick 1998: 85.

21. African National Congress, Mbeki's cabinet statement on HIV/AIDS,

6 May 2002. *ANC Today,* the organization's publication, states that the "government's starting point is based on the premise that HIV causes AIDS" (African National Congress 2002a).

22. African National Congress 2002b.

23. Cameron 2005: 98.

24. Cameron 2005: 99.

25. Le Carré 2001. See also Farber 2006 for a later version of the Duesberg/Rasnick denialist position and Le Carré's worries about the corruption of medicine by drug-industry money. Gallo et al. (2006) present a refutation of Farber's claims.

26. Deane 2005: 543.

27. Cameron 2005: 106, 114.

28. African National Congress 2002b cites the *Sunday Times* of 6 January 2002 as the source of this remark.

29. African National Congress 2002b, chap. 13 (pagination varies in the electronic versions).

30. See Posel 2003b, n. 96, which cites Gazi 2001.

31. Court case: *Costa Gazi versus the Minister of Public Services and Administration; the Director-General: Provincial Administration, Eastern Cape Province, and Magistrate Maqubela;* judgment of 24 March 2006. See TAC electronic newsletter, 30 March 2006, posted online at www.tac.org.za/.

32. Judgment of Judge J. Bertelsman, paragraphs 44 and 45 in *Costa Gazi versus the Minister of Public Services and others,* 24 March 2006. See TAC electronic newsletter, 30 March 2006, posted online at www.tac.org.za/.

33. Cameron 2005: 113

34. Campbell 2003.

35. Treatment Action Campaign press statement, "Day of action, International Human Rights Day," 10 December 1998, posted online at www.tac.org.za/treat.html.

36. Cameron 2005: 162–166; Sidley 2000.

37. Deane 2005: 545; Cameron 2005: 116.

38. Beresford 2006.

39. Leclerc-Madlala 2002.

40. According to the Actuarial Society of South Africa, 2005 model. Press release in TAC electronic newsletter, posted online at www.tac.org.za/ns29_11_2005.htm.

41. South African Government Information Web site (2005); Department of Health, South Africa 2006.

42. South African Institute of Race Relations 2004: 320.

43. South African Institute of Race Relations 2004: 368, "Households with television sets by race, 2001," based on Statistics South Africa 2003, 2004.

44. Butler 2005: 591.

45. Posel 2003b.

46. Salcedo 2004.

47. Moya 2006.

CHAPTER 10

1. I use the phrase *South African culture* with some trepidation and acknowledge a certain lack of exactitude. South Africa, in fact, is as multicultural as most large nations today, if not more so. I simply wish to focus attention on certain aspects that would appear to be common in South African culture since they are treated as such by the public media and in political discourse. Sex and AIDS, and issues that are related to these, seem to have achieved this status of shared national representations and discourses.

2. *Tshepang: The third testament* (Newton 2005) was first performed at the Grahamstown National Arts Festival on 3–5 July 2003, and has been performed several times in South Africa and the United Kingdom. It has been performed, among other places, at the Gate Theatre in London (U.K. premier, 21 September–16 October 2004), at the Dublin Theatre Festival (October 2005), at the Market Theatre, Johannesburg (March 2005), and at the Wits University Theatre (where I saw it).

3. For statistics on rape of children, the category was defined in the police statistics as those less than 18 years of age. Dempster 2001; CNN 2001; Swarns 2002.

4. Ford 2005.

5. This case was observed in Acornhoek, Northern Province, at a 1995 meeting of the Traditional Healers Organisation, led by the organization's founder, Nhlavana Maseko.

6. Wojcicki and Malala 2001.

7. I have tried this. If a small amount of water is put into a condom and it is held up to a strong light, cloudy white streaks that look something like worms can indeed be seen. This may be the result of partial mixing of the lubricant and water that causes differential refraction of sunlight through the swirling mixture, or from reflections from the latex sides of the condom.

8. Collins and Stadler 2001: 333; Stadler 2003.

9. Dempster 2001.

10. Maughan 2006.

11. Soros 2006.

12. The cartoon strip, drawn by Stephen Francis and Rico, is syndicated in many South African newspapers. There is also a spin-off TV weekly sitcom. The basic situation for the comedy is the household of a white upper-middle-class South African family: Madam, the head of the household, her elderly gin-drinking mother, and Eve, her domestic worker, who is also part of the family. Such a situation is not at all uncommon in contemporary South Africa. The strip often offers trenchant but humorous criticism of South African politics, culture, and society. See www.madamandeve.co.za.

13. "UN envoy slams Zuma for hurting AIDS fight," IOL.com, 10 May 2006, posted online at www.iol.co.za/index.php?set_id=1&click_id=3011&art_id= qw114728148499B243.

14. "UN envoy slams Zuma for hurting AIDS fight," IOL.com, 10 May 2006, posted online at www.iol.co.za/index.php?set_id=1&click_id=3011&art_id = qw114728148499B243.

15. For example, Lambeck and Strathern 1998; Strathern 1988.

16. Vance 1999 [1991]: 44–46, 48; Heald 1995.

17. The *hetero-* designation here is neither prescriptive nor descriptive, since I am not certain to what extent what I say here applies equally well to same-sex sexuality. It is clear, however, that same-sex sexuality cannot be entirely classified under the European semantic categories of "homosexual" or "gay," since many people in such relationships do not consider themselves to fall under these categories. Black South African same-sex relationship often adopt the cultural gender patterns of "male" and "female regardless of the biological sex of the participants (e.g., Donham 1998; Moodie, Ndatshe, and Sibuye 1988; Moodie and Ndatshe 1994; Gear 2005: 90; van Onselen 1984; Harries 1994). Whether what I write applies equally to same-sex sex, I cannot say. I leave the question open.

18. Cf. Niehaus 2001: 15.

19. Interview with D. S. Mthembu, traditional doctor, Umnonjaneni section, Tembisa, 10 March 2002.

20. Interview with Nomxolisi Dandaza, nursing sister and *thwasa* (initiate), Pimville Zone 5, Soweto, Johannesburg, 12 March 2002.

21. Collins and Stadler 2001: 330.

22. Collins and Stadler 2001: 331.

23. Jeannerat 1997: 72.

24. In SeSotho, *madi* may also mean "money" (*mali* in Zulu), since the /d/ and /l/ phoneme tend toward the same sound, a rapid alveolar flap, and SeSotho speakers frequently import the Zulu word *mali* into their own lexicons, with sound shifts into the SeSotho sound system. See Niehaus 2001; Ingstad 1990: 34.

25. Caldwell, Caldwell, and Quiggin 1989, 1991; Caldwell, Caldwell, and Orubuloye 1992; Caldwell and Caldwell 1996; Caldwell 2005.

26. The Nguni grouping of South African Bantu languages includes Zulu, Xhosa, and Swazi, while the other major family of languages, Sotho-Tswana, includes the North Sotho (Pedi), the South Sotho, Ndebele, and Tswana. Tsonga (Shangaan) also uses the term *lobolo,* although it is not part of the Nguni grouping.

27. Thornton 2000.

28. Interview with D. S. Mthembu, 10 March 2002.

29. Interview with Makhosi Vikizitha, West Central Jabavu, 6 March 2002.

30. Thornton 2002.

31. Ingstad 1990; Green 1994, 1996a, 1996b, 1999.

32. This system differs in many ways from the Zulu/Xhosa system and that of the highveld Sotho and Tswana cultures, but there are many similarities as well. The following discussion is based primarily on my knowledge of the lowveld systems. People speaking four main languages practice this healing cult: *SiSwati* (Swazi), lowveld *SePedi* or *Pulana* (closely related to the highveld northern Sotho), *XiTsonga* (Shangaan), and *isiZulu* (widely spoken in the region, as it is elsewhere in South Africa). I give linguistic equivalents in the three languages that are spoken widely and that are used by healers in the region.

33. Doke et al. 1990; Doke and Vilakazi 1972.
34. Posel 2003b.
35. Longmore 1959: 22.
36. Longmore 1959: 139.

CHAPTER 11

1. Levi-Strauss 1952: 321.
2. Cameron 2005.
3. Shisana et al. 2005: 70
4. Wellings et al. 2006.
5. This should not be confused with the "Three Ones" goals that the United Nations Program on HIV/AIDS has set for achieving more effective AIDS prevention strategies—that is, one national plan to fight HIV/AIDS, one national coordinating body in each nation, and one national monitoring and evaluation system.

References

Abdool Karim, Salim S. 2005. Introduction. In *HIV/AIDS in South Africa,* edited by Salim S. Abdool Karim and Quarraisha Abdool Karim, 31–36. Cambridge: Cambridge University Press.

Abdool Karim, Salim S., and Quarraisha Abdool Karim, editors. 2005. *HIV/AIDS in South Africa.* Cambridge: Cambridge University Press.

Actuarial Society of South Africa. 2006. Summary of biennial report on the state of the South African HIV/AIDS epidemic (November). Posted online at www.doh.gov.za/docs/reports/2006/summary.html (accessed 20 May 2007).

Adams, Sheena. 2006. Government acts at last on Manto's HIV diet. *The Star* (Johannesburg), 1 November.

African National Congress. 1955. *The freedom charter* (adopted at the Congress of the People, Kliptown, on 26 June). African National Congress, South Africa. Posted online at www.anc.org.za/ancdocs/history/charter.html.

———. 1994. *A national health plan for South Africa.* Maseru: Bahr.

———. 2002a. *ANC Today* 2, no. 16 (19–24 April). Posted online at www.anc.org.za/ancdocs/anctoday/2002/at16.htm.

———. 2002b. Castro Hlongwane, caravans, cats, geese, foot & mouth and statistics, HIV/AIDS and the struggle for the humanisation of the African. Posted online at www.virusmyth.net/aids/data/ancdoc.htm (site last updated 7 July 2003; accessed 30 January 2006).

Anderson, Benedict R. 1983. *Imagined communities: Reflections on the origin and spread of nationalism.* London: Verso.

Anderson, R. M. 1996. The spread of HIV and sexual mixing patterns. In *AIDS in the World II,* edited by J. E. Mann and D. J. M. Tarantola, 71–80. Oxford: Oxford University Press.

Aral, S. O. 1999. Sexual network patterns as determinants of STD rates: Paradigm shift in the behavioural epidemiology of STDs made visible. *Sexually Transmitted Diseases* 26: 262–264.

Asamoah-Odei, Emil, Jesus M. Garcia Calleja, and J. Ties Boerma. 2004. HIV prevalence and trends in sub-Saharan Africa: No decline and large sub-regional differences. *Lancet* 364, no. 9428: 35–40.

Asiimwe, Delius, Richard Kibombo, and Stella Neema. 2003. Focus group discussion on social cultural factors impacting on HIV/AIDS in Uganda (final report, June). Kampala: Makerere Institute of Social Research, for Ministry of Finance, Planning and Economic Development/UNDP. Posted online at www.aidsuganda.org/pdf/social_cultural_factors.pdf.

Asiimwe-Okiror, G., J. Musinguzi, and E. Madraa. 1996. A report on the declining trends in HIV infection rates in sentinel surveillance sites in Uganda. STD/AIDS Control Programme, Ministry of Health, Kampala.

Asiimwe-Okiror, Godwil, Alex A. Opio, Joshua Musinguzi, Elizabeth Madraa, George Tembo, and Michel Caraël. 1997. Change in sexual behaviour and decline in HIV infection among young pregnant women in urban Uganda. *AIDS* 11: 1757–1763.

Baingana, Doreen. 2005. *Tropical fish*. Cape Town: Oshun Books.

Baqwa, Selby A. M. 1996. Investigation of the play Sarafina II (report in terms of Section 8(2) of the Public Protector Act 23 of 1994, Report no. 1 (May). Government of South Africa. Posted online at www.polity.org.za/html/govt/pubprot/report1a.html.

Barabási, A.-L. 2002. *Linked: The new science of networks*. Cambridge, MA: Perseus Publishing.

Barnett, T., and Alan Whiteside. 2002. *AIDS in the twenty-first century: Disease and globalization*. New York: Palgrave and Macmillan.

Baryarama, Fulgentius, Rebecca Bunnell, Willi McFarland, Esther S. Hudes, T. B. Neilands, R. L. Ransom, J Mubongizi, C. Hitimana-Lukanika, and J. H. Mermin. 2007. Estimating HIV incidence in voluntary counseling and testing clients in Uganda (1992–2003). *Journal of Acquired Immune Deficiency Syndromes* 44, no. 1: 99.

Bayley, Anne. 1983. Aggressive Kaposi's sarcoma in Zambia. *Lancet* 323, no. 8390 (16 June): 1318–1320.

Beattie, John. 1971. *The Nyoro state*. Oxford: Oxford University Press.

Beresford, Belinda. 2006. Calls to halt nevirapine. *Mail & Guardian* (South Africa), 15–21 September, 12.

Bessinger, R., P. Akwara, and Daniel Halperin. 2003. Sexual behavior, HIV and fertility trends: A comparative analysis of six countries. Phase I of the ABC Study. Washington, DC: Measure Evaluation/U.S. Agency for Iinternational Development. See the U.S. Agency for International Development Web site, www.usaid.gov/pop_health/aids/Publications/index.html.

Bishai, David, Priya Patil, George Pariyo, and Ken Hill. 2006. The Babel effect: Community linguistic diversity and extramarital sex in Uganda. *AIDS and Behavior* 10, no. 4, doi:10.1007/s10461–006–9118–2.

Bregman, D. J., and A. D. Langmuir. 1990. Farr's law applied to AIDS projections. *Journal of the American Medical Association* 263: 1522–1525.

Brookmeyer, Ron. 1996. AIDS, epidemics, and statistics. *Biometrics* 52, no. 3: 781–796.

Brown, David. 2005. News: Uganda's AIDS decline attributed to deaths. *Washington Post*, 24 February.

Buchanan, Mark. 2002. *Small world: Uncovering nature's hidden networks.* London: Weidenfeld and Nicolson.

Budlender D., N. Chobokoane, and S. Simelane. 2004. Marriage patterns in South Africa: Methodological and substantive issues. *South Africa Journal of Demography* 9, no. 1 (June): 1–25.

Butler, Anthony. 2005. South Africa's HIV/AIDS policy, 1994–2004: How can it be explained? *African Affairs* 104, no. 417: 591–614.

Caldwell, J.C. 2005. Rethinking the African AIDS epidemic. *Population and Development Review* 26, no. 1: 117–135.

Caldwell, J.C., and P. Caldwell. 1996. Toward an epidemiological model of AIDS in sub-Saharan Africa. *Social Science History* 20, no. 4: 559–591.

Caldwell, J.C., P. Caldwell, and I.O. Orubuloye. 1992. The family and sexual networking in sub-Saharan Africa: Historical and regional differences and present-day implications. *Population Studies* 46, no. 3: 385–410.

Caldwell, J.C., P. Caldwell, and P. Quiggin. 1989. The social context of AIDS in sub-Saharan Africa. *Popluation and Development Review* 15, no. 2: 185–234.

———. 1991. The African sexual system: Reply to Le Blanc et al. *Population and Development Review* 17, no. 3: 506–515.

Cameron, Edwin. 2005. *Witness to AIDS.* Cape Town: Tafelberg Publishers.

Campbell, Catherine. 2003. *"Letting them die": Why HIV/AIDS intervention programmes fail.* Oxford: James Currey.

Carswell, J.W., Roy Mugwera, Nelson Sewankambo, Fred Kigozi, and Rick Goodgame. 1986. AIDS in Uganda: A special report by the Clinical Committee on AIDS. *Health Information Quarterly* 2, no. 1: 11–20.

Carswell, J.W., N. Sewankambo, G. Lloyd, and R.G. Downing. 1986. How long has the AIDS virus been in Uganda? (Letter to the editor). *Lancet* 327, no. 8491: 1217.

Centers for Disease Control. 1981. Pneumocystis pneumonia—Los Angeles. *MMWR Weekly* 30, nos. 250–252 (5 June): 1–3.

———. 1982. Current trends update on acquired immune deficiency syndrome (AIDS), United States. *MMWR Weekly,* 24 September, 507–508, 513–514. Posted online at www.cdc.gov/mmwr/preview/mmwrhtml/00001163.htm.

———. 1984. Acquired immunodeficiency syndrome (AIDS). Weekly Surveillance Report, United States AIDS Activity, 31 December. Center for Infectious Diseases, Centers for Disease Control. Posted online at www.cdc.gov/hiv/topics/surveillance/resources/reports/pdf/surveillance84.pdf (accessed 25 January 2008).

Centers for Disease Control and Prevention. 2001. First report of AIDS. *MMWR Weekly,* 1 June, 429. Posted online at www.cdc.gov/mmwr/preview/mmwr html/mm5021a1.htm.

Centre for Development and Enterprise. 2005. *Land reform in South Africa: A 21st century perspective.* Research report no. 14. Johannesburg: Centre for Development and Enterprise (June). Posted online at www.cde.org.za/pdf/Land_Reform.pdf.

Chirambo, K., and M. Caesar, editors. 2003. *AIDS and governance in southern Africa: Emerging theories and perspectives.* Report of the IDASA/UNDP regional governance and AIDS forum (2–4 April). Cape Town: Institute for Democracy in South Africa.

CNN. 2001. South Africa facing child rape crisis. CNN.com, 26 November. Posted online at http://archives.cnn.com/2001/WORLD/africa/11/26/safrica .rape/.

Collins, Terri, and Jonathan Stadler. 2001. Love, passion and play: Sexual meaning among youth in the northern province of South Africa. *Journal des Anthropologues* 82–83: 325–338.

Colvin, M., S. Dawood, I. Kleinschmidt, S. Mullick, and U. Lallo. 2001. Prevalence of HIV and HIV-related diseases in the adult medical wards of a tertiary hospital in Durban, South Africa. *International Journal of STD and AIDS* 12, no. 6: 386–389.

Comaroff, John, and Jean Comaroff. 1992. *Ethnography and the historical imagination: Studies in the ethnographic imagination.* Boulder: Westview Press.

Commission for Africa. 2005. *Our common interest: Report of the Commission for Africa.* London: Commission for Africa (March). Posted online at www .commissionforafrica.org.

Cronje, F. 2005. Bringing capital to life. *Fast Facts,* no. 5/2005 (May): 1. Johannesburg: South Africa Institute of Race Relations.

Cullinan, K. 2006. Manto muscled out in palace coup. *Sunday Times* (South Africa), 5 November, 1.

Deane, Nawaal. 2005. The political history of AIDS treatment. In *HIV/AIDS in South Africa,* edited by Salim S. Karim and Quarraisha Abdool Karim, 538–547. Cambridge: Cambridge University Press.

De Cock, K. M., D. Mbori-Ngacha, and Elisabeth Marum. 2002. Shadow on the continent: Public health and HIV/AIDS in Africa in the 21st century. *Lancet* 360, no. 9326 (6 July): 67–72.

Dempster, Carolyn. 2001. Rape—Silent war on SA women. BBC News, Johannesburg, 9 April. Posted online at www.news.bbc.co.uk/hi/english/world/ africa/newsid_1909000/1909220.stm (accessed 11 May 2006).

Department of Health, South Africa. 2000. *Summary report: 1999 antenatal AIDS survey.* Pretoria: Department of Health, Government of South Africa.

———. 2002. *Summary report: National HIV and syphilis antenatal seroprevalence survey in South Africa.* Pretoria: Department of Health, Government of South Africa.

———. 2006. *Progress report on the declaration of commitment on HIV and AIDS to UNGASS.* Pretoria: Department of Health, Government of South Africa. Posted online at www.doh.gov.za/docs/reports-f.html.

Doherty, T., and M. Colvin. 2004. HIV/AIDS. In *South African health review 2003/04,* chapter 14. Durban: Health Systems Trust. Posted online at www .hst.org.za/publications/423.

Doke, C. M., D. M. Malcolm, J. M. A. Sikakana, and B. W. Vilakazi. 1990. *English-Zulu Zulu-English dictionary.* Johannesburg: University of the Witwatersrand Press.

Doke, C. M., and B. W. Vilakazi. 1972. *Zulu-English dictionary.* Johannesburg: University of the Witwatersrand Press.

Donham, Don L. 1998. Freeing South Africa: The modernization of male-male sexuality in Soweto. *Cultural Anthropology* 13, no. 1: 3–21

Doornbos, Martin R. 2001. *The Ankole kingship controversy: Regalia galore revisited.* Kampala: Fountain Publishers.

Dorrington, Rob, Debbie Bradshaw, and Debbie Budlender. 2002. *HIV/AIDS profile in the provinces of South Africa: Indicators for 2002.* Joint publication by the Centre for Actuarial Research, the Burden of Disease Research Unit (Medical Research Council) and the Actuarial Society of South Africa. Posted online at www.commerce.uct.ac.za/Research_Units/CARE/RESEARCH/Papers/Indicators.pdf.

Dorrington, Rob, Debbie Bradshaw, Leigh Johnson, and Debbie Budlender. 2004. *The demographic impact of HIV/AIDS in South Africa: National indicators for 2004.* Cape Town: Centre for Actuarial Research, South African Medical Council, and Actuarial Society of South Africa. ISBN: 1–920015–17–5. Posted online at www.commerce.uct.ac.za/Research_Units/CARE/Monographs/Monographs/mono08.pdf.

Dorrington, R. E., L. F. Johnson, D. Bradshaw, and D. T. Bradshaw. 2006. *The demographic impact of HIV/AIDS in South Africa: National and provincial indicators for 2006.* Cape Town: Centre for Actuarial Research, South African Medical Research Council, and Actuarial Society of South Africa. Posted online at www.mrc.ac.za/bod (accessed 20 May 2007).

Duesberg, Peter. 2000. The African AIDS epidemic: New and contagious, or, old under a new name? Presentation to President Thabo Mbeki's AIDS panel (22 June).

Duesberg, Peter, and Bryan J. Ellison. 1996. *Inventing the AIDS virus.* Washington, DC: Regnery Publishing.

Duesberg, Peter, and D. Rasnick. 1998. The AIDS dilemma: Drug diseases blamed on a passenger virus. *Genetica* 104: 85–132.

Eglash, Ron. 1999. *African fractals: Modern computing and indigenous design.* New Brunswick, NJ: Rutgers University Press, 1999.

Epstein, Helen. 2005. God and the fight against AIDS. *New York Review of Books* 52, no. 7 (28 April): 47–50.

Evans, Jenni, and Yasheera Rampersadh. 2005. Close watch on Zuma "rape" developments. Mail & Guardian Online, 21 November. Posted online at www.mg.co.za/articlePage.aspx?articleid = 257129&area = /breaking_news/breaking_news__national (accessed 30 January 2006).

Fallers, Lloyd A. 1964. Social stratification in traditional Buganda, In *The king's men: Leadership and status in Buganda on the eve of independence,* 64–117. London: Oxford University Press on behalf of the East African Institute of Social Research.

Faloutsos, Michalis, Petros Faloutsos, and Christos Faloutsos. 1999. On power-law relationships of the Internet topology. *SIGCOMM '99,* 251–262.

Farber, Celia. 2006. Out of control: AIDS and the corruption of medical science. *Harper's Magazine,* May, 37–52. Posted online at www.harpers.org/archive/2006/03/0080961.

Farmer, Paul. 1995. Culture, poverty and HIV transmission in rural Haiti. In *Culture and sexual risk: Anthropological perspectives on AIDS*, edited by Han ten Brummelhuis and Gilbert Herdt, 3–28. Amsterdam: Gordon and Breach.

Farmer, Paul, S. Lindenbaum, and M.D. Good. 1993. Women, poverty and AIDS: An introduction. *Culture, Medicine and Psychiatry* 17, no. 4: 387–397.

Ford, Claudia. 2005. *Why do I scream at God for the rape of babies?* Berkeley, CA: North Atlantic Books & Frog.

Forman, L., Y. Pillay, and L. Sait. 2004. Health legislation, 1994–2003. In *South African health review 2003/04*, chapter 2. Durban: Health Systems Trust. Posted online at www.hst.org.za/publications/423.

Gallo, Robert, Nathan Geffen, Gregg Gonsalves, Richard Jefferys, Daniel R. Kuritzkes, Bruce Mirken, John P. Moore, and Jeffrey T. Safrit. 2006. Errors in Celia Farber's March 2006 article in Harper's Magazine (final version: released 25 March 2006). Posted online at www.aegis.org/files/tac/2006/errorsinfarberarticle.pdf.

Gazi, Costa. 2001. AIDS far deadlier than apartheid. *Mail & Guardian,* 22 March.

Gear, Sasha. 2005. Rules of engagement: Structuring sex and damage in men's prisons and beyond. In *Men behaving differently: South African men since 1994*, edited by Graeme Reid and Liz Walker, 89–109. Cape Town: Double Storey Books.

Geertz, Clifford. 1983. *Local knowledge: Further essays in interpretive anthropology*. New York: Basic Books.

Gladwell, Malcolm. 2000. *The tipping point: How small things make a big difference*. Boston: Little, Brown.

Gluckman, Max. 1963. *Order and rebellion in tribal Africa*. London: Cohen and West.

———. 1965. *Politics, law and ritual in tribal society*. Chicago: Aldine.

Goody, Jack. 1976. *Production and reproduction: A comparative study of the domestic domain*. Cambridge: Cambridge University Press.

Gordin, Jeremy. 2006. Zuma afraid for rape accuser. Agence France Presse, 29 January. Posted online at www.int.iol.co.za/index.php?set_id=1&click_id=3011&art_id=vn20060129081949238C693726 (accessed 29 January 2006).

Gottlieb, M.S., R. Schroff, H.M. Schanker, J.D. Weisman, P.T. Fan, R.A. Wolf, and A. Saxon. 1981. Pneumocystis carinii pneumonia and mucosal candidiasis in previously healthy homosexual men: Evidence of a new acquired cellular immunodeficiency. *New England Journal of Medicine* 305, no. 24 (December): 1425–1431. Unique identifier: AIDSLINE MED/82057985. Posted online at www.aegis.com/aidsline/1982/mar/M8230005.html.

Gouws, Eleanor, and Quarraisha Abdool Karim. 2005. HIV infection in South Africa: The evolving epidemic. In *HIV/AIDS in South Africa*, edited by Salim S. Abdool Karim and Quarraisha Abdool Karim, 48–76. Cambridge: Cambridge University Press.

Gray, R.H., S. Serwadda, G. Kigozi, F. Nalugoda, and M.J. Wawer. 2006. Uganda's HIV prevention success: The role of sexual behavior change and the national response, Commentary on Green et al. (2006). *AIDS and Behavior* 10, no. 4: 347–350.

Green, Edward C. 1994. *AIDS and STDs in Africa: Bridging the gap between traditional healers and modern medicine.* Boulder, CO: Westview Press.

———. 1996a. *Indigenous healers and the African state.* New York: Pact Publications.

———. 1996b. Indigenous knowledge systems and health promotion in Mozambique. In *Indigenous knowledge and its uses in southern Africa,* edited by H. Normann, I. Snyman, and M. Cohen, 51–65. Cape Town: Institute for Indigenous Theory and Practice, Human Sciences Research Council.

——— 1999. *Indigenous theories of contagious disease.* Walnut Creek, CA: Altamira Press, and London: Sage Press.

Green, Edward C., D.T. Halperin, Y. Nantulya, and J. Hogle. 2006. Uganda's HIV prevention success: The role of sexual behavior change and the national response. *AIDS and Behavior* 10, no. 4: 335–346.

Green, Edward C., Vinand Nantulya, Yaa Oppong, and Teresa Harrison. 2003. Literature review and preliminary analysis of "ABC" factors (abstinence, being faithful or partner reduction, condom use) in six developing countries. Harvard Center for Population and Development Studies and U.S. Agency for International Development (draft document, 28 January).

Guérin, J., R. Malebranche, R. Elie, A. Laroche, G. Pierre, E. Arnoux, T. Spira, J. Dupuy, T. Seemayer, and C. Péan-Guichard. 1984. Acquired immune deficiency syndrome: Specific aspects of disease in Haiti. *Annals of the New York Academy of Sciences* 437: 254–261.

Harries, Patrick. 1994. *Work, culture and identity: Migrant labourers in Mozambique and South Africa, c. 1860–1910.* Johannesburg: Witwatersrand University Press.

Hart, Keith. 2004. From bell curve to power law: distributional models between national and world society. *Social Analysis* 48, no. 3: 220–225.

Heald, Suzette. 1995. The power of sex: Some reflections on the Caldwells' "African sexuality" thesis. *Africa* (London) 65, no. 4: 489–505.

———. 2006. Abstain or die: The development of HIV/AIDS policy in Botswana. *Journal of Biosocial Science* 38, doi:10.1017/S0021932005000933.

Heywood, Mark, editor. 2004. From disaster to development: HIV and AIDS in southern Africa. *Development Update* (South Africa) 5, no. 3 (December).

Hogle, Janice A., Edward C. Green, Vinand Nantulya, Rand Stoneburner, and John Stover. 2002. *What happened in Uganda? Declining HIV prevalence, behavior change, and the national response. Project lessons learned case study.* U.S. Agency for International Development, Office of HIV/AIDS, Bureau for Global Health, contract number HRN-C-00-99-00005-00. Posted online at www.usaid.gov/pop_health/aids/Countries/africa/uganda_report.pdf.

Hooper, Edward J. 1990. *Slim: A reporter's own story of AIDS in East Africa.* London: Bodley Head.

Human Sciences Research Council. 2002. *The Nelson Mandela/HSRC study of HIV/AIDS*. Pretoria, South Africa: HSRC Press.

Ijsselmuiden C, C. Evian, J. Matjilla, M. Steinberg, and H. Schneider. 1993. AIDS in South Africa. *AIDS and Society* 4, no. 2 (January–February): 1, 10–11.

Iliffe, John. 1998. *East African doctors: A history of modern medicine*. Kampala: Fountain Publishers.

————. 2006. *The African AIDS epidemic: A history*. Oxford: James Currey.

Ingold, Tim. 1992. Editorial. *Man* (n.s.) 27: 693–696.

Ingstad, Benedicte. 1990. The cultural construction of AIDS and its consequences for prevention in Botswana. *Medical Anthropology Quarterly* 4, no. 1: 28–39.

Integrated Regional Information Network. 2008. Country profile: South Africa. PlusNews: Global HIV/AIDS News and Analysis. Posted online at www.plusnews.org/profiletreatment.aspx?Country=ZA&Region=SAF# (accessed 20 May 2007).

Jeannerat, Caroline. 1997. An anthropology of listening: A study of discourses on tradition, rituals, and the situation of women in Tshiendeuli, Venda, in the early 1990s. MA thesis, Department of Anthropology, University of the Witwatersrand.

Johnson, S., W. Hendson, H. Crewe-Brown, L. Dini, J. Frean, O. Perovic, and E. Vardas. 2000. Effect of human immunodeficiency virus infection on episodes of diarrhea among children in South Africa. *Pediatric Infectious Disease Journal* 19, no. 10: 972–979.

Kagimu, Magid, and Elisabeth Marum. 1996. Review of AIDS prevention and control activities in Uganda. Islamic Medical Association of Uganda (IMAU)/ Makerere University. Unpublished review project supported by the United Nations Programme on HIV/AIDS, the United Nations Development Programme, the World Health Organization, the U.S. Agency for International Development, and the Office of Development Assistance.

Kagimu, Magid, Elisabeth Marum, Fred Wabire-Mangen, Neema Nakyanjo, Yusuf Walakira, and Janice Hogle. 1998. Evaluation of the effectiveness of AIDS health education interventions in the Muslim community in Uganda. *AIDS Education and Prevention* 10, no. 3: 215–228.

Kagwa, Apolo. 1900. *Ekitabo kye basekabaka be Buganda*. Kampala. [Published in translation as *Kings of Buganda*. Edited and translated by M.S.M. Kiwanuka. Eastern and Central African Historical Texts, volume 1. Nairobi: East African Publishing House, 1971].

————. 1905. *Mpisa za Baganda*. London. [Published in the United States as *Customs of the Baganda*. Translated by E.B. Kalibala, edited by M.M. Edel. Columbia University Contributions to Anthropology, vol. 22. New York: Columbia University Press, 1934.]

Kamali, A., L.M. Carpenter, J.A.G. Whitworth, A. Ruberantwari, and A. Ojwiya. 2000. Seven-year trends in HIV-1 infection rates and changes in sexual behaviour among adults in rural Uganda. *AIDS* 14: 427–434.

Kaplan, Esther. 2006. Fairy-tale failure. *American Prospect* 17, no. 7 (July/August): 9.

Karlström, Michael. 2004. Modernity and its aspirants: Moral community and developmental utopianism in Buganda. *Current Anthropology* 45, no. 5: 595–619.

Kauffman, Kyle D., and David L. Lindaur, editors. 2004. *AIDS and South Africa: The social expression of a pandemic*. Houndmills, Basingstoke, Hampshire: Palgrave Macmillan.

Kaufman C. E., T. de Wet, and Jonathan Stadler. 2001. Adolescent pregnancy and parenthood in South Africa. *Studies in Family Planning* 32, no. 2: 147–160.

Kirby, Douglas. 2004. What happened in Uganda: An historical and causal analysis. Unpublished final report, AIDSMark project sponsored by the U.S. Agency for International Development, under the terms of award no. HRN-A-00–97–00021–00 (December).

Kiwawulo, C. 2006. HIV high in Kawempe-Takuba. *New Vision* (Kampala), 6 November. Posted online at http://allafrica.com/stories/200611020229.html (accessed 6 November 2006).

Kohler, Hans-Peter, and Stéphane Helleringer. 2006. The structure of sexual networks and the spread of HIV in sub-Saharan Africa: Evidence from Likoma Island (Malawi). PARC Working Paper Series WPS 06–02. Population Aging Research Center, University of Pennsylvania. Posted online at www.pop.upenn.edu/rc/parc/aging_center/2006/PARCwps06–02.pdf.

Konde-Lule, J. K., M. Musagara, and S. Musgrave. 1993. Focus group interviews about AIDS in Rakai District of Uganda. *Social Science and Medicine* 37, no. 5: 679–684.

Kotwal, Girish J, Jennifer N. Kaczmarek, Steven Leivers, Yohannes T. Ghebremariam, Amod P. Kulkarni, Gabriele Bauer, Corena De Beer, Wolfgang Preiser, and Abdu Rahman Mohamed. 2005. Anti-HIV, anti-poxvirus, and anti-SARS activity of a nontoxic, acidic plant extract from the trifollium species secomet-V/anti-vac suggests that it contains a novel broad-spectrum antiviral. *Natural Products and Molecular Therapy* 1056, doi:10.1196/annals .1352.014. Posted online at www.annalsnyas.org/cgi/reprint/1056/1/293 (accessed 10 June 2007).

Kreiss, J. K., D. Koech, F. A. Plummer, K. K. Holmes, M. Lightfoote, P. Piot, A. R. Ronald, J. O. Ndinya-Achola, L. J. D'Costa, and P. Roberts. 1986. AIDS virus infection in Nairobi prostitutes: Spread of the epidemic to East Africa. *New England Journal of Medicine* 314, no. 7: 414–418. Abstract online at http://content.nejm.org/cgi/content/abstract/314/7/414.

Lambeck, M., and Andrew Strathern. 1988. *Bodies and persons: Comparative perspectives from Africa and Melanesia*. Cambridge: Cambridge University Press.

Le Carré, John. 2001. *The constant gardener*. London: Hodder & Stoughton.

Leclerc-Madlala, Suzanne. 2002. South Africa: Prevention means more than condoms. *Mail & Guardian*, 4 October.

———. 2005. Popular responses to HIV/AIDS and policy. *Journal of Southern African Studies* 31, no. 4, doi:10.1080/03057070500370761.

Lemey, P., O. G. Pybus, B. Wang, N. K. Saksena, M. Salemi, and A-M. Vandamme. 2003. Tracing the origin and history of the HIV-2 epidemic. *Pro-*

ceedings of the National Academy of Science 100, no. 11 (27 May): 6588–6592. Posted online at www.pnas.org_cgi_doi_10.1073_pnas.093 6469100.

Leskovec, Jure, J. Kleinberg, and C. Faloutsos. 2005. Graphs over time: Densification laws, shrinking diameters and possible explanations. In *Proceedings of the conference on knowledge discovery,* 177–187. 11th ACM SIGKDD, Chicago (21–24 August), ACM 1–59593–135-X/05/0008. Posted online at http://portal.acm.org/citation.cfm?id = 1081870.1081893 (accessed 30 May 2007).

Levi-Strauss, Claude. 1952. Social structure. In *Anthropology today,* edited by Sol Tax, 524–553. Chicago: University of Chicago Press.

Liautaud, B., L. Mellon, R. Grand'Pierre, J. Denizé-Vieux, M. Mevs, C. Nolté, and J.W. Pape. 1992. Preliminary data on STDs in Haiti. Abstract PoC 4302, 8th International Conference on AIDS / 3rd STD World Congress, Amsterdam (19–24 July).

Liljeros, F., C.R. Edling, and L.A.N. Amaral. 2003. Sexual networks: Implications for the transmission of sexually transmitted infections. *Microbes and Infection* 5, no. 2: 189–196.

Loconte, Joseph. 2003. The White House initiative to combat AIDS: Learning from Uganda. Heritage Foundation Backgrounder and Executive Summary no. 1692 (29 September). Domestic Policy Studies Department, Heritage Foundation, Washington, DC. Posted online at www.heritage.org/research/africa/bg1692.cfm.

Longmore, Laura. 1959. *The dispossessed: A study of the sex-life of Bantu women in and around Johannesburg.* London: Jonathan Cape.

Low-Beer, Daniel, and Rand L. Stoneburner. 1997. An age- and sex-structured HIV epidemiological model: Features and applications. *Bulletin of the World Health Organisation* 75, no. 3: 213–221.

———. 2003. Behaviour and communication change in reducing HIV: Is Uganda unique? *African Journal of AIDS Research* 2003 2, no. 1: 9–12.

Lwanga, John Baptist, and Catherine Othieno. 2005. Childhood sexuality: Knowledge, attitudes, practices and behavior in Mayuge District (Uganda). Uganda Youth Anti AIDS Association in Collaboration with International Solidarity Foundation. Posted online at www.finsolid.fi/easydata/customers/finsolid/files/Pdf/Uganda_Childhood_Sexuality.pdf.

Lyons, Maryinez. 1996. *AIDS Prevention and Control Project: Was it effective, is it replicable?* Final report prepared for World Learning and U.S. Agency for International Development (27 March).

Mann, Jonathan M. 1989. AIDS: A worldwide pandemic. In *Current topics in AIDS,* volume 2, edited by M.S. Gottlieb, D.J. Jeffries, D. Mildvan, A.J. Pinching, and T.C. Quinn, 1–10. Hoboken, NJ: John Wiley & Sons.

Mann, Jonathan M., Thomas W. Netter, and Daniel Tarantola, editors. 1992. *AIDS in the world.* Cambridge, MA: Harvard University Press.

Maquet, Jacques J. 1961. *The premise of inequality in Ruanda.* London: Oxford University Press for the International Africa Institute.

Marks, Shula. 2002. An epidemic waiting to happen. *African Studies* 61, no. 1: 16.

Marx, Jean L. 1982. New disease baffles medical community. *Science* (n.s.) 217, no. 4560: 618–621.

Masur, H., M.A. Michelis, J.B. Greene, I. Onorato, R.A. Stouwe, R.S. Holzman, G. Wormser, L. Brettman, M. Lange, H.W. Murray, and S. Cunningham-Rundles. 1981. An outbreak of community-acquired Pneumocystis carinii pneumonia: Initial manifestation of cellular immune dysfunction. *New England Journal of Medicine* 305, no. 24: 1431–1438. Abstract posted online at www.ncbi.nlm.nih.gov/entrez/query.fcgi?cmd=Retrieve&db=PubMed&list_uids=6975437&dopt=Abstract.

Maughan, Karyn. 2006. Zuma stands his ground on shower comment. IOL. com, 10 May. Posted online at www.iol.co.za/index.php?set_id=1&click_id=3011&art_id=vn20060510004406115C497518; also published in *The Star* (Johannesburg), 10 May, 1.

Mbeki, Thabo. 1998. The ANC has no financial stake in Virodene. (March). Posted online at the official Web site of the African National Congress, www .anc.org.za/ancdocs/history/mbeki/1998/virodene.html.

Measure DHS+. 1998. *South Africa demographic and health survey, 1998: Full report*. Publication ID FR131. Pretoria: South Africa Department of Health and Measure DHS+, and Calverton, MD: ORC Macro. Posted online at www.measuredhs.com/pubs/pub_details.cfm?ID=360&ctry_id=55&SrchTp=ctry (accessed 26 January 2008).

———. 2002. *Uganda demographic and health survey, 2000/01: Final report*. Publication ID: FR128. Entebbe: Uganda Bureau of Statistics, and Calverton, MD: ORC Macro. Posted online at www.measuredhs.com/pubs/pub_details. cfm?ID=346&ctry_id=44&SrchTp=ctry (accessed 26 January 2008).

Merson, M. 2006. Uganda's HIV/AIDS epidemic: Guest editorial. *AIDS and Behavior* 10, no. 4, doi:10.1007/s10461-006-9120-8.

Meyer, Birgit. 2004. Christianity in Africa: From African independent to Pentecostal-charismatic churches. *Annual Review of Anthropology* 33, doi:10.1146/annurev.anthro.33.070203.143835.

Meyers, T.M., J.M. Pettifor, G.E. Gray, H. Crewe-Brown, and J.S. Galpin. 2000. Pediatric admissions with human immunodeficiency virus infection at a regional hospital in Soweto, South Africa. *Journal of Tropical Pediatrics* 46, no. 4: 224–230.

Ministry of Health, Uganda. 1992–2002. *HIV/AIDS Surveillance Report*. STD/AIDS Control Programme [for each of the years 1992–2002].

———. 2002a. Condom distribution plan (draft). Condom Coordination Unit, STD/AIDS Control Programme, Uganda Ministry of Health, Kampala (September). Unpublished document provided by Product Coordinator/Protector & Clear Seven, Commercial Market Strategies, CMS Project, Kampala.

Ministry of Health, Uganda, and ORC Macro. 2006. *Uganda HIV/AIDS serobehavioural survey 2004/2005*. Kampala: Ministry of Health, and Calverton, MD: ORC Macro.

Monare, M., and L. Daniels. 2006. Deputy president urges unity in fight against AIDS. *The Star* (Johannesburg), 20 September, 3.

Moodie, T. Dunbar, and V. Ndatshe. 1994. *Going for gold*. Johannesburg: Witwatersrand University Press.

Moodie, T. Dunbar, Vivienne Ndatshe, and British Sibuyi. 1988. Migrancy and male sexuality on the South African gold mines. *Journal of Southern African Studies* 14, no. 2: 228–256 (special issue on culture and consciousness in southern Africa).

Morris, Martina. 1997. Sexual networks and HIV. *AIDS* 11: 209–216.

Morris, Martina, Nelson Sewankambo, Maria Wawer, David Serwada, and Bongs Lainjo. 1995. Concurrent partnerships and HIV transmission in Rakai District, Uganda. Abstract TuC105, 9th International Conference on AIDS and STDs in Africa, Kampala (10–14 December).

Motsei, Mmatshilo. 2007. *The kanga and the kangaroo court: Reflections on the rape trial of Jacob Zuma.* Auckland Park, Johannesburg: Jacana Press.

Moya, Fikile-Ntsikelelo. 2006. 100% Zuluboy. *Mail & Guardian* (South Africa), 6 April. Posted online at www.mg.co.za/articlePage.aspx?articleid= 268739&area=/insight/insight__national/.

Mukyala-Mukiika, Rebecca. 2000. Traditional leaders and decentralisation. In *Decentralisation and civil society in Uganda: The quest for good governance,* edited by Apolo Nsibambi, 96–109. Kampala: Fountain Publishers.

Mulondo, E. 2006. Complacence worsens AIDS prevalence. *The Monitor* (Kampala), 9 October. Posted online at http://allafrica.com/stories/200610090159 .html (accessed 6 November 2006).

Museveni, Yoweri. 1997. *Sowing the mustard seed: The struggle for freedom and democracy in Uganda.* Oxford: Macmillan.

Nattrass, Nicoli. 2004. *The moral economy of AIDS in South Africa.* Cambridge: Cambridge University Press.

Newton, Laura Foot. 2005. *Tshepang: The third testament* (drama script). Johannesburg: Wits University Press.

Niehaus, Isak. 2001. *Witchcraft, power and politics: Exploring the occult in the South African lowveld.* London: Pluto Press, and Cape Town: David Phillip Publishers.

Pape, J.W., and W. Johnson. 1988. Epidemiology of AIDS in the Carribean. *Baillière's Clinical Tropical Medicine and Communicable Diseases* 3, no. 1: 31–42.

Parkhust, Justin O., and Louisiana Lush. 2004. The political environment of HIV: Lessons from a comparison of Uganda and South Africa. *Social Science and Medicine* 59: 1913–1924.

Parry, Eldryd O.H., editor. 1984. *Principles of medicine in Africa,* 2nd edition. Oxford: Oxford University Press.

Pillay, K., M. Colvin, R. Williams, and H. M. Coovadia. 2001. Impact of HIV-1 infection in South Africa. *Archives of Disease in Childhood* 85, no. 1: 50–51.

Posel, Deborah. 2003a. Getting the nation talking about sex: Reflections on the politics of sexuality and "nation-building" in post-apartheid South Africa. Wits Institute for Social and Economic Research, University of the Witwatersrand, Johannesburg, South Africa (February).

———. 2003b. A matter of life and death: Revisiting "modernity" from the vantage point of the "new" South Africa. Wits Institute for Social and Economic Research, University of the Witwatersrand, Johannesburg, South Africa (November).

Rasebotsa, Nobantu, Meg Samuelson, and Kylie Thomas. 2004. *Nobody ever said AIDS: Stories and poems from southern Africa.* Cape Town: Kwela Press.

Reid, Richard. 2002. *Political power in pre-colonial Buganda.* Oxford: James Currey.

Rice, Andrew. 2004. Enemy's enemy: Evangelicals v. Muslims in Africa. *New Republic,* 8 September, 18–21.

Richards, A.D. 1966. *The changing structure of a Ganda village.* Kampala: Makerere Institute of Social Research.

Roberts, A.D. 1962. The sub-imperialism of the Baganda. *Journal of African History* 3: 435–450.

Rothenberg, Richard B., David M. Long, Claire E. Sterk, Albert Pach, John J. Potterat, Sephen Muth, Julie A. Baldwin, and Robert T. Trotter. 2000. The Atlanta Urban Networks Study: A blueprint for endemic transmission. *AIDS* 14: 2191–2200.

Rothenberg, R.B., J.J. Potterat, D.E. Woodhouse, S.Q. Muth, W.W. Darrow, and A.S. Klovdahl. 1998. Social network dynamics and HIV transmission. *AIDS* 12: 1529–1536.

Sahlins, Marshall. 1981. *Historical metaphors and mythical realities.* Ann Arbor: University of Michigan Press.

———. 1983. Other times, other customs: The anthropology of history. *American Anthropologist* 85, no. 3: 517–544.

———. 1985. *Islands of history.* Chicago: University of Chicago Press.

Salcedo, Marcela Ospina. 2004. Discourse and disease: An analysis of Thabo Mbeki's position on AIDS, 2000–2004. MA thesis, Department of Sociology, University of the Witwatersrand.

Schopper, Doris, Serge Douissantousse, Natal Ayiga, Geroges Ezatirale, William Jean Idro, and Jacques Homsy. 1995. Village-based AIDS prevention in a rural district in Uganda. *Health Policy and Planning* 10, no. 2: 171–180.

Seidel, G. 1996. Confidentiality and HIV status in Kwazulu-Natal, South Africa: Implications, resistances and challenges. *Health Policy Planning* 11, no. 4: 418–427.

Seligmann, M., L.Chess, J.L. Fahey, A.S. Fauci, P.J. Lachmann, J. L'Age-Stehr, J. Ngu, A.J. Pinching, F.S. Rosen, and T.J. Spira. 1984. AIDS—An immunologic reevaluation. *New England Journal of Medicine* 311: 1286–1292.

Serwadda, D., N.K. Sewankambo, J.W. Carswell, A.C. Bayley, R.S. Tedder, R.A. Weiss, R.D. Mugerwa, A. Lwegaba, G.B. Kirya, R.G. Downing, S.A. Clayden, and A.G. Dalgleish. 1985. Slim disease: A new disease in Uganda and its association with HTLV-III infection. *Lancet* 326, no. 8460: 849–852. doi:10.1016/S0140-6736(85)90122-9.

Sewankambo, N., R.D. Mugerwa, R. Goodgame, J.W. Carswell, A. Moody, G. Lloyd, and S.B. Lucas. 1987. Enteropathic AIDS in Uganda: An endoscopic, histological and microbiological study. *AIDS* 1: 9–13.

Shafer, Leigh Ann, S. Birarol, A. Kamalil, H. Grosskurthl, W. Kirungi, E. Madraa, and A. Opio. 2006. HIV prevalence and incidence are no longer falling in Uganda—A case for renewed prevention efforts: Evidence from a rural population cohort, 1989–2005, and from ANC surveillance. Abstract no. ThLBo108, 16th International AIDS Conference, Toronto (13–18 August).

Shilts, Randy. 2001. *And the band played on.* New York: St. Martin's Press.

Shisana O., T. Rehle, et al. 2005. *South African national HIV prevalence, HIV incidence, behaviour and communication survey, 2005.* Cape Town: HSRC Press. Posted online at www.hsrc.ac.za/research/output/outputDetail.php?id =2093.

Sidley, Pat. 2000. AIDS patients in South Africa to get free drug. *British Medical Journal* 320: 1095. doi:10.1136/bmj.320.7242.1095/a.

Soros, Eugene. 2006. Zuma trial heightens rape awareness. Worldpress.com, 29 April. Posted online at www.worldpress.org/Africa/2329.cfm#down.

South African Communication Service. 1996. Zuma's response to Sarafina II. Posted online at www.doh.gov.za/docs/pr/1996/pro605.html (accessed 26 January 2008).

South African Government. 2000. HIV/AIDS/STD strategic plan for South Africa, 2000–2005. Department of Health, South Africa (February). Posted online at www.info.gov.za/otherdocs/2000/aidsplan2000.pdf and www.doh .gov.za/docs/policy/aids-plan00–05.pdf.

South African Government Information Web site. 2005. Implementation of the comprehensive plan on prevention, treatment, and care of HIV and AIDS: Fact sheet (23 November). Posted online at www.info.gov.za/issues/hiv/ implementation2006.htm.

South African Institute of Race Relations. 2002. *South Africa survey, 2001/2002.* Johannesburg: South African Institute of Race Relations.

———. 2003. *South Africa survey, 2002/2003.* Johannesburg: South African Institute of Race Relations.

———. 2004. *South Africa survey, 2003/2004.* Johannesburg: South African Institute of Race Relations.

———. 2005a. *Fast Facts,* no. 2/2005 (February). Johannesburg: South African Institute of Race Relations.

———. 2005b. *South Africa survey, 2004/2005.* Johannesburg: South African Institute of Race Relations.

———. 2006. *Fast Facts,* no. 1/2006 (January). Johannesburg: South African Institute of Race Relations.

———. 2007. *Fast Facts,* nos. 4–5/2007 (April–May). Johannesburg: South African Institute of Race Relations.

Ssewanyana, Sarah, and Stephen D. Younger. 2005. Infant mortality in Uganda: Determinants, trends, and the millennium development goals. Economic Policy Research Centre, Cornell University (January). Posted online at www .cfnpp.cornell.edu/images/wp186.pdf#search = %22Uganda%20infant%20 mortality%22.

Stadler, Jonathan. 2003. Rumour, gossip and blame: Implications for HIV/AIDS prevention in the the South African lowveld. *AIDS Education and Prevention* (special issue, HIV/AIDS prevention and education in context: Current perspectives, future challenges) 15, no. 4: 357–368.

Stanton, David. 2006. Evidence vs. conventional wisdom: AIDS prevention in the 21st century. Unpublished PowerPoint presentation. U.S. Agency for International Development, Office of HIV/AIDS (13 March).

Statistics South Africa. 1998. *Marriages and divorces, 1996* (Statistical release P0307). Pretoria, South Africa: Statistics South Africa (17 December).

————. 2003. *Census 2001: Census in brief.* Report no: 03–02–03(2001). Pretoria: Statistics South Africa. Posted online at www.statssa.gov.za/census01/html/C2001publications.asp (accessed 25 January 2008).

————. 2004. *Census 2001: Primary tables South Africa: Census '96 and 2001 compared.* Report no. 03/02/04. Pretoria: Statistics South Africa. Posted online at www.statssa.gov.za/census01/html/C2001publications.asp (accessed 25 January 2008).

————. 2005. *Mortality and causes of death in South Africa, 1997–2003: Findings from death notification* (Statistical release P0309.3). Pretoria: Statistics South Africa. Posted online at www.statssa.gov.za/publications/P03093/P03093.pdf (accessed 20 May 2007).

Stoneburner, Rand L., M. Carballo, R. Bernstein, and T. Saidel. 1998. Simulation of HIV incidence dynamics in the Rakai population-based cohort, Uganda. *AIDS* 12, no. 2: 226–228.

Stoneburner, Rand L., and Daniel Low-Beer. 2004. Population-level HIV declines and behavioural risk avoidance in Uganda. *Science* 304, no. 5671: 714–718.

Stoneburner, Rand L., Daniel Low-Beer, George S. Tembo, Thierry E. Mertens, and Godwill Asiimwe-Okiror. 1996. Human immunodeficiency virus infection dynamics in East Africa deduced from surveillance data. *American Journal of Epidemiology* 144, no. 7: 682–695.

Strathern, Marilyn. 1988. *The gender of the gift: Problems with women and problems with society in Melanesia.* Berkeley and Los Angeles: University of California Press.

Strogatz, Steven. 2003. *Sync: The emergence of spontaneous order.* London: Penguin Books.

Swarns, Rachel L. 2002. Grappling with South Africa's alarming increase in the rapes of children. *New York Times,* 29 January.

Thornton, Robert J. 1994. South Africa: Countries, boundaries, enemies and friends. *Anthropology Today* 10, no. 6: 7–15.

————. 2000. The "landspace": Land and landscapes in contemporary South Africa. In *Sociocultural anthropology at the turn of the century: Voices from the periphery,* edited by Peter Skalník, 133–164. Prague Studies in Sociocultural Anthropology, no. 1. Prague: Set Out Press.

————. 2001. "Traditional authority" and governance in the Emjindini Royal Swazi Chiefdom, Barberton, Mpumalanga: An empirical study. Unpublished research paper.

————. 2002. Traditional healers, medical doctors and HIV/AIDS in Gauteng and Mpumalanga provinces, South Africa. Unpublished report to the Margaret Sanger Institute and Medical Care Development International.

————. 2003a. The "ABC" field study in Uganda. Unpublished report for AIDS-Mark project sponsored by the U.S. Agency for International Development, under the terms of award no. HRN-A-00–97–00021–00 (September).

———. 2003b. Chiefs: Power in a political wilderness. In *Grassroots governance: Chiefs in Africa and the Afro-Caribbean,* edited by Donald Ray, 123–144. Calgary, Canada: International Association of Schools and Institutes of Administration and University of Calgary Press.

———. 2005. Four principles of South African political culture at the local level. *Anthropology Southern Africa* 28, nos. 1–2: 22–30.

Tshabalala-Msimang, Manto. 2004. Towards greater equity in health care. Speech by Dr. Manto Tshabalala-Msimang, minister of health (11 June). Posted online at the South African Department of Health Web site, www .doh.gov.za/docs/sp/2004/sp0611a.html (accessed 6 June 2007).

Turner, Victor. 1969. *The ritual process: Structure and anti-structure.* Chicago: Aldine.

Turyasingura, Godwin B. 1989. Sexual behaviour and contraceptive knowledge: Attitudes and practice among youths of Jinja District, Uganda. MA thesis, Department of Demography, Makerere University.

Udjo, E. O. 1998. Marital patterns and fertility in South Africa: The evidence from the 1996 population census. Pretoria: Statistics South Africa. Posted online at www.iussp.org/Brazil2001/s40/S43_P01_Udjo.pdf.

Uganda AIDS Commission. 1993. AIDS control in Uganda: The multi-sectoral approach. Principle planning document for MACA [multi-sectoral AIDS control approach] (February). Kampala: Uganda AIDS Commission.

———. 2002. *Twenty years of HIV/AIDS in the world: Evolution of the epidemic and response in Uganda.* 8-page brochure. Kampala: Uganda AIDS Commission (September). Posted online at www.aidsuganda.org.

United Nations Development Programme. 2002. *Uganda human development report 2002: The challenge of HIV/AIDS: Maintaining the momentum of success.* Kampala: United Nations Development Programme.

United Nations Programme on HIV/AIDS (UNAIDS). 2002. Epidemiological fact sheets on HIV/AIDS and sexually transmitted infections: South Africa, 2002 update. Posted online at www.aegis.org/files/unaids/june2000/SouthAfrica_en.pdf (accessed 26 January 2008).

———. 2006. UNAIDS/WHO AIDS epidemic update: December 2006. Posted online at www.unaids.org/en/HIV_data/epi2006/ (accessed 20 May 2007).

United Nations, Uganda. 2005. High HIV/AIDS levels among fishing communities. Office for the Coordination of Humanitarian Affairs, Integrated Regional Information Network. Posted online at www.plusnews.org/AIDSreport .asp?ReportID = 5044&SelectRegion = East_Africa&SelectCountry = UGANDA.

Vance, Carole S. 1999 [1991]. Anthropology rediscovers sexuality: A theoretical comment. In *Culture, society and sexuality: A reader,* edited by Richard Parker and Peter Aggleton, 39–54. London: UCL Press [Originally published in *Social Science and Medicine* 33, no. 8 (1991).]

van der Vliet, Virgina. 1994. Apartheid and the politics of AIDS. In *Global AIDS policy,* edited by D. A. Feldman, 107–128. Westport, CT: Bergin & Garvey.

———. 1996. *The politics of AIDS.* London: Bowerdean.

————. 2001. AIDS: Losing "the new struggle"? *Daedalus* 130, no. 1 (Winter): 151–186.

————. 2004. South Africa divided against AIDS: A crisis in leadership. In *AIDS and South Africa: The social expression of a pandemic,* edited by Kyle D. Kauffman and David Lindauer, 48–96. Houndmills, Hampshire, UK: Palgrave/Macmillan.

van Dijk, Rijk A. 2000. Christian fundamentalism in sub-Saharan Africa: The case of Pentecostalism. Occasional Paper, Centre of African Studies University of Copenhagen. ISBN 87–986741–2-9. Posted online at www.teol.ku .dk/cas/nyhomepage/mapper/Occasional%20Papers/Occ_Van%20Dikj%20 (internet%20ver).doc (accessed 30 May 2007).

van Onselen, Charles. 1984. *The small matter of a horse: The life of "Nongoloza" Mathebula, 1867–1948.* Johannesburg: Ravan Press.

Wakabi, W. 2006. Condoms still contentious in Uganda's struggle over AIDS. *Lancet* 367, no. 9520: 1387–1388.

Wasswa, Henry. 2005. Survey: Uganda HIV prevalence rate high. *Washington Post* (via *Associated Press*), 3 May. Posted online at www.washingtonpost .com/wp-dyn/content/article/2005/05/03/AR2005050300658.html or www .body1.com/news/index.cfm/2/13566/1 (accessed 12 May 2005).

Watts, Duncan. 2003. *Six degrees: The science of a connected age.* London: Heinemann.

Wawer, M. J., D. Serwadda, S. D. Musgrave, J. K. Konde-Lule, M. Musagara, and N. Sewankambo. 1991. Dynamics of HIV-1 infection in a rural district of Uganda. *British Medical Journal* 383: 1303–1308.

Weber, Max. 1979. *Economy and society: An outline of interpretive sociology.* 2 volumes. Edited by Guenther Roth and Claus Wittich, translated by E. Fischoff et al. Berkeley and Los Angeles: University of California Press.

Wellings, Kaye, Martine Collumbien, Emma Slaymaker, Susheela Singh, Zoé Hodges, Dhaval Patel, and Nathalie Bajos. 2006. Sexual behaviour in context: A global perspective. *Lancet* 368: 1706–1728.

Westhead, R., C. Carter, and E. Momberg. 2006. Manto's HIV salad gets dressing down. *Sunday Independent* (South Africa), 20 August, 1.

Whiteside, A. 1993. First step to a multi-racial black-and-white policy on AIDS. Report from South Africa 1. *AIDS Analysis Africa* 3, no. 6 (November–December): 2.

Whitworth, J. A. G., C. Mahe, S. M. Mbulaiteye, J. Nakiyingi, A. Ruberantwari, A. Ojwiya, and A. Kamali. 2002. HIV-1 epidemic trends in rural south-west Uganda over a 10-year period. *Tropical Medicine and International Health* 7, no. 12: 1047–1052.

Wilkinson, D., N. F. Wilkinson, and C. Connolly. 1999. HIV infection among women admitted to the gynaecology service of a district hospital in South Africa. *International Journal of STD and AIDS* 10, no. 11: 735–737.

Wohlfeiler, D., and J. Potterat. 2003. How do sexual networks affect HIV/STD prevention? Fact sheet. Center for AIDS Prevention Studies and the AIDS Research Institute, University of California, San Francisco.

Wojcicki, Janet, and Josephine Malala. 2001. Condom use, power and HIV/

AIDS risk: Sex-workers bargain for survival in Hillbrow/Joubert Park/Berea, Johannesburg. *Social Science and Medicine* 53: 99–121.

Wrigley, C. C. 1996. *Kingship and state: The Buganda dynasty.* Cambridge: Cambridge University Press 1996.

Zhu, Tuofu, Bette T. Korber, André J. Nahinias, Edward Hooper, Paul M. Sharp, and David D. Ho. 1998. An African HIV-1 sequence from 1959 and implications for the origin of the epidemic. *Nature* 391, no. 6667: 594. Abstract posted online at www.aegis.com/news/ads/1998/ad980242.html (accessed 30 May 2007).

Index

ABC prevention model, 56, 83–89, 92, 131, 139–44, 165, 221–34; "ABCD," or ABC + death, 78, 81, 82, 84; definition of, 87, 228; USAID "ABC" study (2002–2003), 93

abstinence, sexual: in AIDS policy, 21, 56, 78, 80, 84, 87, 91, 221–25, 232–33; and causality, 86, 90; epidemiological irrelevance, 91, 226–32; and religion, 19, 91, 226–28; South Africa, 74, 176; Uganda, 19, 78, 83, 86–87, 103–9, 131, 165, 228; and zero grazing, 19

Abuja Declaration (2001), 172

Achmat, Zackie, 184–85. See also Treatment Action Campaign (TAC)

ACP. See AIDS Control Program (Uganda)

African experience of AIDS, 82–84, 99, 190

Africanist ideology and AIDS, 151, 172, 176–79, 189, 194, 217. See also African solution to African problems

African National Congress (ANC), 10, 39, 152–53, 158–69, 174–94, 196

African sexuality thesis, 12, 85, 103, 157, 176, 180, 193, 202, 208. See also sexuality: African cultural practices

African solution to African problems, 149, 166, 172, 175–76, 189

African Union (AU), 171, 172, 175

AIDS: activists, 3, 59, 200; and the body, 192, 223–24; cause of, 37, 38, 39, 40, 110–14, 115–20, 125–26, 177–78, 201, 225, 237; community of, xx, xxi, 171, 217; complexity of, 4, 23–25, 26 (Fig. 2), 43–49, 79, 94, 101, 194, 216, 224; in daily life, xx, 1, 4, 26, 151; deaths, 2, 79, 89–90, 120–23, 133, 147, 150, 182–84, 235–36, 249; debate in South Africa, 150, 176–78, 183, 195, 201, 222; debate in Uganda, 91–92, 115–26; desire for a cure, 2, 166, 173, 193, 197, 201; as disease of knowledge, 221–23; dissidents, 39, 193; as imagined community, xx, 29, 208, 217; legislation, 168–72, 216; as local knowledge, 31, 115; medicalization of, 131, 155, 202, 224; as moral mystery, xix; and poverty, 79, 174, 180, 231, 240; as social imaginary, 26, 151, 171, 190–94, 198, 205, 207, 215; "success story" in Uganda, 84, 88, 85–95, 97, 101; time of, 26 (Fig. 2), 206–9; as unimagined community, xx, 208. See also denialism; human rights; indigenization of AIDS as native medical category; siliimu

AIDS Charter (South Africa), 158–60

AIDS Consortium, 154–58, 168, 184–86

AIDS Control Programme (Uganda), 91–101, 129–38, 143

AIDS education campaigns, 3, 57, 81, 92, 112, 126, 132–35, 154, 153–55, 161, 172, 225, 230–32

AIDS epidemic: in Africa, xx, 15, 40, 59, 82, 102, 146, 220; different from other epidemics, 37–39; heterosexual

AIDS epidemic *(continued)*
  in Africa, 25, 39, 58, 85, 119, 126,
  160; and property regimes, 61, 62; as
  temporal process, 22–28, 26 (Fig. 2),
  42, 43
AIDS Law Project (ALP), 154, 168, 172,
  178, 184–86
AIDS Support Organization, The
  (TASO), Uganda, 132, 142–48
ALP. *See* AIDS Law Project (ALP)
AMREF, 145
Anan, Kofi, Secretary General of the
  UN, 38, 172, 174
ANC. *See* African National Congress
  (ANC)
ancestors and AIDS (South Africa), 150,
  151, 176, 206, 204–7, 209–13, 209
  (Fig. 19). *See also* traditional healers
  (South Africa)
Anderson, Benedict, xx
anthropological approach to AIDS, xvii,
  xviii, 1–4, 18, 28, 31, 186, 195–202,
  224–28
antiretroviral medications (ARVs), 3, 21,
  27, 37, 39, 146, 162, 167, 172–75,
  180–87, 193, 221–25; provision of,
  187. *See also* AZT; Mbeki, Thabo,
  President; pharmaceutical companies; Treatment Action Campaign;
  Tshabalala-Msimang, Manto;
  Virodene scandal
apartheid (South Africa), xviii , 9–16,
  62, 72–76, 79, 125, 151–68, 176, 182–
  84, 189–94, 200
ARVs. *See* antiretroviral medications
  (ARVs)
AZT (antiretroviral medication), 38,
  122, 177, 183–85. *See also* antiretroviral medications (ARVs)

Baby Tshepang, 196–98, 200, 216, 218,
  254
behavior change, 1, 36, 50, 54, 59, 86,
  96, 133, 225; and HIV prevalence, 27–
  30, 56–59, 80–95; linked to national
  development strategy in Uganda, 139–
  42; policy in Uganda, 95, 137–43, 231
Bhengu, Nosipho, death of, 173
Biko, Steve, 183
blood: cultural meanings, 196–99, 204–
  15, 206 (Fig. 18)
body: cultural meanings in South Africa,
  31, 195–219, 213 (Fig. 20). *See also*
  semen; sex; sexual behavior
Buganda kingdom, 5–7, 61, 64–70, 75,
  114–16, 242; King's council chamber,
  67 (Fig. 8)

Bush, George W., President, 19, 21, 85,
  86

Cameron, Edwin, 158, 178
Campbell, Catherine, 183
CARE, 145
"Castro Hlongwane" (document), 11,
  178–82, 193
catastrophe event (complexity theory),
  49, 53, 66, 84
CBOs. *See* community-based
  organizations
CDC. *See* Centers for Disease Control
  and Prevention (CDC), U.S.
Centers for Disease Control and Prevention (CDC), U.S., 25, 133, 137
Centre for Applied Legal Studies, 158
chiefs. *See* traditional society
Christianity. *See* abstinence, sexual: and
  religion; religion: Christianity; sex:
  and religion
circumcision. *See* cultural practices:
  circumcision
civil society, 10; and AIDS, 24, 59, 68;
  and culture of conflict in South Africa,
  192–93; exponential growth in
  Uganda, 148; in South Africa, 57, 153,
  168, 182–90; in Uganda, 81–83, 91–
  104, 123, 130–41, 147–48. *See also*
  prevention of AIDS: civil society in;
  Truth and Reconciliation Commission
Clinton, Bill, President (U.S.), 38–39
CODESA. *See* Convention for a Democratic South Africa (CODESA)
community, xxi, 136, 138, 142, 147,
  234; and care for orphans, 145; political, 190, 192; theater, 31, 154, 165,
  197. *See also* AIDS: as imagined
  community
community-based organizations (CBOs),
  59, 81, 93, 101, 131; South Africa,
  189; Uganda, 147. *See also*
  community
comparative approach, 1, 15, 56, 102,
  156, 235
comparison: of Ugandan and South African trends, 34, 41–48, 42 (Fig. 4), 43,
  56; validity of, xvii, 2, 88, 156, 235
condoms, 63, 69, 78, 83, 95, 96, 103,
  123, 145; as part of ABC strategy, 56,
  57, 228; availability (Uganda), 144;
  effectiveness of, 57, 59, 90, 231; social
  marketing of, 95; South African attitudes toward, 176, 198, 199, 203,
  210, 229; South African policy, 165,
  175; Ugandan policy, 22, 131, 133,
  142–44; Ugandan policy influenced

by American conservatism, 84, 86, 87, 92, 143
Convention for a Democratic South Africa (CODESA), 152–56
Cuba, 110, 132, 152
cultural meanings of HIV/AIDS, 1, 23–29, 123, 153, 171, 194–95, 202–5, 216–20, 224. *See also* body; semen
cultural practices: burial of dead, 89; change in, 101, 140; circumcision, 66, 81, 104, 140, 212; multiple sexual partners, 145; sexual, 140; sexual cleansing rites, 104; sexual, in Uganda, 140–43; uvulectomy (Uganda), 140; wife inheritance, 66, 90, 108; wife sharing, 61, 66, 81, 92, 104

denialism, xix, xx, 29, 161; of AIDS in South Africa, 3, 2–3, 11, 12, 18, 151, 167, 171, 175, 173–91, 222, 239; of AIDS in Uganda, 124. *See also* Bhengu, Nozipho, death of; Duesberg, Peter; Rasnick, David; Sonnabend, Dr. Joe
development, socio-economic: linked to AIDS prevention in Uganda, 12, 85, 105, 120–23, 134–39, 143–48; not linked to AIDS prevention in South Africa, 151, 168, 181, 190. *See also* prevention of AIDS: linked to nation building in Uganda
disclosure of HIV status, 220, 223; human rights argument against, 155, 160; public health benefits of, 221. *See also* knowledge of HIV/AIDS; stigma
Dlamini-Zuma, Nkosizana, 161–64, 166–68, 183–84
Drum Magazine, 8, 15
Duesberg, Peter, 38–39, 191, 239; influence on Mbeki's AIDS policy, 38, 177–78, 239

ecological approach to AIDS, 1, 28–32, 48–50, 57–58, 69–71, 86–87
education. *See* AIDS education campaigns; media
epidemiology: compared with anthropology, xvii, 1, 22–24, 35; exponential growth curves, 51 (box), 52 (Fig. 7); model of HIV prevalence (Stoneburner & Low-Beer), 35; network or power law model, 42 (Fig. 4), 49; standard model, xvii, 35, 36, 37, 35–38, 43, 51 (box), 52 (Fig. 7), 52–58, 78, 88, 230, 238, 241
ethnicity, 156; and HIV transmission, 60, 102, 231; South Africa, 12, 15, 71–72, 194; Uganda, 5, 8, 64–65, 68, 242

European Community, 164
exponential growth curves, 51 (box)

faith-based organizations (FBOs), 91, 95, 131, 168, 228; in South Africa, 189; in Uganda, 147
faithfulness (in marriage). *See* marriage: fidelity and faithfulness
family, 2, 127, 136, 191; caring for members with AIDS, 89, 132; role of sex in, 196, 205, 234
family planning, 134
family structures: and AIDS, 33, 59, 82, 139, 209; and orphans, 27, 90, 145; in South Africa, 71–79, 150, 157, 207–16; in Uganda, 59–71, 90, 146
FBOs. *See* faith-based organizations
fertility, 208, 216; in South Africa, 74, 226; in Uganda, 86, 102, 226. *See also* total fertility rate (TFR)
Foucault, Michel, 195
Freedom Charter, 158, 159

Gauteng Province, South Africa, 169, 186
Gemeinschaft für technische Zusammenarbeit (GtZ), 96, 133
gender and HIV/AIDS, 60, 174. *See also* women and HIV/AIDS
gift: in bride-wealth, 61; as exchange, 196, 209 (Fig. 19); as flow of bodily fluids, 203–16; and sex, 195
Gluckman, Max, 31
governance, 68. *See also* civil society; Mbeki, Thabo; Museveni, Yoweri; political leadership on AIDS
GtZ. *See* Gemeinschaft für technische Zusammenarbeit

Heritage Foundation (U.S.), 85, 143
HIV exceptionalism, 160
HIV prevalence: change as "phase transition" in complex system, 49 (Fig. 6), 54, 63–66, 84; change as property of social whole, 79; change in, 2, 4, 17, 18, 41, 54, 66, 77, 80, 87, 95–99, 156–57, 188; determined by sexual networks, 1, 32, 48, 55–59, 78–80, 226, 231; in Kampala, change in, 49 (Fig. 6); modeling, 33–39, 93; in South Africa, 10–12, 33, 50–52, 149, 153–57, 165, 169, 173; in Uganda, 7, 22, 35–37, 44–48, 49 (Fig. 6), 78, 81, 83, 89–98, 130–36, 143–48, 236, 243; USAID pamphlet *What happened in Uganda?*, 36, 87, 88, 94, 98
homosexuality, 17, 25, 37, 110, 111, 151, 157, 160, 172

human rights, 191, 208; and South African AIDS policy, 155, 156–62, 189–92; and Ugandan AIDS policy, 91, 108, 139

Idi Amin, President (Uganda), 6–8, 62, 68–69, 77, 105–8, 115, 134
IEC. *See* Information, Education and Communication (IEC)
indigenization of AIDS as native medical category, 31, 114–26, 135–36, 148
Information, Education and Communication (IEC), 92, 96, 132, 133, 135, 142
Islam. *See* religion

KABP. *See* knowledge, attitudes, beliefs, practice
Kamondo, Mr., 20, 89, 90 (Fig. 10)
Kenya, 5, 9, 18, 69, 119, 201
knowledge of HIV/AIDS, 11, 24, 27, 28, 57, 91, 115, 127, 139, 145, 212, 224; anxiety caused by, xix, xx, 220; first in Uganda, 91–99, 110. *See also* indigenization of AIDS as native medical category
knowledge, attitudes, beliefs, practice (KABP), 40
Kreditanstalt für Wiederaufbau, 144

land tenure systems: South Africa, 13–14, 60–62, 72–76; Uganda, 60–70
language diversity and HIV transmission, 65
Le Carré, John (*The Constant Gardener*), 11, 179, 180
Leclerc-Madlala, Suzanne, 169, 186
Levi-Strauss, Claude, 220
Lewis, Stephen, UN Special Envoy for HIV/AIDS in Africa, 174, 201
LoveLife, 3, 154, 155, 188
Low-Beer, Daniel, 34–36, 42, 45, 58, 80

MACA. *See* Multisectoral AIDS Control Approach (MACA) in Uganda
Madlala-Routledge, Nozizwe, 174–75
Mandela, Nelson, President, 10–11, 18, 149–55, 158–67, 191–93, 226
Marie Stopes International, 144
marriage: age at first, in South Africa, 74, 77; age at first, in Uganda, 71, 92; bride-price in South Africa, 61, 195, 210, 216; bride-price in Uganda, 61; and fertility in South Africa, 74, 212; fidelity and faithfulness, 56, 66, 69, 86–87, 92, 175, 228, 232; polyandry (wife sharing), 66; polygamous, 65–

66, 73, 87; low prevalence in South Africa, 73; in sexual networks, 41, 162, 229, 233; in South Africa, 71, 73–74; in Uganda, 66, 91, 104; wife inheritance, 66, 90, 104, 108
Mbeki, Thabo, President, 2, 11, 39, 166–67, 174–77; Africanist ideology and AIDS, 177, 181, 189, 194; attitude to ARVs, 157, 166; denialism, 18, 38, 150, 155, 175–78, 182–83, 193, 201; and Parks Mankanhlana, 181; policy on AIDS, 173–78, 182, 191; role in Africa, 171; views on AIDS, 12, 38–39, 85, 155, 167–71, 177–84, 222; and Virodene scandal, 166, 193. *See also* Africanist ideology and AIDS; denialism; pharmaceutical companies: suspicion of
MCC. See Medicines Control Council
media, 141; "edutainment" in South African AIDS prevention, 154; mass advertising, 3, 29, 128, 154, 188; *Munno* (newspaper, Uganda), 116–23, 128; *New Vision* (newspaper, Uganda), 122, 128; popular press and newspapers, 102–4, 120–21, 151, 198; posters, 127–28; radio, 99, 197, 199, 202; South African Broadcasting Corporation, 150–51; *The Sun* (newspaper, South Africa), 197. *See also* LoveLife; Sarafina scandal; Soul City
medical pluralism in South Africa, 177, 222
Medicines Control Council (South Africa), 166, 187
methodology, xvii–xviii, xviii–xix, 238
Mlambo-Ngcuka, Phumzile, 174–75
mobility of population, 82; South Africa, 14, 71–77, 159, 188, 215, 230; Uganda, 69, 139–40, 231
mother-to-child transmission (MTCT), 146, 181, 185, 187. See also Nevirapine
Mozambique, 82
Mpumalanga Province, South Africa, 165
MTCT. *See* mother-to-child transmission (MTCT)
Multisectoral AIDS Control Approach (MACA) in Uganda, 134–41, 143, 148
Museveni, Janet, 130
Museveni, Yoweri, President, 7–8, 11, 19, 62–68, 77, 91, 99, 105–10, 120–26, 130, 143, 155; early intervention against AIDS, 123, 128; first knowledge of AIDS, 110; personal history, 8; policy on AIDS, 8, 19–21, 59, 85, 91, 101–4, 118, 138; political leadership against AIDS, 131, 137, 139; poli-

tics of AIDS, 31; restoration of Ugandan kingships, 64, 68

NACOSA. *See* National AIDS Committee of South Africa (NACOSA)
National AIDS Committee of South Africa (NACOSA), 154, 156, 157
National Party (South Africa), 9, 14, 176; merger with ANC, 152
National Resistance Army (NRA), Uganda, 7, 8, 108
National Resistance Movement (NRM), Uganda, 122–23, 127–29
native medical category, AIDS as. *See* indigenization of AIDS as native medical category; *siliimu*
networks: clustered, 49–53, 63–65, 71, 77–80, 230–31; configuration (topology) of, 1, 33, 58, 63, 70–71, 78, 230; fractal structures, 43–44, 49, 77; power-law model of, 47–50; small world, 63, 80; social, xviii, 4, 16, 41, 205; social determinants of configuration, 32–33, 41–48, 51, 52–82; theory of, 40–53, 84. *See also* power law
networks, sexual: configuration of, 1, 81; density of, 77, 148, 193; dynamics of, 46, 53, 96, 104; empirical data lacking, 40, 54, 79, 240; and family property regimes, 62–79; HIV trends a property of, 80; importance in South African society, 196–219; methodology, xviii; and prevention of HIV/AIDS, 232–33; and race, 77; and self-organizing behavior, 56, 85; as social structures, xix, 28–34, 40, 59, 102–4, 192, 206–9, 229; and transmission of HIV, 1, 19, 27, 32–36, 40, 80–82, 139, 194, 229–32; as unimagined community, xviii, xx, 208
Nevirapine (antiretroviral medication), 146, 162, 181, 185. *See also* antiretroviral medications (ARVs)
nongovernmental organizations (NGOs). *See names of specific organizations*
NRA. *See* National Resistance Army (NRA), Uganda
NRM. *See* National Resistance Movement (NRM), Uganda
Nyerere, Julius, 6–7

Obote, Milton, President (Uganda), 6–7, 68–69, 77, 91, 99, 105, 129
Okello, Tito, 8, 77, 91, 108, 120, 123, 127, 129
Okware, Dr. Samuel, 91, 98, 101–4, 113, 117–18, 123, 129, 244

orphans, 90, 130–34, 145. *See also* family structures

Pathfinder International, 144
Paton, Alan (*Cry the Beloved Country*), 10
people living with AIDS (PLWA), 132, 135, 143, 147, 187, 191. *See also* The AIDS Support Organization (TASO), Uganda
PEPFAR. *See* President's Emergency Program for AIDS Relief (PEPFAR)
pharmaceutical companies: Boehringer Ingelheim, 180, 184; Bristol Meyers Squibb, 184; Glaxo Wellcome PLC, 184; Merck, 184; Pfizer, 184, 185; provision of ARVs, 122; reduction of ARV prices, 146, 162, 181–185; Roche, 184; suspicion of, 2, 11, 121, 157, 162, 176, 179–84, 189, *See also* Treatment Action Campaign (TAC); Nevirapine; Tshabalala-Msimang, Manto, Minister of Health (South Africa)
PLWA. *See* people living with AIDS (PLWA)
political leadership on AIDS, 101, 151, 222–23; African, 201; global, 38, 146, 149; Mbeki and Museveni compared, 155; in South Africa, 4, 11, 12, 18, 59, 162, 167, 178, 183, 193–94; in Uganda, 91, 121, 155. *See also* African National Congress (ANC); Museveni, Yoweri, President; Mbeki, Thabo, President; National Resistance Movement (NRM), Uganda; Sarafina scandal; Virodene scandal; Zuma, Jacob
polygamy. *See* marriage
Population Services International, 144
poverty. *See* AIDS: and poverty; Mbeki, Thabo, President: views on AIDS
power law: curves associated with network structures, 43–58; mathematical explanation, 46 (box), 47–50; model of HIV prevalence, 34, 41–45, 43 (Fig. 5), 44 (box), 78, 83–84; model of HIV prevalence, South Africa, 50 (box)
President's Emergency Program for AIDS Relief (PEPFAR), 85, 92
prevalence. *See* HIV prevalence
prevention of AIDS: assessment of effectiveness, 56, 188; change over time, 24, 28; civil society in, 68, 98, 122, 129, 136, 139, 154; frequent failure of, 3, 18, 29, 81, 154, 169, 183, 194, 198, 221–26; integrated approach, 12, 27,

prevention of AIDS *(continued)*
  81–82, 93, 138; linked to nation building in Uganda, 122–28, 148, 192; new
  strategy, 55, 232–34; "One, One,
  One" approach, 234; PEPFAR, 85;
  role of sexual networks in, 54, 220–
  30; in South Africa, 162–69, 184–88;
  in Uganda, 144, 155
prostitution, 22, 77–78, 103, 119, 212,
  215–16, 231. *See also* sex:
  transactional

race, 9–10, 11–12, 77, 156–58, 171–81,
  193; methodological approach to,
  xviii. *See also* apartheid (South Africa)
Rakai District, Uganda, 7, 111, 113,
  115–25, 133–34
Rakai Project, 70, 133, 145
Ramphele, Dr. Mamphela, 183
rape, 4, 7, 101–8, 139, 180–82, 187,
  196–97, 201; of children, 196–99,
  216–18; of children as cure for AIDS,
  198; Zuma, Jacob, 199–201, 216
Rasnick, David, 238–39. *See also* Duesberg, Peter
Rath, Matthias, 173, 177, 187, 238, 251;
  illegal drug trials, 173
religion: Christianity, 8, 18, 21, 65, 83,
  91–92, 105, 137, 177–79, 225–28;
  Islam, 16, 60, 65–66, 91–92, 105, 137,
  172, 177, 225; leadership on AIDS
  prevention in, 92–95, 123. *See also*
  faith-based organizations; abstinence,
  sexual: and religion
religion, African traditional. *See* ancestors and AIDS (South Africa); traditional healers (South Africa); traditional society
response to AIDS: adversarial in South
  Africa, 157, 192, 191–94, 223
risk, sexual, 3, 86, 139, 186, 201; and
  cultural practices, 140–142, 218–19;
  factors of, 40; focus on behavior, 55,
  80; of HIV infection, 39; reduction of,
  145, 234; shift from focus on individual risk, 82

SABC. *See* media: South African Broadcasting Corporation
sangoma. See traditional healers (South
  Africa)
Sarafina scandal 162–65, 176, 193
Save the Children, 134
semen: cultural meanings, 198, 199,
  204–7. *See also* blood; sexual substance, flows of
sex: and healing, 141, 196–202, 214–22,
  230; meanings of, 30, 104, 194–95,
  211, 202–21; and religion, 112, 226–
  28; as social action, xix, 29, 30, 218–
  19, 207–12, 217–19, 234; as social
  relation, 31, 207, 228; theory of, 28–
  32, 195, 202, 216–26; transactional,
  77, 207, 212, 216
sexual attitudes (South Africa), 197,
  204, 208
sexual behavior, 18, 27, 28, 31, 34, 56,
  195; and network theory, 40–49, 63,
  79, 80, 93; social control of, 60–61,
  74–75, 86, 101–9, 127, 143–45, 201,
  221–27
sexual debut, 92; age of, in South Africa,
  73, 77; age of, in Uganda, 70, 127;
  delay of, 90, 92
sexuality: African cultural practices,
  140–45, 202; theater of, 30. *See also*
  African sexuality thesis
sexually transmitted infection/disease
  (STI or STD), 132, 133, 139, 142, 145,
  146, 163, 165, 211, 226
sexual substance, flows of, 31, 195–218
  (Figs. 18, 19)
SIDA (French acronym for AIDS), 117
siliimu (name for AIDS in Uganda), 7,
  91, 100, 111–12, 124; as Ugandan
  native medical category, 31, 100, 108,
  115–29
slim disease (name for AIDS in Uganda),
  7, 111–27. *See also siliimu*
social action, 26, 28, 123, 194. *See also*
  sex: as social action
social imaginary, 171, 192. *See* AIDS: as
  social imaginary
social structure, 23–27; of HIV transmission, 31–34, 40, 82, 218, 227; and
  sexual networks, xix, 41, 81. *See also*
  networks, sexual: as social structures
Sonnabend, Dr. Joe, 39
Soul City, 154, 155, 188
South Africa: society and history, xviii,
  8–11, 12–18, 27, 62, 71–75, 152–53,
  254. *See also* African National Congress (ANC); HIV prevalence: in
  South Africa; Mandela, Nelson,
  President; Mbeki, Thabo, President
South African Medical Association, 187
STD. *See* sexually transmitted infection/
  disease (STI or STD)
STI. *See* sexually transmitted infection/
  disease (STI or STD)
stigma, xx, 160, 170, 191; a problem of
  knowledge, 24, 29, 95, 220; Uganda,
  132; Uganda and South Africa compared, 115

Stoneburner, Rand L., 34–36, 42–45, 58, 80
Strategic Plan for South Africa, 2000–2005, 169
Strogatz, Steve, 49
Swedish International Development Cooperation Agency, 133

TAC. See Treatment Action Campaign (TAC)
Tanzania, 6–8, 15–16, 34, 69, 100, 105–7, 111–15, 119–25, 228
TASO. See The AIDS Support Organization (TASO), Uganda
TB. See tuberculosis
testing (HIV), 110, 113, 118, 122, 153; argument for mandatory, 152, 160. See also voluntary counseling and testing (VCT)
Thailand, 18, 185, 231
The AIDS Support Organization (TASO), Uganda, 132, 142–48
THETA. See Traditional and Modern Health Practitioners Together against AIDS (THETA)
total fertility rate (TFR): South Africa, 33; Uganda, 33–36
Traditional and Modern Health Practitioners Together against AIDS (THETA), 130, 142; pamphlet, 141 (Fig. 13)
traditional healers (South Africa), 18, 31, 59, 150, 168, 176, 198–215: model of the body, 213 (Fig. 20); in Uganda, 81, 121, 140–42. See also indigenization of AIDS as native medical category; Traditional and Modern Health Practitioners Together against AIDS (THETA)
traditional society: chiefship in South Africa, 12, 13, 71, 75, 208; in Uganda, 5, 64–68, 81, 103–8, 116
Treatment Action Campaign (TAC), 154, 168, 172–75, 183–87, 193
Truth and Reconciliation Commission (South Africa), 190; as model for AIDS response, 149, 188
Tshabalala-Msimang, Manto, Minister of Health (South Africa), 2, 161–62, 167–68, 173–77, 183–87, 201, 222, 237
tuberculosis, xix, 112, 126, 173

UAC. See Uganda AIDS Commission (UAC)
ubuntu (humanity), 217
Uganda, society and history, 5–7, 244

Uganda AIDS Commission (UAC), 104, 132, 135–40
ukimwi (KiSwahili name for AIDS), 112, 117
UNAIDS. See United Nations Program on HIV/AIDS (UNAIDS)
UNDP. See United Nations Development Program (UNDP)
UNGASS. See United Nations General Assembly Special Session on HIV/AIDS (UNGASS)
UNICEF. See United Nations Children's Fund (UNICEF)
unimagined community: as unseen structure of sexual networks, 208
United Nations Children's Fund (UNICEF), 132
United Nations Development Program (UNDP), 135, 145
United Nations General Assembly Special Session on HIV/AIDS (UNGASS), 172, 173, 174, 186
United Nations Program on HIV/AIDS (UNAIDS), 145, 169, 184
United States Agency for International Development (USAID), 18–19, 36, 87–89, 93–101, 108, 127, 131–35, 143–46, 228
urbanization: in South Africa, 8, 13–16, 70, 75–77, 168; in Uganda, 62, 69–70, 96, 131, 139
USAID. See United States Agency for International Development (USAID)

VCT. See Voluntary counseling and testing (VCT)
violence, xix, 4, 10, 69; and AIDS, xix, 7; coercive, 60; and gender, 60, 101, 106, 197, 216; political, 152–56
virginity: belief in cure by sex with virgin, 197–98; as identity, 212; as value, 30, 218, 226
Virodene scandal, 166–68, 173, 176, 193
voluntary counseling and testing (VCT), 36, 78, 93, 95, 134, 142–46, 169, 221; discouraged in South Africa, 155

Wawer, Maria, 70
WHO. See World Health Organization (WHO)
witchcraft, 5, 68, 112, 13, 124–27, 176–77, 203, 211
women and HIV/AIDS, 10, 35–36, 66, 78, 95, 103, 106; in South Africa, 165–68, 170, 180–85, 198–211, 212–18; in Uganda, 106–13, 126, 130, 138, 141. See also cultural practices: wife

women and HIV/AIDS *(continued)*
  inheritance; cultural practices: wife
  sharing
World Bank, 136, 145, 147, 183, 184
World Health Organization (WHO),
  11, 101, 117, 131, 132, 133, 136, 143,
  146, 169
World Learning, 145

World Vision, 145

zero grazing, 83; defined, 19
Zimbabwe, 18, 76, 82, 172
Zuma, Jacob, 161, 169, 174, 194–96,
  199–202, 208, 218–19; accused of
  rape, 3, 201, 236; political views of,
  194.

Text: 10/13 Sabon
Display: Sabon
Compositor: BookMatters, Berkeley
Illustrator: BookMatters, Berkeley
Printer and binder: Thomson-Shore, Inc.